THE 2021 COM[...]
MEDITERRANEAN COOKBOOK

2 BOOKS IN 1 | 500+ RECIPES FOR EVERYDAY COOKING | A MEDITERRANEAN DIET MADE EASY | START TO EAT HEALTHY AND LOSE WEIGHT | FOR BEGINNERS AND NOT

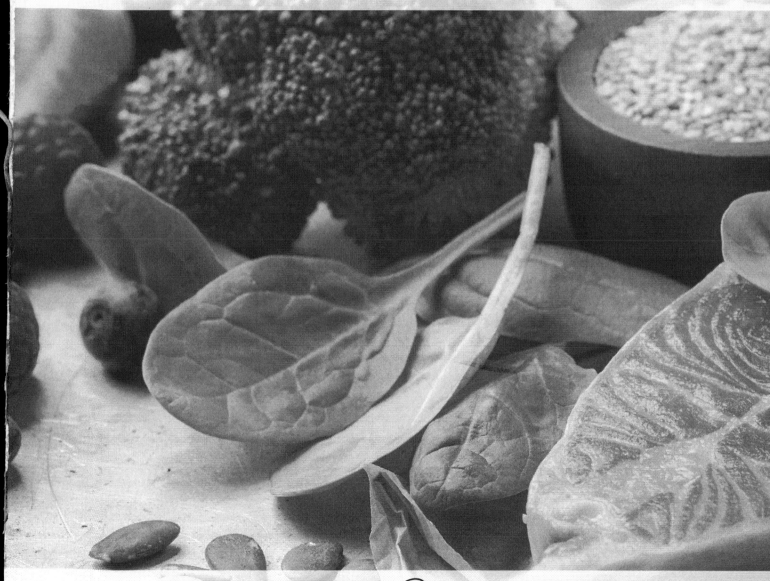

Jennifer Paul

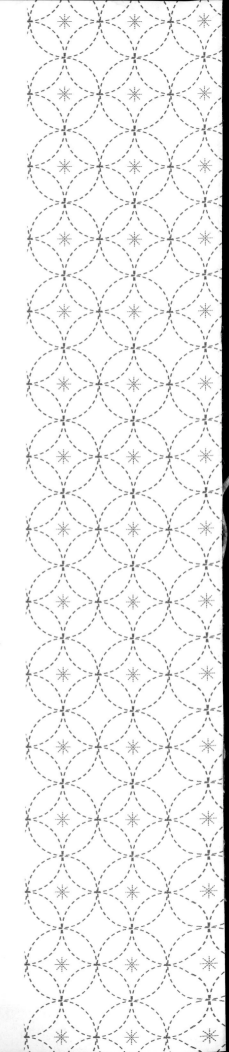

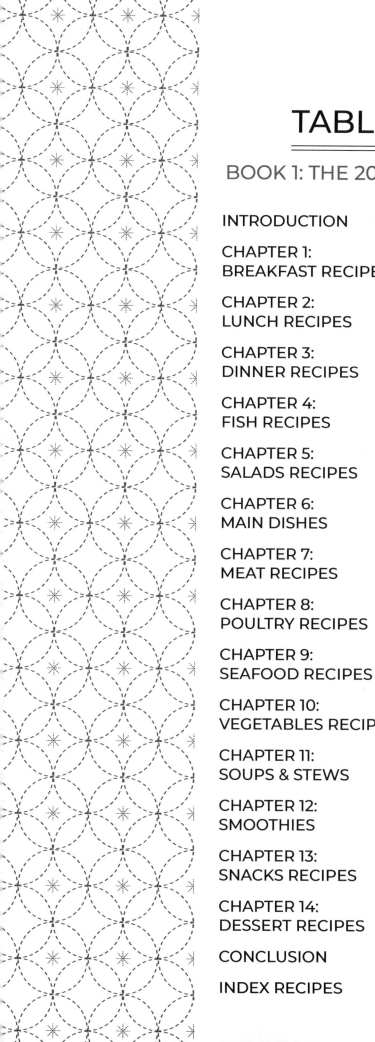

TABLE OF CONTENTS

BOOK 1: THE 2021 COMPLETE MEDITERRANEAN COOKBOOK

INTRODUCTION	7
CHAPTER 1: BREAKFAST RECIPES	9
CHAPTER 2: LUNCH RECIPES	37
CHAPTER 3: DINNER RECIPES	59
CHAPTER 4: FISH RECIPES	81
CHAPTER 5: SALADS RECIPES	105
CHAPTER 6: MAIN DISHES	121
CHAPTER 7: MEAT RECIPES	141
CHAPTER 8: POULTRY RECIPES	157
CHAPTER 9: SEAFOOD RECIPES	179
CHAPTER 10: VEGETABLES RECIPES	201
CHAPTER 11: SOUPS & STEWS	215
CHAPTER 12: SMOOTHIES	225
CHAPTER 13: SNACKS RECIPES	241
CHAPTER 14: DESSERT RECIPES	267
CONCLUSION	291
INDEX RECIPES	293

BOOK 2: THE 2021 COMPLETE MEDITERRANEAN COOKBOOK

INTRODUCTION   301

CHAPTER 1:
BREAKFAST RECIPES   303

CHAPTER 2:
LUNCH RECIPES   343

CHAPTER 3:
DINNER RECIPES   381

CHAPTER 4:
DESSERT RECIPES   479

CHAPTER 5:
SNACK RECIPES   529

CHAPTER 6:
FISH AND SEAFOOD RECIPES   549

CONCLUSION   575

INDEX RECIPES   577

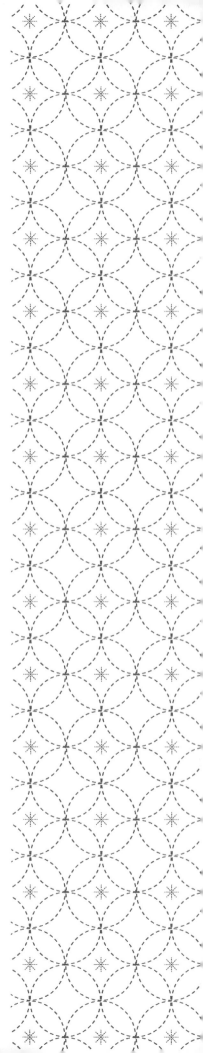

THE 2021 COMPLETE MEDITERRANEAN COOKBOOK

RESET YOUR METABOLISM AND START TO EAT HEALTHY WITH THE MEDITERRANEAN DIET | 250+ QUICK AND EASY RECIPES FOR WEIGHT LOSS | LIFELONG TRANSFORMATION | FEEL BETTER

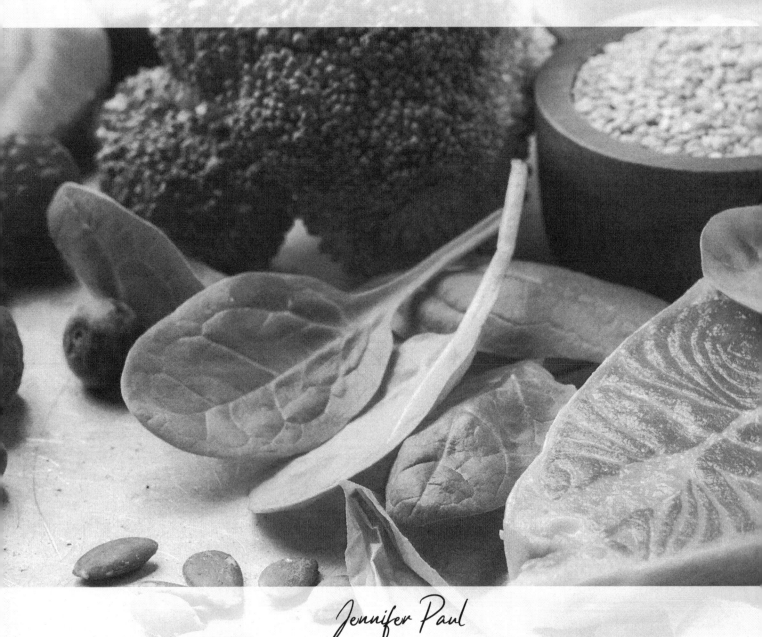

Jennifer Paul

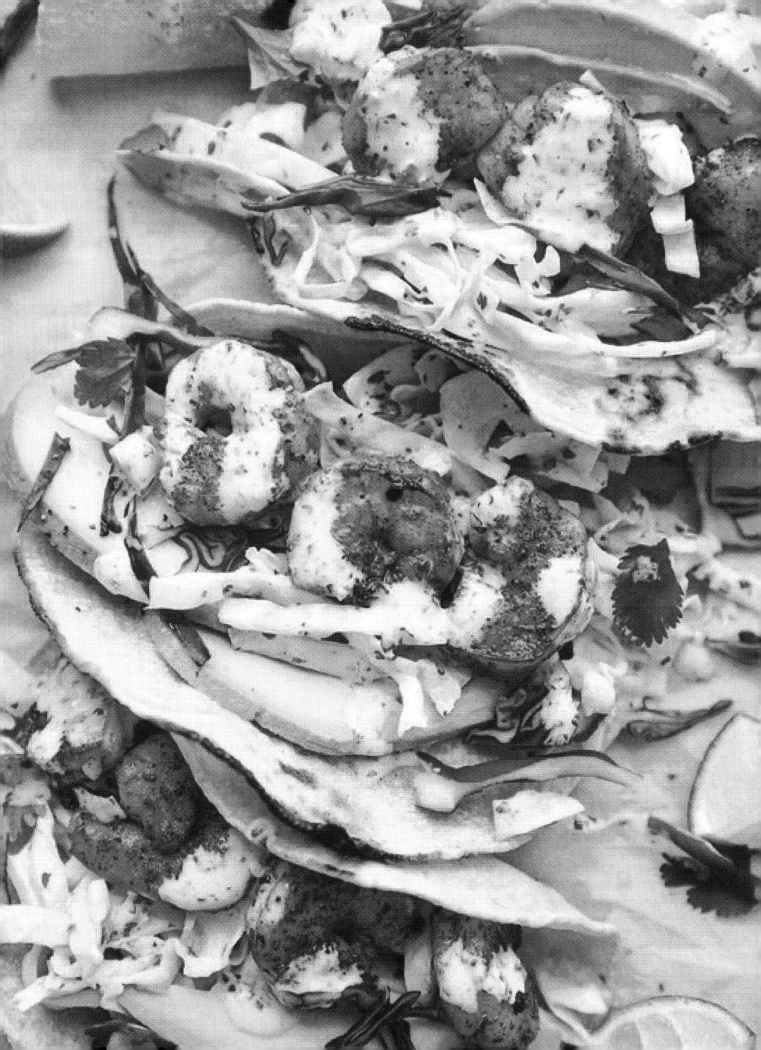

INTRODUCTION

What is Mediterranean Diet?

The Mediterranean diet is a pattern of eating that is closely linked with the food cultures of countries bordering the Mediterranean Sea. It is based on the simple premise that by eating in a healthy way, you can prevent illness and promote better health. While there are several versions of this diet, all include eating plenty of vegetables, fruits, whole grains, beans and legumes; using olive oil as the basic fat for cooking; and choosing healthy fats from fish and nuts (instead of butter). The Mediterranean diet also emphasizes low consumption of red meat (especially processed meat) and sugar-free desserts.

What evidence does it offer?

In people with heart disease or diabetes: These studies have found that those who follow a Mediterranean-type diet have lower blood pressure (about 3/2 mmHg), lower levels of cholesterol (3 to 4 percent) and less inflammation than those who don't follow the diet. They also are less likely to develop heart disease or diabetes.

How do you follow it?

The Mediterranean-style eating pattern is most closely linked with the following countries: France; Spain; Italy; Greece; and coastal areas of North Africa (Morocco, Tunisia, Egypt). These dietary patterns spread through migration and expanded rapidly northward toward the sea as healthy people migrated away from island regions. The traditional Mediterranean diet shares features with some of the diets that evolve from ancient times in these areas. Rich in legumes, whole grains, vegetables and fruits (few dairy products and meat) and low in red meat, sugar and energy dense foods were early characteristics of this dietary pattern. Recently however many of these diets

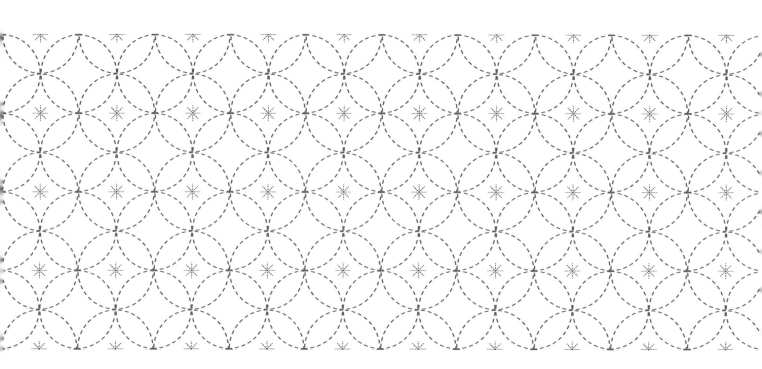

have changed to include various amounts of LAFA (Local Food Agricultural) foods (supplements), such as milk products, fish several times per week (depending on the region), kilos of sugar per year from fruits among other changes.

Is it sustainable?

It is difficult to sustain a Mediterranean-type pattern over time. The lack of meat and dairy products may lead to lower intakes of these nutrients if replacements are not made for these items in the diet. People with chronic disease may be unable to tolerate high intakes of legumes, grains and vegetables because of side effects from their conditions. A recent study found that health problems such as early death or frequent hospitalizations were more likely in this group than in those who had followed other diets over long periods.

What are the benefits of Mediterranean Diet?

Minimize risk factors for chronic diseases (heart disease/cancer/diabetes) Improve weight status by lowering caloric intake and increasing physical activity. Increase consumption of vegetables, fruits, whole grains, nuts and legumes Decrease intake of red meat and dairy products. Decrease bad fats while increasing good fats, such as olive oil and avocados.

Meals based on the Mediterranean diet are very high in carbohydrates and fiber. Getting too much of these can raise triglyceride levels in people who have diabetes or heart disease. The diet is also low in protein, which can lead to ketoacidosis in people with diabetes.

This book will help you with your Mediterranean Diet. Let us start?

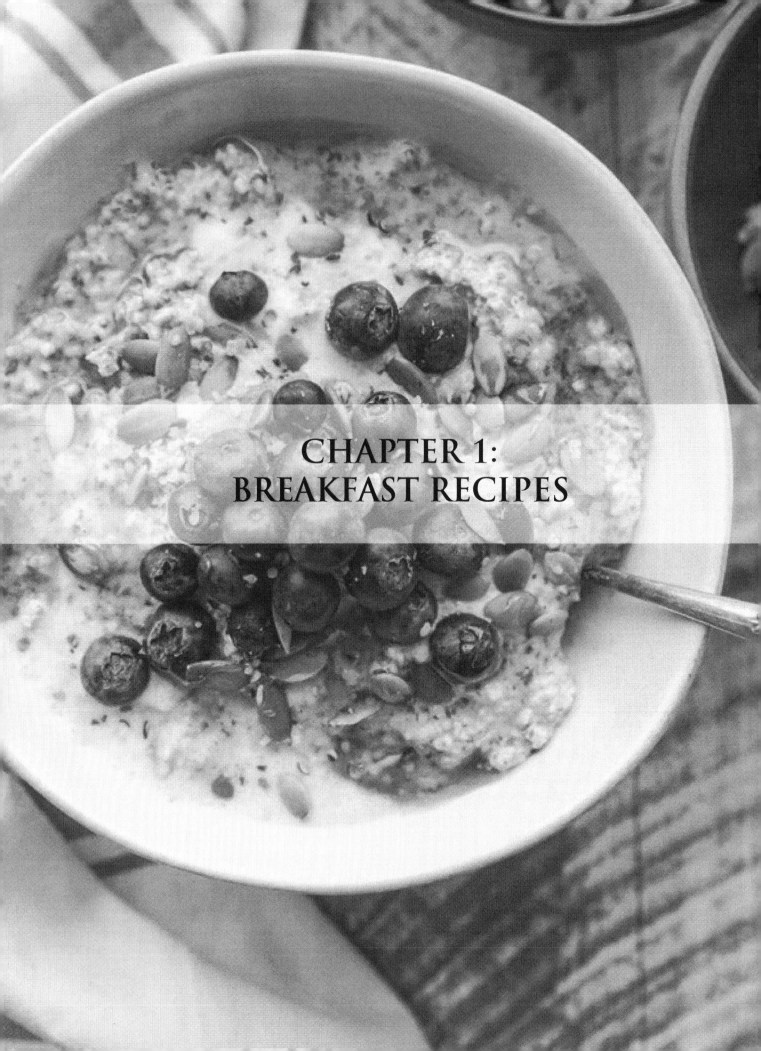

CHAPTER 1:
BREAKFAST RECIPES

1. BASIC CREPES

PREPARATION	COOKING	SERVES
15 MIN	4 MIN	2

INGREDIENTS

- 2 eggs
- 1 cup all-purpose flour
- ½ cup of water
- ½ cup milk
- ¼ cup of salt
- 2 tbsp melted butter

DIRECTIONS

1. Whisk the flour and eggs together. Slowly blend in the milk and water. Fold in the butter and salt. Whisk until smooth.
2. Warm-up a skillet or griddle using the medium-high temperature setting. Lightly oil the griddle.
3. Pour 1/4 cup of the batter for each crepe. Tilt and swirl the pan to prepare the crepe until the first side is lightly browned within 2 minutes. Gently flip and cook the second side. Enjoy hot.

NUTRITIONS

- Calories: 216
- Carbs: 25.5 g
- Protein: 7.4 g
- Fat: 9.2 g

2. BREAKFAST EGG MUFFINS

PREPARATION	COOKING	SERVES
15 MIN	15-20 MIN	3

INGREDIENTS

- cooking oil spray, as needed
- 3 large eggs
- 2 tbsp skimmed milk
- 4 tbsp grated parmesan cheese
- ¼ cup leek
- ¾ cup baby spinach
- ¼ cup red pepper
- 1 tomato, seeds removed
- also needed:
- 6-count silicone or aluminum muffin tin

DIRECTIONS

1. Spritz the muffin tin with cooking oil as needed. Warm the oven to 375° Fahrenheit before baking time.
2. Whisk the parmesan cheese, eggs, and milk together in a pouring jug. Finely chop the spinach, leek, red pepper, and tomato.
3. Mix all the veggies into a bowl and portion into the six muffin cups. Pour the egg batter into each cup, then mix it in with the chopped vegetables. Bake until the egg is set or approximately 15 to 20 minutes.

NUTRITIONS

- *Calories: 308*
- *Carbs: 8.7 g*
- *Protein: 24.4 g*
- *Fat: 19.4 g*

3. BROCCOLI & CHEESE OMELET

PREPARATION	COOKING	SERVES
15 MIN	20 MIN	4

INGREDIENTS

- 2 ½ cups fresh broccoli florets
- 6 large eggs
- ½ cup 2% milk
- ½ tsp salt
- ¼ tsp pepper
- 1/3 cup grated Romano cheese
- 1/3 cup sliced pitted Greek olives
- 1 tbsp olive oil

Optional garnish:
- Romano cheese shaved
- fresh parsley, minced

Also needed:
- 10-inch ovenproof skillet

DIRECTIONS

1. Set the oven temperature to broil. Arrange a steamer basket in a saucepan. Put 1 inch of water, then toss the broccoli into the basket. Wait for it to boil.
2. Lower the heat to simmer for 4 to 6 minutes with a lid. Whisk the milk, eggs, pepper, and salt. Toss in the broccoli, olives, and grated cheese into the mixture.
3. Prepare the skillet using the medium heat setting and add the oil. Dump in the egg mixture, then simmer for 6 minutes.
4. Place the skillet in the oven approximately 3 to 4 inches from the heat. Bake until the eggs are set or for 2 to 4 minutes.
5. Move the skillet to the countertop to cool for about 5 minutes. Slice into wedges. Sprinkle using the parsley and shaved cheese.

NUTRITIONS

- Calories: 229
- Carbs: 5 g
- Protein: 15 g
- Fat: 17 g

4. CHIA BERRY OVERNIGHT OATS

PREPARATION	COOKING	SERVES
OVERNIGHT	0 MIN	1

INGREDIENTS

- ¼ cup chia seeds
- ½ cup Quaker oats rolled oats
- 1 pinch salt
- 1 cup water or milk
- 1 pinch cinnamon
- maple syrup or another sweetener to your liking
- 1 cup of frozen berries of choice

Optional toppings:
- yogurt
- berries

DIRECTIONS

1. Use a jar with a lid, and add the salt, milk, seeds, oats, and cinnamon. Store in the fridge overnight.
2. Puree the berries and combine them with the oats. Top it off with yogurt and more berries, honey, nuts, or other toppings of choice.

NUTRITIONS

- *Calories: 526*
- *Carbs: 78.8 g*
- *Protein: 15.3 g*
- *Fat: 17g*

5. CRUSTLESS SPINACH QUICHE

PREPARATION	COOKING	SERVES
15 MIN	30 MIN	6

INGREDIENTS

- 1 tbsp vegetable oil
- 1 onion, chopped
- 10 oz frozen chopped spinach
- 5 eggs, beaten
- 3 cups shredded muenster cheese
- ¼ tsp salt
- ¼ tsp ground black pepper

Also needed:
- 9-inch pie pan

DIRECTIONS

1. Lightly grease the pan. Thaw and drain the spinach. Warm-up the oven to reach 350 Fahrenheit. Warm up the oil in a skillet using the medium-high temperature setting.
2. Toss in the onions. Sauté until they're are softened. Stir occasionally. Toss the spinach into the mixture, then simmer until the excess moisture has evaporated.
3. In another container, whisk the shredded cheese with the pepper, salt, and eggs. Fold in the spinach mixture, stirring well. Scoop into the pie pan.
4. Bake until the eggs are set within 30 minutes. Cool the quiche for about 10 minutes and serve.

NUTRITIONS

- Calories: 309
- Carbs: 4.8 g
- Protein: 20.4 g
- Fat: 23.7 g

6. DEEP DISH SPINACH QUICHE

PREPARATION	COOKING	SERVES
15 MIN	1 H 5 MIN	6

INGREDIENTS

- ½ cup butter
- 3 garlic, chopped
- 1 small onion, chopped
- 10 oz frozen chopped spinach
- 4 ½ oz mushrooms
- 6 oz crumbled herb and garlic feta
- 8 oz shredded cheddar cheese
- salt & black pepper
- 9-inch deep-dish pie crust, unbaked
- 4 eggs
- 1 cup milk

DIRECTIONS

1. Heat the oven to 375° Fahrenheit. Thaw and drain the spinach and mushrooms. Put the butter in the skillet, then dissolve using the medium temperature heat setting.
2. Sauté the onions and garlic for about 7 minutes until lightly browned. Fold in the feta, mushrooms, spinach, 1/2 cup of cheese, pepper, and salt. Scoop into the pie crust.
3. Whisk the eggs and milk. Dump into the pastry shell and blend with the spinach mixture.
4. Set the timer for 15 minutes. Add the remainder of the cheddar cheese. Bake within 35-45 minutes. Wait for approximately 10 minutes before serving. Enjoy.

NUTRITIONS

- Calories: 613
- Carbs: 23.9 g
- Protein: 22.9 g
- Fat: 48.2 g

7. DELICIOUS SCRAMBLED EGGS

PREPARATION	COOKING	SERVES
15 MIN	5 MIN	2

INGREDIENTS

- 1 tbsp oil
- 1 yellow pepper
- 8 cherry tomatoes
- 2 spring onions
- 1 tbsp capers
- 2 tbsp black olives
- 4 eggs
- ¼ tsp dried oregano
- black pepper

Optional for serving:
- Fresh parsley

DIRECTIONS

1. Warm up the oil in a pan using the medium temperature setting. Dice the bell pepper and spring onions. Add to the skillet and sauté for a few minutes until slightly soft.
2. Quarter the tomatoes, and slice the olives and capers. Toss into the skillet, then sauté for 1 more minute. Break the eggs into your skillet and scramble.
3. Sprinkle with the black pepper and the oregano. Keep stirring until the eggs are done. Serve warm, topped with a portion of fresh parsley.

NUTRITIONS

- Calories: 249
- Carbs: 13 g
- Protein: 14 g
- Fat: 17 g

8. EGG WHITE SCRAMBLE WITH CHERRY TOMATOES & SPINACH

PREPARATION	COOKING	SERVES
5 MIN	5 MIN	4

INGREDIENTS

- 1 tbsp olive oil
- 1 whole & 10 white eggs
- ½ tsp salt
- 1 minced garlic clove
- ¼ tsp black pepper
- 2 cups halved cherry tomatoes
- 2 cups packed fresh baby spinach
- ½ cup light cream, half & half
- ¼ cup finely grated parmesan cheese

DIRECTIONS

1. Whisk the eggs, pepper, salt, and milk. Prepare a skillet using the medium-high heat setting. Toss in the garlic when the pan is hot. Sauté for approximately 30 seconds.
2. Fold in the spinach and tomatoes. Continue sautéing for one additional minute.
3. Add the egg batter into the pan using the medium heat setting. Fold the egg gently as it cooks for about 2 to 3 minutes. Remove from the burner and sprinkle with the cheese.

NUTRITIONS

- *Calories: 142*
- *Carbs: 7 g*
- *Protein: 15 g*
- *Fat: 5 g*

9. EGGS BAKED IN TOMATOES

PREPARATION	COOKING	SERVES
10 MIN	15 MIN	4

INGREDIENTS

- 2 tbsp olive oil
- 8 large eggs
- 8 medium tomatoes
- ¼ cup milk
- ¼ cup grated parmesan cheese
- black pepper & salt (as desired)
- 4 tbsp freshly chopped herbs, e.g., parsley, thyme, rosemary, or a mixture

DIRECTIONS

1. Warm up the oven to 375° Fahrenheit. Grease a large oven-safe skillet using olive oil. Prepare the tomatoes. Remove the stem and scoop out all the insides.
2. Place the tomato shells in the prepared skillet. Crack an egg into over the tomatoes. Top it off with salt, pepper, and 1 tablespoon each of the milk and parmesan.
3. Bake until the tomatoes are tender, the yolks are still a little jiggly, and the egg whites are set within 15 minutes. Let it cool for about 5 minutes. Garnish with the fresh herbs. Serve immediately.

NUTRITIONS

- Calories: 288
- Carbs: 12 g
- Protein: 18 g
- Fat: 19 g

10. FETA FRITTATA

PREPARATION	COOKING	SERVES
15 MIN	15 MIN	2

INGREDIENTS

- 1 green onion
- 1 small garlic clove
- 2 large eggs
- ½ cup egg substitute
- 4 tbsp crumbled feta cheese, divided
- 1/3 cup plum tomato
- 4 avocados, thinly sliced
- 2 tbsp reduced-fat sour cream
- 1 mozzarella cheese

Also needed:
- 6-inch nonstick skillet

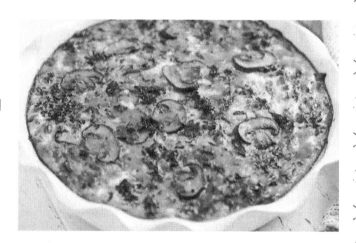

DIRECTIONS

1. Peel the avocado. Thinly slice the avocado and onions. Mince the garlic, and chop the tomatoes. Warm up the pan using the medium temperature setting and lightly spritz it with cooking oil.
2. Whisk the egg substitute, eggs, and 3 tablespoons of feta cheese. Empty into the skillet, then simmer for 4 to 6 minutes.
3. Toss in the rest of the feta cheese and tomato. Place the top back on the skillet. Simmer until the eggs are set.
4. Put 1 slice of mozzarella on top of the prosciutto, and spread 1/4 of the avocado slices into each wrap.
5. Garnish each of the wraps with one sliced tomato and about 1/4 cup of lettuce leaves, torn apart. Let it rest within 5 minutes before cutting it into halves. Serve with a portion of the avocado and sour cream.

NUTRITIONS

- Calories: 203
- Carbs: 7 g
- Protein: 17 g
- Fat: 12 g

11. TASTY BREAKFAST DONUTS

PREPARATION	COOKING	SERVES
5 MIN	5 MIN	4

INGREDIENTS

- 43 grams of cream cheese
- 2 eggs
- 2 tablespoons almond flour
- 2 tablespoons erythritol
- 1 ½ tablespoons coconut flour
- ½ teaspoon baking powder
- ½ teaspoon vanilla extract
- 5 drops Stevia (liquid form)
- 2 strips bacon, fried until crispy

DIRECTIONS

1. Rub coconut oil over donut maker and turn on. Mix all ingredients except bacon in a blender or food processor until smooth within 1 minute.
2. Pour batter into donut maker, leaving 1/10 in each round for rising. Leave for 3 minutes before flipping each donut. Leave for another 2 minutes or until a fork comes out clean when piercing them.
3. Take donuts out and let cool. Repeat all steps until all batter is used. Crumble bacon into bits and use to top donuts.

NUTRITIONS

- *Calories: 60*
- *Fat: 5 g*
- *Carbs: 1 g*
- *Fiber: 0 g*
- *Protein: 3 g*

12. CHEESY SPICY BACON BOWLS

PREPARATION	COOKING	SERVES
10 MIN	22 MIN	12

INGREDIENTS

- 6 strips bacon, pan-fried until cooked but still malleable
- 4 eggs
- 60 grams' cheddar cheese
- 40 grams' cream cheese, grated
- 2 Jalapenos, sliced and seeds removed
- 2 tablespoons coconut oil
- ¼ teaspoon onion powder
- ¼ teaspoon garlic powder
- Dash of salt and pepper

DIRECTIONS

1. Warm oven to 375 degrees F. In a bowl, beat together eggs, cream cheese, jalapenos (minus 6 slices), coconut oil, onion powder, garlic powder, and salt and pepper.
2. Using leftover bacon grease on a muffin tray, rubbing it into each insert. Place bacon-wrapped inside the parameters of each insert.
3. Pour beaten mixture halfway up each bacon bowl. Garnish each bacon bowl with cheese and leftover jalapeno slices (placing one on top of each).
4. Leave in the oven for about 22 minutes, or until the egg is thoroughly cooked and cheese is bubbly. Remove from oven and let cool until edible. Enjoy!

NUTRITIONS

- *Calories: 259*
- *Fat: 24g*
- *Carbs: 1g*
- *Protein: 10g*

13. GOAT, CHEESE, ZUCCHINI, AND KALE QUICHE

PREPARATION	COOKING	SERVES
35 MIN	1H 10 MIN	4

INGREDIENTS

- 4 large eggs
- 8 ounces fresh zucchini, sliced
- 10 ounces kale
- 3 garlic cloves (minced)
- 1 cup of soy milk
- 1-ounce goat cheese
- 1 cup grated parmesan
- 1 cup shredded cheddar cheese
- 2 teaspoons olive oil
- Salt and pepper, to taste

DIRECTIONS

1. Warm oven to 350 F, then heat 1 tsp of olive oil in a saucepan over medium-high heat. Sauté garlic for 1 minute until flavored.
2. Add the zucchini and cook again within 5-7 minutes until soft. Beat the eggs, and then add a little milk and parmesan cheese.
3. Meanwhile, heat-up the rest of the olive oil in another saucepan and add the kale. Cover and cook for 5 minutes until dry.
4. Slightly grease a baking dish with cooking spray and spread the kale leaves across the bottom. Add the zucchini and top with goat cheese.
5. Pour the egg, milk, and parmesan mixture evenly over the other ingredients. Top with cheddar cheese.
6. Bake for 50–60 minutes until golden brown. Check the center of the quiche; it should have a solid consistency. Let chill for a few minutes before serving.

NUTRITIONS

- Calories: 290
- Carbohydrates: 15g
- Carbs: 13 g
- Protein: 19 g
- Fat: 18 g

14. CREAM CHEESE EGG BREAKFAST

PREPARATION	COOKING	SERVES
5 MIN	5 MIN	4

INGREDIENTS

- 2 eggs, beaten
- 1 tablespoon butter
- 2 tablespoons soft cream cheese with chives

DIRECTIONS

1. Dissolve the butter in a small skillet, then add the eggs and cream cheese. Stir and cook to desired doneness.

NUTRITIONS

- *Calories: 341*
- *Fat: 31 g*
- *Protein: 15 g*
- *Carbohydrate: 0 g*

15. AVOCADO RED PEPPERS ROASTED SCRAMBLED EGGS

PREPARATION	COOKING	SERVES
10 MIN	12 MIN	3

INGREDIENTS

- 1/2 tablespoon butter
- 2 eggs
- 1/2 roasted red pepper, about 1 1/2 ounces
- 1/2 small avocado, coarsely chopped, about 2 1/4 ounces
- Salt, to taste

DIRECTIONS

1. In your nonstick skillet, heat-up butter over medium heat. Break your eggs and break their yolks with a spoon into the pan. Sprinkle with a little salt.
2. Stir to stir and continue stirring until the eggs start to come out. Quickly add the bell peppers and avocado. Cook and stir until the eggs suit your taste. Adjust the seasoning, if necessary.

NUTRITIONS

- *Calories: 317*
- *Fat: 26g*
- *Protein: 14g*
- *Carbs: 4g*

16. MUSHROOM QUICKIE SCRAMBLE

PREPARATION	COOKING	SERVES
10 MIN	10 MIN	4

INGREDIENTS

- 3 small-sized eggs, whisked
- 4 pcs. Bella mushrooms
- ½ cup of spinach
- ¼ cup of red bell peppers
- 2 deli ham slices
- 1 tablespoon of ghee or coconut oil
- Salt and pepper to taste

DIRECTIONS

1. Chop the ham and veggies. Put half a tbsp of butter in a frying pan and heat until melted. Sauté the ham and vegetables in a frying pan, then set aside.
2. Get a new frying pan and heat the remaining butter. Add the whisked eggs into the second pan while stirring continuously to avoid overcooking.
3. When the eggs are done, sprinkle with salt and pepper to taste. Add the ham and veggies to the pan with the eggs. Mix well. Remove and transfer to a plate, then serve.

NUTRITIONS

- *Calories: 350*
- *Fat: 29 g*
- *Protein: 21 g*
- *Carbs: 5 g*

17. COCONUT COFFEE AND GHEE

PREPARATION	COOKING	SERVES
10 MIN	10 MIN	5

INGREDIENTS

- ½ tbsp of coconut oil
- ½ tbsp of ghee
- 1-2 cups of preferred coffee (or rooibos or black tea, if desired)
- 1 tbsp of coconut or almond milk

DIRECTIONS

1. Place the almond (or coconut) milk, coconut oil, ghee, and coffee in a blender. Mix for around 10 seconds or until the coffee turns creamy and foamy. Pour contents into a coffee cup. Serve immediately and enjoy.

NUTRITIONS

- *Calories: 150*
- *Fat: 15 g*
- *Protein: 0 g*
- *Carbs: 0 g*

18. YUMMY VEGGIE WAFFLES

PREPARATION	COOKING	SERVES
10 MIN	9 MIN	3

INGREDIENTS

- 3 cups raw cauliflower, grated
- 1 cup cheddar cheese
- 1 cup mozzarella cheese
- ½ cup parmesan
- 1/3 cup chives, finely sliced
- 6 eggs
- 1 teaspoon garlic powder
- 1 teaspoon onion powder
- ½ teaspoon chili flakes
- Dash of salt and pepper

DIRECTIONS

1. Turn the waffle maker on. In a bowl, mix all the listed fixings very well until incorporated. Once the waffle maker is hot, distribute the waffle mixture into the insert.
2. Let cook for about 9 minutes, flipping at 6 minutes. Remove from waffle maker and set aside. Serve and enjoy!

NUTRITIONS

- Calories: 390
- Fat: 28 g
- Carbs: 6 g
- Protein: 30 g

19. OMEGA 3 BREAKFAST SHAKE

PREPARATION	COOKING	SERVES
5 MIN	5 MIN	2

INGREDIENTS

- 1 cup vanilla almond milk (unsweetened)
- 2 tablespoons blueberries
- 1 ½ tablespoons flaxseed meal
- 1 tablespoon MCT Oil
- ¾ tablespoon banana extract
- ½ tablespoon chia seeds
- 5 drops Stevia (liquid form)
- 1/8 tablespoon Xanthan gum

DIRECTIONS

1. In a blender, mix vanilla almond milk, banana extract, Stevia, and three ice cubes. When smooth, add blueberries and pulse.
2. Once blueberries are thoroughly incorporated, add flaxseed meal and chia seeds. Let sit for 5 minutes. After 5 minutes, pulse again until all ingredients are nicely distributed. Serve and enjoy.

NUTRITIONS

- *Calories: 264*
- *Fats: 25 g*
- *Carbs: 7 g*
- *Protein: 4 g*

20. LIME BACON THYME MUFFINS

PREPARATION	COOKING	SERVES
10 MIN	20 MIN	3

INGREDIENTS

- 3 cups of almond flour
- 4 medium-sized eggs
- 1 cup of bacon bits
- 2 tsp. of lemon thyme
- ½ cup of melted ghee
- 1 tsp. of baking soda
- ½ tsp. of salt, to taste

DIRECTIONS

1. Pre-heat oven to 3500 F. Put ghee in the mixing bowl and melt. Add baking soda and almond flour.
2. Put the eggs in. Add the lemon thyme (if preferred, other herbs or spices may be used). Drizzle with salt. Mix all ingredients well.
3. Sprinkle with bacon bits. Line the muffin pan with liners. Spoon mixture into the pan, filling the pan to about ¾ full.
4. Bake for about 20 minutes. Test by inserting a toothpick into a muffin. If it comes out clean, then the muffins are done. Serve immediately.

NUTRITIONS

- *Calories: 300*
- *Fat: 28 g*
- *Protein: 11 g*
- *Carbs: 6 g*

21. AMARANTH PORRIDGE

PREPARATION	COOKING	SERVES
5 MIN	30 MIN	2

INGREDIENTS

- 2 cups of coconut milk
- 2 cups alkaline water
- 1 cup amaranth
- 2 tbsps. coconut oil
- 1 tbsp. ground cinnamon

DIRECTIONS

1. In a saucepan, mix the milk with water, then boil the mixture. Stir in the amaranth, then reduce the heat to medium.
2. Cook on medium heat, then simmers for at least 30 minutes as you stir it occasionally. Turn off the heat. Add in cinnamon and coconut oil, then stir. Serve.

NUTRITIONS

- *Calories: 434*
- *Fat: 35g*
- *Carbs: 27g*
- *Protein: 6.7g*

22. GLUTEN-FREE PANCAKES

PREPARATION	COOKING	SERVES
5 MIN	2 MIN	2

INGREDIENTS

- 6 eggs
- 1 cup low-fat cream cheese
- 1 1/12; teaspoons baking powder
- 1 scoop protein powder
- 1/4 cup almond meal
- ¼ teaspoon salt

DIRECTIONS

1. Combine dry ingredients in a food processor. Add the eggs one after another and then the cream cheese. Mix it well.
2. Lightly grease a skillet with cooking spray and place over medium-high heat. Pour the batter into the pan. Turn the pan gently to create round pancakes.
3. Cook within 2 minutes on each side. Serve pancakes with your favorite topping.

NUTRITIONS

- *Calories: 288*
- *Carbs: 5 g*
- *Protein: 25 g*
- *Fat: 14 g*

23. MUSHROOM & SPINACH OMELET

PREPARATION	COOKING	SERVES
20 MIN	20 MIN	3

INGREDIENTS

- 2 tablespoons butter, divided
- 6-8 fresh mushrooms, sliced, 5 ounces
- Chives, chopped, optional
- Salt and pepper, to taste
- 1 handful baby spinach, about 1/2 ounce
- Pinch garlic powder
- 4 eggs, beaten
- 1-ounce shredded Swiss cheese

DIRECTIONS

1. In a large saucepan, sauté the mushrooms in one tablespoon of butter until soft—season with salt, pepper, and garlic.
2. Remove and keep warm—heat-up the remaining tablespoon of butter in the same skillet over medium heat.
3. Beat the eggs with salt plus pepper and add to the hot butter. Turn the pan over to coat the entire bottom of the pan with an egg. Once the egg is almost out, place the cheese over the middle of the tortilla.
4. Fill the cheese with spinach leaves and hot mushrooms. Let cook for about a minute for the spinach to start to wilt.
5. Fold the tortilla's empty side carefully over the filling and slide it onto a plate and sprinkle with chives, if desired.
6. Alternatively, you can make two tortillas using half the mushroom, spinach, and cheese filling in each.

NUTRITIONS

- *Calories: 321*
- *Fat: 26 g*
- *Protein: 19 g*
- *Carbohydrate: 4 g*

24. WHOLE-WHEAT BLUEBERRY MUFFINS

PREPARATION	COOKING	SERVES
5 MIN	25 MIN	8

INGREDIENTS

- 1/2 cup plant-based milk
- 1/2 cup unsweetened applesauce
- 1/2 cup maple syrup
- 1 teaspoon vanilla extract
- 2 cups whole-wheat flour
- 1/2 teaspoon baking soda
- 1 cup blueberries

DIRECTIONS

1. Preheat the oven to 375°F. Mix the milk, applesauce, maple syrup, and vanilla in a large bowl. Mix in the flour plus baking soda until no dry flour is left, and the batter is smooth.
2. Fold in the blueberries throughout the batter. In a muffin tin, fill eight muffin cups with three-quarters full of batter.
3. Bake within 25 minutes, or until you can stick a knife into the center of a muffin and it comes out clean. Allow cooling before serving.

NUTRITIONS

- *Calories: 288*
- *Fat: 1 g*
- *Carbohydrates: 45 g*
- *Protein: 4 g*

25. HEMP SEED PORRIDGE

PREPARATION	COOKING	SERVES
5 MIN	5 MIN	6

INGREDIENTS

- 3 cups cooked hemp seed
- 1 packet Stevia
- 1 cup of coconut milk

DIRECTIONS

1. In a saucepan, mix the rice and the coconut milk over moderate heat for about 5 minutes as you stir it frequently. Remove, then put the Stevia. Stir. Serve in 6 bowls.

NUTRITIONS

- *Calories: 236*
- *Fat: 1.8 g*

- *Carbs: 48.3 g*
- *Protein: 7 g*

26. WALNUT CRUNCH BANANA BREAD

PREPARATION	COOKING	SERVES
5 MIN	1H 30 MIN	1

INGREDIENTS

- 4 ripe bananas
- 1/4 cup maple syrup
- 1 tablespoon apple cider vinegar
- 1 teaspoon vanilla extract
- 1 1/2 cups whole-wheat flour
- 1/2 teaspoon ground cinnamon
- 1/2 teaspoon baking soda
- 1/4 cup walnut pieces (optional)

DIRECTIONS

1. Warm oven to 350 F. In a large bowl, use a fork or mixing spoon to mash the bananas until they reach a puréed consistency.
2. Mix in your maple syrup, apple cider vinegar, plus vanilla. Stir in the flour, cinnamon, and baking soda. Fold in the walnut pieces (if using).
3. Pour the batter into your loaf pan, filling it no more than three-quarters of the way full. Bake for 1 hour, or you can stick a knife into the middle, and it comes out clean.
4. Remove, and allow cooling on the countertop for a minimum of 30 minutes before serving.

NUTRITIONS

- Calories: 125
- Fat: 1g
- Carbohydrates: 40 g
- Protein: 4 g

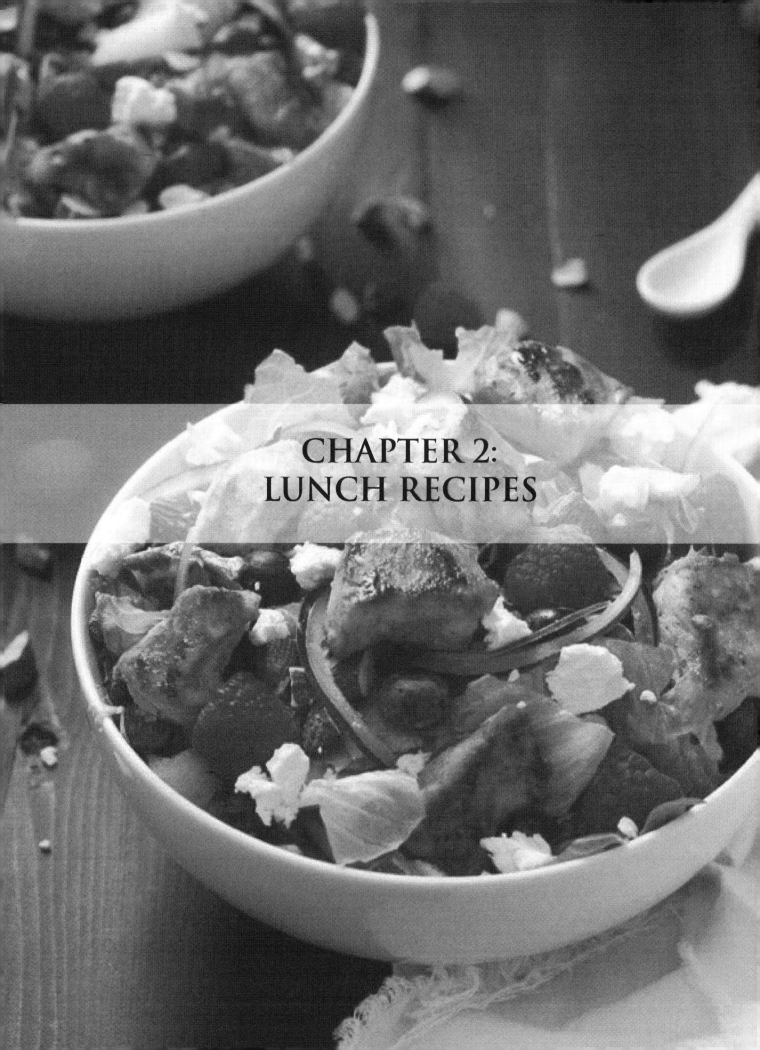

CHAPTER 2:
LUNCH RECIPES

27. STRAWBERRY & ASPARAGUS SALAD

PREPARATION	COOKING	SERVES
15 MIN	3 MIN	8

INGREDIENTS

- 2 pounds fresh asparagus, trimmed and sliced
- 3 cups fresh strawberries, hulled and sliced
- ¼ cup extra-virgin olive oil
- ¼ cup balsamic vinegar
- 2 tablespoons maple syrup
- Salt and ground black pepper, as required

DIRECTIONS

1. In a pan of water, add the asparagus over medium-high heat and bring to a boil. Boil the asparagus for about 2-3 minutes or until al dente.
2. Drain the asparagus and immediately transfer it into a bowl of ice water to cool completely. Strain the asparagus, then pat-dry with paper towels.
3. Put the asparagus and strawberries in a large bowl, and mix. Put the olive oil, vinegar, honey, salt, and black pepper in a small bowl, and beat until well blended.
4. Place the dressing over the asparagus strawberry mixture and gently toss to coat. Refrigerate for about 1 hour before serving.

NUTRITIONS

- *Calories: 109*
- *Fat: 6.6g*
- *Carbohydrates: 12g*
- *Protein: 2.9g*

28. BERRIES & SPINACH SALAD

PREPARATION	COOKING	SERVES
15 MIN	0 MIN	4

INGREDIENTS

For the Salad:
- 6 cups fresh baby spinach
- ¾ cup fresh strawberries, hulled and sliced
- ¾ cup fresh blueberries
- ¼ cup onion, sliced
- ¼ cup almond, sliced
- ¼ cup feta cheese, crumbled

For Dressing:
- 1/3 cup olive oil
- 2 tablespoons fresh lemon juice
- ¼ teaspoon liquid stevia
- 1/8 teaspoon garlic powder
- Salt, as required

DIRECTIONS

1. For the salad, add the spinach, berries, onion, and almonds and mix in a bowl. For the dressing, add all the fixings in another small bowl and beat until well blended. Place the dressing over salad and gently toss to coat well. Serve immediately.

NUTRITIONS

- *Calories: 97*
- *Fat: 5.3g*
- *Carbohydrates: 10g*
- *Protein: 4.4g*

29. EGGS & VEGGIE SALAD

PREPARATION	COOKING	SERVES
15 MIN	0 MIN	8

INGREDIENTS

For Salad:
- 2 large English cucumbers, sliced thinly sliced
- 2 cups tomatoes, chopped
- 8 hard-boiled eggs, peeled and sliced
- 8 cups fresh baby spinach

For Dressing:
- 4 tablespoons olive oil
- 2 tablespoons balsamic vinegar
- 1 tablespoon fresh lemon juice
- Salt and ground black pepper, as required

DIRECTIONS

1. For the salad, mix the cucumbers, onion, and dill in a salad bowl. For the dressing, mix all the fixings in a small bowl. Place the dressing over the salad and toss to coat well. Serve immediately.

NUTRITIONS

- *Calories: 150*
- *Fat: 11.7g*
- *Carbohydrates: 6g*
- *Protein: 7.3g*

30. CHICKEN STUFFED AVOCADO

PREPARATION	COOKING	SERVES
15 MIN	0 MIN	2

INGREDIENTS

- 1 cup cooked chicken, shredded
- 1 avocado, halved and pitted
- 1 tablespoon fresh lime juice
- ¼ cup yellow onion, chopped finely
- ¼ cup low-fat plain Greek yogurt
- Pinch of cayenne pepper
- Salt and ground black pepper, as required

DIRECTIONS

1. With a small scooper, scoop out the flesh from the middle of each avocado half and transfer it into a bowl. In the avocado flesh bowl, add the lime juice, and with a fork, mash until well blended.
2. Add remaining ingredients and stir to combine. Divide the chicken mixture into avocado halves evenly and serve immediately.

NUTRITIONS

- Calories: 281
- Fat: 16g
- Carbohydrates: 9g
- Protein: 23.7g

31. CHICKEN LETTUCE WRAPS

PREPARATION	COOKING	SERVES
15 MIN	15 MIN	5

INGREDIENTS

For Chicken:
- 2 tablespoons avocado oil
- 1 small onion, chopped finely
- 1 teaspoon fresh ginger, minced
- 2 garlic cloves, minced
- 1¼ pounds grass-fed ground chicken
- Salt and ground black pepper, as required

For Wraps:
- 10 romaine lettuce leaves
- 1½ cups carrot, peeled and julienned
- 2 tablespoons fresh parsley, chopped finely
- 2 tablespoons fresh lime juice

DIRECTIONS

1. In a large nonstick pan, heat the avocado oil over medium heat and sauté the onion, ginger, and garlic for about 4-5 minutes.
2. Add the ground chicken, salt, and black pepper, and cook over medium-high heat for about 7-9 minutes.
3. Remove the pan of the chicken mixture from the heat and set aside to cool. Arrange the lettuce leaves onto serving plates.
4. Place the cooked chicken over each lettuce leaf and top with carrot and cilantro. Drizzle with lime juice and serve immediately.

NUTRITIONS

- Calories: 246
- Fat: 9g
- Carbohydrates: 5.8g
- Protein: 33.5g

32. CHICKEN BURGERS

PREPARATION	COOKING	SERVES
15 MIN	10 MIN	4

INGREDIENTS

For Burgers:
- 1¼ pounds ground chicken
- 1 egg
- ½ of yellow onion, grated
- Salt and ground black pepper, as required
- 1 teaspoon dried thyme
- 2 tablespoons olive oil

For Serving:
- 4 cups fresh arugula
- 1 cup tomato, chopped

DIRECTIONS

1. For the burgers, add all the ingredients in a bowl and mix until well blended. Make 8 small equal-sized patties from the mixture.
2. Warm-up oil over medium heat in a large frying pan, and cook the patties within 4-5 minutes per side or until done completely.
3. Divide the arugula and tomato onto serving plates and top each with 2 burgers. Serve hot.

NUTRITIONS

- Calories: 298
- Fat: 19g
- Carbohydrates: 4.1g
- Protein: 27.2g

33. BEEF BURGERS

PREPARATION	COOKING	SERVES
15 MIN	12 MIN	4

INGREDIENTS

For Burgers:
- 1-pound lean ground beef
- 1 cup fresh baby spinach leaves, chopped
- ½ of small yellow onion, chopped
- ¼ cup sun-dried tomatoes, chopped
- 1 egg, beaten
- ¼ cup feta cheese, crumbled
- Salt and ground black pepper, as required
- 2 tablespoons olive oil

For Serving:
- 4 cups fresh spinach, torn
- 1 large tomato, sliced

DIRECTIONS

1. For burgers, add all ingredients except for oil in a large bowl, and mix until well blended. Make 4 equal-sized patties from the mixture.
2. In a pan, heat the oil over medium-high heat and cook the patties for about 5-6 minutes per side or until desired doneness.
3. Divide the spinach and tomato slices and onto serving plates. Top each plate with 1 burger and serve.

NUTRITIONS

- *Calories: 244*
- *Fat: 19g*
- *Carbohydrates: 4.9g*
- *Protein: 15g*

34. MEATBALLS WITH SALAD

PREPARATION	COOKING	SERVES
20 MIN	15 MIN	4

INGREDIENTS

For Meatballs:
- 1-pound lean ground turkey
- 1 cup chopped spinach, squeezed
- ½ cup feta cheese, crumbled
- ½ teaspoon dried oregano
- Salt and ground black pepper, as required
- 2 tablespoons olive oil

For Salad:
- 4 cups fresh baby spinach
- 1 cup cherry tomatoes, halved

DIRECTIONS

1. For meatballs, place all ingredients except for oil in a bowl and mix until well blended. Make 12 equal-sized meatballs from the mixture.
2. Warm-up olive oil over medium heat in a large nonstick pan, and cook the meatballs for about 10-15 minutes or until done completely, flipping occasionally.
3. With a slotted spoon, place the meatballs onto a plate. Meanwhile, in a large salad bowl, add all ingredients and toss to coat well for the salad. Divide meatballs and salad onto serving plates and serve.

NUTRITIONS

- *Calories: 289*
- *Fat: 19g*
- *Carbohydrates: 4g*
- *Protein: 26.4g*

35. STUFFED BELL PEPPERS

PREPARATION	COOKING	SERVES
20 MIN	40 MIN	5

INGREDIENTS

- 5 large bell peppers, tops, and seeds removed
- 1 tablespoon olive oil
- ½ of a large onion, chopped
- ½ teaspoon dried oregano
- ½ teaspoon dried thyme
- Salt and ground black pepper, as required
- 1-pound grass-fed ground beef
- 1 large zucchini, chopped
- 3 tablespoons homemade tomato paste

DIRECTIONS

1. Warm your oven to 350 degrees F. Grease a small baking dish. In a large pan of boiling water, place the bell peppers and cook for about 4-5 minutes.
2. Remove from the water and place onto a paper towel, cut side down. Meanwhile, in a large nonstick pan, heat the olive oil over medium heat and sauté onion for about 3-4 minutes.
3. Add the ground beef, oregano, salt, and pepper, and cook for about 8-10 minutes. Add the zucchini and cook for about 2-3 minutes.
4. Remove from the heat and drain any juices from the beef mixture. Put the tomato paste, then stir to combine. Arrange the bell peppers into the prepared baking dish, cut side upward.
5. Stuff the bell peppers using the beef batter evenly—Bake for approximately 15 minutes. Serve warm.

NUTRITIONS

- *Calories: 241*
- *Fat: 8.8g*
- *Carbohydrates: 11g*
- *Protein: 29.9g*

36. SHRIMP WITH ZOODLES

PREPARATION	COOKING	SERVES
20 MIN	8 MIN	4

INGREDIENTS

- 2 tablespoons olive oil
- 1 garlic clove, minced
- ¼ teaspoon red pepper flakes, crushed
- 1-pound shrimp, peeled and deveined
- Salt and ground black pepper, as required
- 1/3 cup low-sodium chicken broth
- 2 medium zucchinis, spiralized with blade C

DIRECTIONS

1. In a large nonstick pan, warm-up olive oil over medium heat and sauté garlic and red pepper flakes for about 1 minute.
2. Put the shrimp, salt, plus black pepper and cook for about 1 minute per side. Add the broth and zucchini noodles and cook for about 3-4 minutes. Serve hot.

NUTRITIONS

- *Calories: 213*
- *Fat: 9.1g*
- *Carbohydrates: 5.4g*
- *Protein: 27.3g*

37. SHRIMP WITH ASPARAGUS

PREPARATION	COOKING	SERVES
15 MIN	10 MIN	4

INGREDIENTS

- 2 tablespoons olive oil
- 1-pound asparagus, trimmed
- 1-pound shrimp, peeled and deveined
- 4 garlic cloves, minced
- 2 tablespoons fresh lemon juice
- 1/3 cup chicken broth
- Salt and ground black pepper, as required

DIRECTIONS

1. In a large pan, warm-up oil over medium-high heat, then add all the ingredients except for broth and cook for about 2 minutes, without stirring.
2. Stir the mixture and cook for about 3-4 minutes, stirring occasionally. Stir in the broth, salt, and black pepper and cook for about 2-4 more minutes. Serve hot.

NUTRITIONS

- *Calories: 227*
- *Fat: 9.3g*
- *Carbohydrates: 7.4g*
- *Protein: 29g*

38. SHRIMP WITH BELL PEPPERS

PREPARATION	COOKING	SERVES
20 MIN	10 MIN	6

INGREDIENTS

- ½ cup low-sodium soy sauce
- 2 tablespoons balsamic vinegar
- 2 tablespoons Erythritol
- 1 tablespoon arrowroot starch
- 1 tablespoon fresh ginger, minced
- ½ teaspoon red pepper flakes, crushed
- 3 tablespoons olive oil
- ½ of small red bell pepper, seeded and cut into thin strips
- ½ of small yellow bell pepper, seeded and cut into thin strips
- ½ of small red bell pepper, seeded and cut into thin strips
- ½ of small green bell pepper, seeded and cut into thin strips
- 1 small onion, cut into thin strips
- 1 fresh red chili, chopped
- 1½ pounds shrimp, peeled and deveined
- Freshly ground black pepper, as required

DIRECTIONS

1. Place the soy sauce, vinegar, Erythritol, arrowroot starch, ginger, and red pepper flakes and mix well in a bowl. Set aside.
2. In a large high-sided pan, warm-up the oil over high heat and stir fry the bell peppers, onion, and red chili for about 1-2 minutes.
3. With the spoon, push the pepper mixture to the edge of the pan to create a center space. Put the shrimp in a single layer and cook within 1-2 minutes in the pan's center.
4. Stir the shrimp with bell pepper mixture and cook for about 2 minutes. Stir in the sauce and cook for about 2-3 minutes, stirring frequently. Stir in the black pepper and remove from the heat. Serve hot.

NUTRITIONS

- Calories: 221
- Fat: 9g
- Carbohydrates: 7.5g
- Protein: 27.6g

39. SHRIMP WITH SPINACH

PREPARATION	COOKING	SERVES
15 MIN	10 MIN	4

INGREDIENTS

- 3 tablespoons olive oil
- 1-pound medium shrimp, peeled and deveined
- 1 medium onion, chopped
- 4 garlic cloves, chopped finely
- 1-pound fresh spinach, chopped
- ¼ cup chicken broth
- Salt and ground black pepper, as required

DIRECTIONS

1. In a large nonstick pan, warm-up 1 tablespoon of the oil over medium-high heat and cook the shrimp within 2 minutes per side.
2. With a slotted spoon, transfer the shrimp onto a plate. Warm-up the rest of your oil over medium heat in the same pan, and sauté the garlic and red chili for about 1 minute.
3. Add the spinach and broth and cook for about 3-4 minutes, stirring occasionally. Stir in the cooked shrimp, salt, and black pepper and cook for about 1 minute. Serve hot.

NUTRITIONS

- Calories: 240
- Fat: 12.3g
- Carbohydrates: 7.7g
- Protein: 28.2g

40. SCALLOPS WITH BROCCOLI

PREPARATION	COOKING	SERVES
15 MIN	9 MIN	2

INGREDIENTS

- 1 tablespoon olive oil
- 1 cup broccoli, cut into small pieces
- 1 garlic clove, crushed
- ½ pound scallops
- 1 teaspoon fresh lemon juice
- Salt, as required

DIRECTIONS

1. In a large nonstick pan, heat-up oil over medium heat and cook the broccoli and garlic for about 3-4 minutes, stirring occasionally.
2. Put in the scallops and cook within 3-4 minutes, flipping occasionally. Stir in the lemon juice and salt and remove from the heat. Serve hot.

NUTRITIONS

- *Calories: 178*
- *Fat: 8g*
- *Carbohydrates: 6.3g*
- *Protein: 20.4g*

41. CAULIFLOWER WITH PEAS

PREPARATION	COOKING	SERVES
15 MIN	15 MIN	4

INGREDIENTS

- 2 medium tomatoes, chopped
- ¼ cup of water
- 2 tablespoons olive oil
- 3 garlic cloves, minced
- ½ tablespoon fresh ginger, minced
- 1 teaspoon ground cumin
- 2 teaspoons ground coriander
- 1 teaspoon cayenne pepper
- ¼ teaspoon ground turmeric
- 2 cups cauliflower, chopped
- 1 cup fresh green peas, shelled
- Salt and ground black pepper, as required
- ½ cup of warm water

DIRECTIONS

1. In a blender, add tomato and ¼ cup of water and pulse until a smooth puree forms. Set aside. In a large pan, warm-up oil over medium heat and sauté the garlic, ginger, green chilies, and spices for about 1 minute.
2. Add the cauliflower, peas, and tomato puree and cook, stirring for about 3-4 minutes. Add the warm water and bring to a boil.
3. Adjust the heat to medium-low and cook, covered for about 8-10 minutes or until vegetables are done completely. Serve hot.

NUTRITIONS

- *Calories: 123*
- *Fat: 7.6g*
- *Carbohydrates: 12g*
- *Protein: 3.8g*

42. BROCCOLI WITH BELL PEPPERS

PREPARATION	COOKING	SERVES
15 MIN	10 MIN	6

INGREDIENTS

- 2 tablespoons olive oil
- 4 garlic cloves, minced
- 1 large white onion, sliced
- 2 cups small broccoli florets
- 3 red bell peppers, seeded and sliced
- ¼ cup vegetable broth
- Salt and ground black pepper, as required

DIRECTIONS

1. In a large pan, warm-up oil over medium heat and sauté the garlic for about 1 minute. Add the onion, broccoli, and bell peppers and cook for about 5 minutes, stirring frequently.
2. Stir in the broth and cook for about 4 minutes, stirring frequently. Stir in the salt plus black pepper and remove from the heat. Serve hot.

NUTRITIONS

- *Calories: 84*
- *Fat: 5g*
- *Carbohydrates: 9.6g*
- *Protein: 2.1g*

43. 3-VEGGIES COMBO

PREPARATION	COOKING	SERVES
15 MIN	25 MIN	4

INGREDIENTS

- 1 tablespoon olive oil
- 1 small yellow onion, chopped
- 1 teaspoon fresh thyme, chopped
- 1 garlic clove, minced
- 8 ounces fresh button mushroom, sliced
- 1-pound Brussels sprouts, trimmed and halved
- 3 cups fresh spinach
- Salt and ground black pepper, as required

DIRECTIONS

1. In a large pan, warm-up oil over medium heat and sauté the onion for about 3-4 minutes. Add the thyme and garlic and sauté for about 1 minute.
2. Add the mushrooms and cook for about 15 minutes or until caramelized. Put the Brussels sprouts and cook within 2-3 minutes.
3. Add in the spinach and cook for about 3-4 minutes. Stir in the salt plus black pepper and remove from the heat. Serve hot.

NUTRITIONS

- Calories: 84
- Fat: 3.3g
- Carbohydrates: 12g
- Protein: 5.2g

44. TOFU WITH BROCCOLI

PREPARATION	COOKING	SERVES
10 MIN	25 MIN	4

INGREDIENTS

For Tofu:
- 14 ounces firm tofu, drained, pressed, and cut into 1-inch slices
- 1/3 cup arrowroot starch, divided
- ¼ cup olive oil
- 1 teaspoon fresh ginger, grated
- 1 medium onion, sliced thinly
- 3 tablespoons low-sodium soy sauce
- 2 tablespoons balsamic vinegar
- 1 tablespoon maple syrup

- ½ cup of water

For Steamed Broccoli:
- 2 cups broccoli florets

DIRECTIONS

1. In a shallow bowl, place ¼ cup of the arrowroot starch. Add the tofu cubes and coat with arrowroot starch. In a cast-iron pan, heat the olive oil over medium heat and cook the tofu cubes for about 8-10 minutes or until golden from all sides.
2. With a slotted spoon, transfer the tofu cubes onto a plate. Set aside. In the same pan, add ginger and sauté for about 1 minute.
3. Add the onions and sauté for about 2-3 minutes. Add the soy sauce, vinegar, and maple syrup and bring to a gentle simmer.
4. Dissolve the remaining arrowroot starch in a small bowl with water. Slowly, add the arrowroot starch mixture into the sauce, stirring continuously.
5. Stir in the cooked tofu and cook for about 1 minute. Meanwhile, in a large pan of water, arrange a steamer basket and bring to a boil.
6. Adjust the heat to medium-low. Put the broccoli florets in your steamer and steam, covered for about 5-6 minutes.
7. Remove from the heat and drain the broccoli thoroughly. Transfer the broccoli into the pan of tofu and stir to combine. Serve hot.

NUTRITIONS

- *Calories: 230*
- *Fat: 17g*
- *Carbohydrates: 13g*
- *Protein: 10.9g*

45. TOFU WITH KALE

PREPARATION	COOKING	SERVES
15 MIN	10 MIN	2

INGREDIENTS

- 1 tablespoon extra-virgin olive oil
- ½ pound tofu, pressed, drained, and cubed
- 1 teaspoon fresh ginger, minced
- 1 garlic clove, minced
- ¼ teaspoon red pepper flakes, crushed
- 6 ounces fresh kale, tough ribs removed and chopped finely
- 1 tablespoon low-sodium soy sauce

DIRECTIONS

1. In a large nonstick pan, warm-up olive oil over medium-high heat and stir-fry the tofu for about 5 minutes.
2. Put the ginger, garlic, plus red pepper flakes and cook for about 1 minute, stirring continuously. Stir in the kale and soy sauce and stir-fry for about 4-5 minutes. Serve hot.

NUTRITIONS

- *Calories: 190*
- *Fat: 11.8g*
- *Carbohydrates: 12.5g*
- *Protein: 12.5g*

46. TOFU WITH PEAS

PREPARATION	COOKING	SERVES
15 MIN	20 MIN	5

INGREDIENTS

- 2 tablespoons olive oil, divided
- 1 package extra-firm tofu, drained, pressed, and cubed
- 1 cup yellow onion, chopped
- 1 tablespoon fresh ginger, minced
- 2 garlic cloves, minced
- 1 tomato, chopped finely
- 2 cups frozen peas, thawed
- ¼ cup of water
- 2 tablespoons fresh cilantro, chopped

DIRECTIONS

1. In a nonstick pan, warm-up 1 tablespoon of the oil over medium-high heat and cook the tofu for about 4-5 minutes or until browned completely, stirring occasionally. Transfer the tofu into a bowl.
2. Heat-up the rest of your oil over medium heat in the same pan and sauté the onion for about 3-4 minutes. Put the ginger plus garlic and sauté for about 1 minute.
3. Add the tomatoes and cook for about 4-5 minutes, crushing with the back of a spoon. Stir in the peas and broth and cook for about 2-3 minutes.
4. Stir in the tofu and cook for about 1-2 minutes. Serve hot with the garnishing of cilantro.

NUTRITIONS

- *Calories: 198*
- *Fat: 11.4g*
- *Carbohydrates: 14g*
- *Protein: 12.8g*

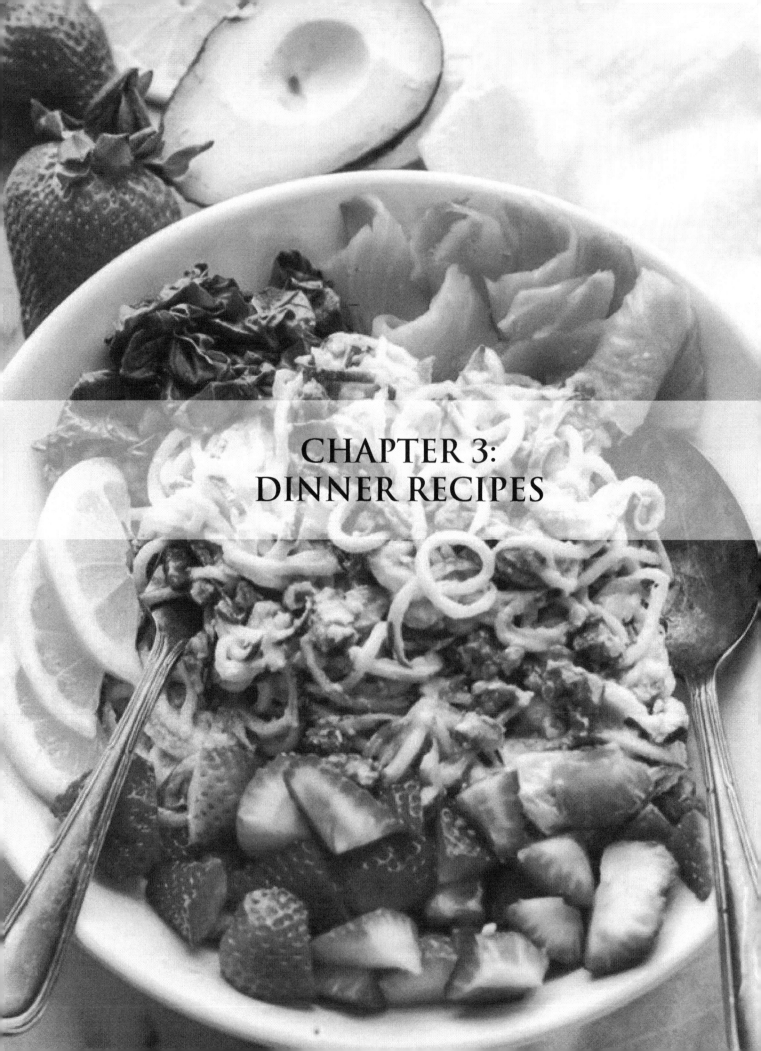

CHAPTER 3:
DINNER RECIPES

47. ZUCCHINI SALMON SALAD

PREPARATION	COOKING	SERVES
5 MIN	10 MIN	3

INGREDIENTS

- 2 salmon fillets
- 2 tablespoons soy sauce
- 2 zucchinis, sliced
- Salt and pepper to taste
- 2 tablespoons extra virgin olive oil
- 2 tablespoons sesame seeds
- Salt and pepper to taste

DIRECTIONS

1. Drizzle the salmon with soy sauce. Heat-up a grill pan over a medium flame. Cook salmon on the grill on each side for 2-3 minutes.
2. Flavor the zucchini with salt plus pepper and place it on the grill as well. Cook on each side until golden.
3. Place the zucchini, salmon, and the rest of the ingredients in a bowl. Serve the salad fresh.

NUTRITIONS

- Calories: 224
- Fat: 19g
- Protein: 18g
- Carbohydrates: 0g

48. PAN-FRIED SALMON

PREPARATION	COOKING	SERVES
5 MIN	20 MIN	4

INGREDIENTS

- 4 salmon fillets
- Salt and pepper to taste
- 1 teaspoon dried oregano
- 1 teaspoon dried basil
- 3 tablespoons extra virgin olive oil

DIRECTIONS

1. Season the fish with salt, pepper, oregano, and basil. Heat the oil in a pan and place the salmon in the hot oil, with the skin facing down.
2. Fry on each side within 2 minutes until golden brown and fragrant. Serve the salmon warm and fresh.

NUTRITIONS

- *Calories: 327*
- *Fat: 25g*
- *Protein: 36g*
- *Carbohydrates: 0.3g*

49. GRILLED SALMON WITH PINEAPPLE SALSA

PREPARATION	COOKING	SERVES
5 MIN	30 MIN	4

INGREDIENTS

- 4 salmon fillets
- Salt and pepper to taste
- 2 tablespoons Cajun seasoning
- 1 fresh pineapple, peeled and diced
- 1 cup cherry tomatoes, quartered
- 2 tablespoons chopped cilantro
- 2 tablespoons chopped parsley
- 1 teaspoon dried mint
- 2 tablespoons lemon juice
- 2 tablespoons extra virgin olive oil
- 1 teaspoon honey

- Salt and pepper to taste

DIRECTIONS

1. Add salt, pepper, and Cajun seasoning to the fish. Heat-up a grill pan over a medium flame. Cook fish on the grill on each side for 3-4 minutes.
2. For your salsa, mix the pineapple, tomatoes, cilantro, parsley, mint, lemon juice, and honey in a bowl—season with salt and pepper. Serve the grilled salmon with the pineapple salsa.

NUTRITIONS

- *Calories: 332*
- *Fat: 12g*

- *Protein: 34g*
- *Carbohydrates: 0g*

50. MEDITERRANEAN CHICKPEA SALAD

PREPARATION	COOKING	SERVES
5 MIN	20 MIN	6

INGREDIENTS

- 1 can chickpeas, drained
- 1 fennel bulb, sliced
- 1 red onion, sliced
- 1 teaspoon dried basil
- 1 teaspoon dried oregano
- 2 tablespoons chopped parsley
- 4 garlic cloves, minced
- 2 tablespoons lemon juice
- 2 tablespoons extra virgin olive oil
- Salt and pepper to taste

DIRECTIONS

1. Combine the chickpeas, fennel, red onion, herbs, garlic, lemon juice, and oil in a salad bowl. Add salt and pepper and serve the salad fresh.

NUTRITIONS

- *Calories: 200*
- *Fat: 9g*
- *Protein: 4g*
- *Carbohydrates: 28g*

51. WARM CHORIZO CHICKPEA SALAD

PREPARATION	COOKING	SERVES
5 MIN	20 MIN	6

INGREDIENTS

- 1 tablespoon extra-virgin olive oil
- 4 chorizo links, sliced
- 1 red onion, sliced
- 4 roasted red bell peppers, chopped
- 1 can chickpeas, drained
- 2 cups cherry tomatoes
- 2 tablespoons balsamic vinegar
- Salt and pepper to taste

DIRECTIONS

1. Heat-up oil in a skillet and add the chorizo. Cook briefly just until fragrant, then add the onion, bell peppers, and chickpeas and cook for 2 additional minutes.
2. Transfer the mixture to a salad bowl, then add the tomatoes, vinegar, salt, and pepper. Mix well and serve the salad right away.

NUTRITIONS

- *Calories: 359*
- *Fat: 18g*
- *Protein: 15g*
- *Carbohydrates: 21g*

52. GREEK ROASTED FISH

PREPARATION	COOKING	SERVES
5 MIN	30 MIN	4

INGREDIENTS

- 4 salmon fillets
- 1 tablespoon chopped oregano
- 1 teaspoon dried basil
- 1 zucchini, sliced
- 1 red onion, sliced
- 1 carrot, sliced
- 1 lemon, sliced
- 2 tablespoons extra virgin olive oil
- Salt and pepper to taste

DIRECTIONS

1. Add all the ingredients to a deep-dish baking pan. Season with salt and pepper and cook in the preheated oven at 350F for 20 minutes. Serve the fish and vegetables warm.

NUTRITIONS

- *Calories: 328*
- *Fat: 13g*
- *Protein: 38g*
- *Carbohydrates: 8g*

53. TOMATO FISH BAKE

PREPARATION	COOKING	SERVES
5 MIN	30 MIN	4

INGREDIENTS

- 4 cod fillets
- 4 tomatoes, sliced
- 4 garlic cloves, minced
- 1 shallot, sliced
- 1 celery stalk, sliced
- 1 teaspoon fennel seeds
- 1 cup vegetable stock
- Salt and pepper to taste

DIRECTIONS

1. Layer the cod fillets and tomatoes in a deep-dish baking pan. Add the rest of the ingredients and add salt and pepper—Cook in the preheated oven at 350F for 20 minutes. Serve the dish warm or chilled.

NUTRITIONS

- *Calories: 299*
- *Fat: 3g*
- *Protein: 64g*
- *Carbohydrates: 2g*

54. GARLICKY TOMATO CHICKEN CASSEROLE

PREPARATION	COOKING	SERVES
5 MIN	50 MIN	4

INGREDIENTS

- 4 chicken breasts
- 2 tomatoes, sliced
- 1 can diced tomatoes
- 2 garlic cloves, chopped
- 1 shallot, chopped
- 1 bay leaf
- 1 thyme sprig
- ½ cup dry white wine
- ½ cup chicken stock
- Salt and pepper to taste

DIRECTIONS

1. Combine the chicken and the remaining ingredients in a deep-dish baking pan. Adjust the taste with salt and pepper and cover the pot with a lid or aluminum foil—Cook in the preheated oven at 330F for 40 minutes. Serve the casserole warm.

NUTRITIONS

- *Calories: 313*
- *Fat: 8g*
- *Protein: 47g*
- *Carbohydrates: 6g*

55. CHICKEN CACCIATORE

PREPARATION	COOKING	SERVES
5 MIN	45 MIN	6

INGREDIENTS

- 2 tablespoons extra virgin olive oil
- 6 chicken thighs
- 1 sweet onion, chopped
- 2 garlic cloves, minced
- 2 red bell peppers, cored and diced
- 2 carrots, diced
- 1 rosemary sprig
- 1 thyme sprig
- 4 tomatoes, peeled and diced
- ½ cup tomato juice
- ¼ cup dry white wine
- 1 cup chicken stock
- 1 bay leaf
- Salt and pepper to taste

DIRECTIONS

1. Heat the oil in a heavy saucepan. Cook chicken on all sides until golden. Stir in the onion plus garlic and cook within 2 minutes.
2. Stir in the rest of the fixings and season with salt and pepper. Cook on low heat for 30 minutes. Serve the chicken cacciatore warm and fresh.

NUTRITIONS

- *Calories: 363*
- *Fat: 14g*
- *Protein: 42g*
- *Carbohydrates: 9g*

56. FENNEL WILD RICE RISOTTO

PREPARATION	COOKING	SERVES
5 MIN	35 MIN	6

INGREDIENTS

- 2 tablespoons extra virgin olive oil
- 1 shallot, chopped
- 2 garlic cloves, minced
- 1 fennel bulb, chopped
- 1 cup wild rice
- ¼ cup dry white wine
- 2 cups chicken stock
- 1 teaspoon grated orange zest
- Salt and pepper to taste

DIRECTIONS

1. Heat the oil in a heavy saucepan. Add the garlic, shallot, and fennel and cook for a few minutes until softened.
2. Stir in the rice and cook within 2 additional minutes, then add the wine, stock, and orange zest, with salt and pepper to taste. Cook on low heat for 20 minutes. Serve the risotto warm and fresh.

NUTRITIONS

- *Calories: 162*
- *Fat: 2g*
- *Protein: 8g*
- *Carbohydrates: 20g*

57. WILD RICE PRAWN SALAD

PREPARATION	COOKING	SERVES
5 MIN	35 MIN	6

INGREDIENTS

- ¾ cup wild rice
- 1¾ cups chicken stock
- 1-pound prawns
- Salt and pepper to taste
- 2 tablespoons lemon juice
- 2 tablespoons extra virgin olive oil
- 2 cups arugula

DIRECTIONS

1. Combine the rice and chicken stock in a saucepan and cook until the liquid has been absorbed entirely. Transfer the rice to a salad bowl.
2. Flavor the prawns with salt plus pepper and drizzle them with lemon juice and oil—warm grill pan over a medium flame.
3. Place the prawns on the hot pan and cook on each side for 2-3 minutes. For the salad, combine the rice with arugula and prawns and mix well. Serve the salad fresh.

NUTRITIONS

- Calories: 207
- Fat: 4g
- Protein: 20.6g
- Carbohydrates: 17g

58. CHICKEN BROCCOLI SALAD WITH AVOCADO DRESSING

PREPARATION	COOKING	SERVES
5 MIN	40 MIN	6

INGREDIENTS

- 2 chicken breasts
- 1-pound broccoli, cut into florets
- 1 avocado, peeled and pitted
- ½ lemon, juiced
- 2 garlic cloves
- ¼ teaspoon chili powder
- ¼ teaspoon cumin powder
- Salt and pepper to taste

DIRECTIONS

1. Cook the chicken in a large pot of salty water. Drain and cut the chicken into small cubes—place in a salad bowl. Add the broccoli and mix well.
2. Combine the avocado, lemon juice, garlic, chili powder, cumin powder, salt, and pepper in a blender. Pulse until smooth. Spoon the dressing over your salad and mix well. Serve the salad fresh.

NUTRITIONS

- *Calories: 195*
- *Fat: 11g*
- *Protein: 14g*
- *Carbohydrates: 3g*

59. SEAFOOD PAELLA

PREPARATION	COOKING	SERVES
5 MIN	45 MIN	8

INGREDIENTS

- 2 tablespoons extra virgin olive oil
- 1 shallot, chopped
- 2 garlic cloves, chopped
- 1 red bell pepper, cored and diced
- 1 carrot, diced
- 2 tomatoes, peeled and diced
- 1 cup wild rice
- 1 cup tomato juice
- 2 cups chicken stock
- 1 chicken breast, cubed
- Salt and pepper to taste

- 2 monkfish fillets, cubed
- ½ pound fresh shrimps, peeled and deveined
- ½ pound prawns
- 1 thyme sprig
- 1 rosemary sprig

DIRECTIONS

1. Heat-up oil in a skillet and stir in the shallot, garlic, bell pepper, carrot, and tomatoes, then cook within few minutes until softened.
2. Stir in the rice, tomato juice, stock, chicken, salt, and pepper, and cook on low heat for 20 minutes. Put the rest of the fixings and cook for 10 additional minutes. Serve the paella warm and fresh.

NUTRITIONS

- *Calories: 245*
- *Fat: 8g*
- *Protein: 27g*
- *Carbohydrates: 20.6g*

60. HERBED ROASTED CHICKEN BREASTS

PREPARATION	COOKING	SERVES
5 MIN	50 MIN	4

INGREDIENTS

- 2 tablespoons extra virgin olive oil
- 2 tablespoons chopped parsley
- 2 tablespoons chopped cilantro
- 1 teaspoon dried oregano
- 1 teaspoon dried basil
- 2 tablespoons lemon juice
- Salt and pepper to taste
- 4 chicken breasts

DIRECTIONS

1. Combine the oil, parsley, cilantro, oregano, basil, lemon juice, salt, and pepper in a bowl. Spread this mixture over the chicken and rub it well into the meat.
2. Place in a deep-dish baking pan and cover with aluminum foil. Cook in the preheated oven at 350F for 20 minutes, then remove the foil and cook for 25 additional minutes. Serve the chicken warm and fresh with your favorite side dish.

NUTRITIONS

- *Calories: 330*
- *Fat: 15g*
- *Protein: 40.7g*
- *Carbohydrates: 1g*

61. MARINATED CHICKEN BREASTS

PREPARATION	COOKING	SERVES
5 MIN	2 HOURS	4

INGREDIENTS

- 4 chicken breasts
- Salt and pepper to taste
- 1 lemon, juiced
- 1 rosemary sprig
- 1 thyme sprig
- 2 garlic cloves, crushed
- 2 sage leaves
- 3 tablespoons extra virgin olive oil
- ½ cup buttermilk

DIRECTIONS

1. Boil the chicken with salt and pepper and place it in a resealable bag. Add remaining ingredients and seal bag. Refrigerate for at least 1 hour.
2. After 1 hour, heat a roasting pan over medium heat, then place the chicken on the grill. Cook on each side for 8-10 minutes or until juices are gone. Serve the chicken warm with your favorite side dish.

NUTRITIONS

- *Calories: 371*
- *Fat: 21g*
- *Protein: 46g*
- *Carbohydrates: 2g*

62. BALSAMIC BEEF AND MUSHROOMS MIX

PREPARATION	COOKING	SERVES
5 MIN	8 HOURS	4

INGREDIENTS

- 2 pounds' beef, cut into strips
- ¼ cup balsamic vinegar
- 2 cups beef stock
- 1 tablespoon ginger, grated
- Juice of ½ lemon
- 1 cup brown mushrooms, sliced
- A pinch of salt and black pepper
- 1 teaspoon ground cinnamon

DIRECTIONS

1. Mix all the ingredients in your slow cooker, cover, and cook on low for 8 hours. Divide everything between plates and serve.

NUTRITIONS

- *Calories: 446*
- *Fat: 14 g*
- *Carbs 2.9 g*
- *Protein 70.8 g*

63. OREGANO PORK MIX

PREPARATION	COOKING	SERVES
5 MIN	7H 6 MIN	4

INGREDIENTS

- 2 pounds' pork roast
- 7 ounces' tomato paste
- 1 yellow onion, chopped
- 1 cup beef stock
- 2 tablespoons ground cumin
- 2 tablespoons olive oil
- 2 tablespoons fresh oregano, chopped
- 1 tablespoon garlic, minced
- ½ cup fresh thyme, chopped

DIRECTIONS

1. Heat-up a sauté pan with the oil over medium-high heat, add the roast, brown it for 3 minutes per side, then move it to your slow cooker.
2. Add the rest of the ingredients, toss a bit, cover and cook on low for 7 hours. Slice the roast, divide it between plates and serve.

NUTRITIONS

- *Calories: 623*
- *Fat: 30.1 g*
- *Carbs 19.3 g*
- *Protein 69.2 g*

64. SIMPLE BEEF ROAST

PREPARATION	COOKING	SERVES
10 MIN	8 HOURS	8

INGREDIENTS

- 5 pounds' beef roast
- 2 tablespoons Italian seasoning
- 1 cup beef stock
- 1 tablespoon sweet paprika
- 3 tablespoons olive oil

DIRECTIONS

1. In your slow cooker, mix all the ingredients, cover, and cook on low for 8 hours. Carve the roast, divide it between plates and serve.

NUTRITIONS

- *Calories: 587*
- *Fat: 24.1 g*
- *Carbs 0.9 g*
- *Protein 86.5 g*

65. CHICKEN BREAST SOUP

PREPARATION	COOKING	SERVES
5 MIN	4 HOURS	4

INGREDIENTS

- 3 chicken breasts, skinless, boneless, cubed
- 2 celery stalks, chopped
- 2 carrots, chopped
- 2 tablespoons olive oil
- 1 red onion, chopped
- 3 garlic cloves, minced
- 4 cups chicken stock
- 1 tablespoon parsley, chopped

DIRECTIONS

1. In your slow cooker, mix all the ingredients except the parsley, cover, and cook on high for 4 hours. Add the parsley, stir, ladle the soup into bowls and serve.

NUTRITIONS

- *Calories: 445*
- *Fat: 21.1 g*
- *Carbs 7.4 g*
- *Protein 54.3 g*

66. CAULIFLOWER CURRY

PREPARATION	COOKING	SERVES
5 MIN	5 HOURS	4

INGREDIENTS

- 1 cauliflower head, florets separated
- 2 carrots, sliced
- 1 red onion, chopped
- ¾ cup of coconut milk
- 2 garlic cloves, minced
- 2 tablespoons curry powder
- A pinch of salt and black pepper
- 1 tablespoon red pepper flakes
- 1 teaspoon garam masala

DIRECTIONS

1. In your slow cooker, mix all the ingredients. Cover, cook on high for 5 hours, divide into bowls and serve.

NUTRITIONS

- *Calories: 160*
- *Fat: 11.5 g*
- *Carbs 14.7 g*
- *Protein 3.6 g*

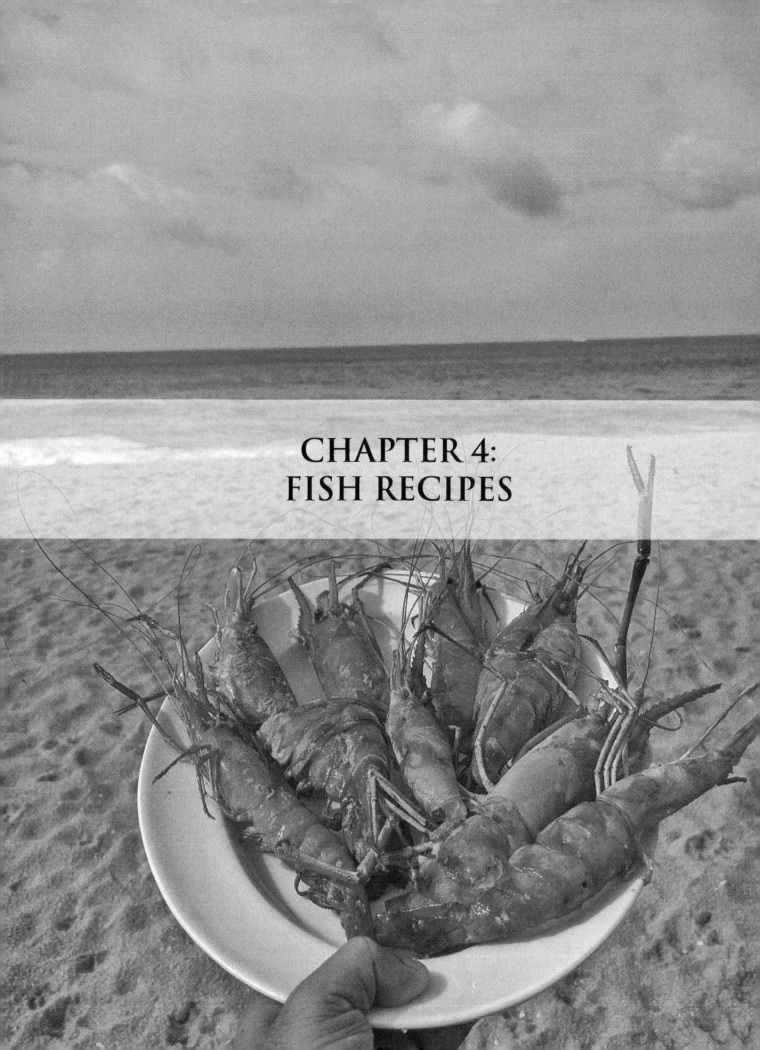

CHAPTER 4:
FISH RECIPES

67. PISTACHIO-CRUSTED WHITEFISH

PREPARATION	COOKING	SERVES
10 MIN	20 MIN	2

INGREDIENTS

- ¼ cup shelled pistachios
- 1 tablespoon fresh parsley
- 1 tablespoon grated Parmesan cheese
- 1 tablespoon panko bread crumbs
- 2 tablespoons olive oil
- ¼ teaspoon salt
- 10 ounces skinless whitefish (1 large piece or 2 smaller ones)

DIRECTIONS

1. Preheat the oven to 350°F and set the rack to the middle position. Line a sheet pan with foil or parchment paper.
2. Combine all of the ingredients except the fish in a mini food processor, and pulse until the nuts are finely ground.
3. Alternatively, you can mince the nuts with a chef's knife and combine the ingredients by hand in a small bowl.
4. Place the fish on the sheet pan. Spread the nut mixture evenly over the fish and pat it down lightly.
5. Bake the fish for 20 to 30 minutes, depending on the thickness, until it flakes easily with a fork.
6. Keep in mind that a thicker cut of fish takes a bit longer to bake. You'll know it's done when it's opaque, flakes apart easily with a fork, or reaches an internal temperature of 145°F

NUTRITIONS

- *Calories – 185,*
- *Carbs - 23.8 g,*
- *Protein - 10.1 g,*
- *Fat - 5.2 g*

68. GRILLED FISH ON LEMONS

PREPARATION	COOKING	SERVES
10 MIN	10 MIN	2

INGREDIENTS

- 4 (4-ounce) fish fillets, such as tilapia, salmon, catfish, cod, or your favorite fish
- Nonstick cooking spray
- 3 to 4 medium lemons
- 1 tablespoon extra-virgin olive oil
- ¼ teaspoon freshly ground black pepper
- ¼ teaspoon kosher or sea salt

DIRECTIONS

1. Using paper towels pat the fillets dry and let stand at room temperature for 10 minutes.
2. Meanwhile, coat the cold cooking grate of the grill with nonstick cooking spray, and preheat the grill to 400°F, or medium-high heat. Or preheat a grill pan over medium-high heat on the stove top.
3. Cut one lemon in half and set half aside. Slice the remaining half of that lemon and the remaining lemons into ¼-inch-thick slices. (You should have about 12 to 16 lemon slices.)
4. Into a small bowl, squeeze 1 tablespoon of juice out of the reserved lemon half.
5. Add the oil to the bowl with the lemon juice, and mix well.
6. Brush both sides of the fish with the oil mixture, and sprinkle evenly with pepper and salt.
7. Carefully place the lemon slices on the grill (or the grill pan), arranging 3 to 4 slices together in the shape of a fish fillet, and repeat with the remaining slices
8. Place the fish fillets directly on top of the lemon slices, and grill with the lid closed. (If you're grilling on the stove top, cover with a large pot lid or aluminum foil.)
9. Turn the fish halfway through the cooking time only if the fillets are more than half an inch thick.
10. The fish is done and ready to serve when it just begins to separate into flakes (chunks) when pressed gently with a fork

NUTRITIONS

- Calories – 185,
- Carbs - 23.8 g,
- Protein - 10.1 g,
- Fat - 5.2 g

69. WEEKNIGHT SHEET PAN FISH DINNER

PREPARATION	COOKING	SERVES
10 MIN	10 MIN	2

INGREDIENTS

- Nonstick cooking spray
- 2 tablespoons extra-virgin olive oil
- 1 tablespoon balsamic vinegar
- 4 (4-ounce) fish fillets, such as cod or tilapia (½ inch thick)
- 2½ cups green beans (about 12 ounces)
- 1-pint cherry or grape tomatoes (about 2 cups)

DIRECTIONS

1. Preheat the oven to 400°F. Coat two large, rimmed baking sheets with nonstick cooking spray.
2. In a small bowl, whisk together the oil and vinegar. Set aside. Place two pieces of fish on each baking sheet.
3. In a large bowl, combine the beans and tomatoes. Pour in the oil and vinegar, and toss gently to coat.
4. Pour half of the green bean mixture over the fish on one baking sheet, and the remaining half over the fish on the other.
5. Turn the fish over, and rub it in the oil mixture to coat. Spread the vegetables evenly on the baking sheets so hot air can circulate around them.
6. Bake for 5 to 8 minutes, until the fish is just opaque and not translucent. The fish is done and ready to serve when it just begins to separate into flakes (chunks) when pressed gently with a fork.

NUTRITIONS

- *Calories – 185,*
- *Carbs - 23.8 g,*
- *Protein - 10.1 g,*
- *Fat - 5.2 g*

70. CRISPY POLENTA FISH STICKS

PREPARATION	COOKING	SERVES
15 MIN	10 MIN	2

INGREDIENTS

- 2 large eggs, lightly beaten 1 tablespoon 2% milk
- 1-pound skinned fish fillets (cod, tilapia, or other white fish) about ½ inch thick, sliced into 20 (1-inch-wide) strips
- ½ cup yellow cornmeal
- ½ cup whole-wheat panko bread crumbs or whole-wheat bread crumbs
- ¼ teaspoon smoked paprika
- ¼ teaspoon kosher or sea salt
- ¼ teaspoon freshly ground black pepper
- Nonstick cooking spray

DIRECTIONS

1. Place a large, rimmed baking sheet in the oven. Preheat the oven to 400°F with the pan inside. In a large bowl, mix the eggs and milk.
2. Using a fork, add the fish strips to the egg mixture and stir gently to coat.
3. Put the cornmeal, bread crumbs, smoked paprika, salt, and pepper in a quart-size zip-top plastic bag.
4. Using a fork or tongs, transfer the fish to the bag, letting the excess egg wash drip off into the bowl before transferring. Seal the bag and shake gently to completely coat each fish stick.
5. With oven mitts, carefully remove the hot baking sheet from the oven and spray it with nonstick cooking spray.
6. Using a fork or tongs, remove the fish sticks from the bag and arrange them on the hot baking sheet, with space between them so the hot air can circulate and crisp them up.
7. Bake for 5 to 8 minutes, until gentle pressure with a fork causes the fish to flake, and serve

NUTRITIONS

- *Calories – 185,*
- *Carbs - 23.8 g,*
- *Protein - 10.1 g,*
- *Fat - 5.2 g*

71. CRISPY HOMEMADE FISH STICKS RECIPE

PREPARATION	COOKING	SERVES
10 MIN	15 MIN	2

INGREDIENTS

- ½ cup of flour
- 1 beaten egg
- 1 cup of flour
- ½ cup of parmesan cheese
- ½ cup of bread crumbs.
- Zest of 1 lemon juice
- Parsley
- Salt
- 1 teaspoon of black pepper
- 1 tablespoon of sweet paprika
- 1 teaspoon of oregano
- 1 ½ lb. of salmon
- Extra virgin olive oil

DIRECTIONS

1. Preheat your oven to about 450 degrees F. Get a bowl, dry your salmon and season its two sides with the salt.
2. Then chop into small sizes of 1½ inch length each. Get a bowl and mix black pepper with oregano.
3. Add paprika to the mixture and blend it. Then spice the fish stick with the mixture you have just made. Get another dish and pour your flours.
4. You will need a different bowl again to pour your egg wash into. Pick yet the fourth dish, mix your breadcrumb with your parmesan and add lemon zest to the mixture.
5. Return to the fish sticks and dip each fish into flour such that both sides are coated with flour. As you dip each fish into flour, take it out and dip it into egg wash and lastly, dip it in the breadcrumb mixture.
6. Do this for all fish sticks and arrange on a baking sheet. Ensure you oil the baking sheet before arranging the stick thereon and drizzle the top of the fish sticks with extra virgin olive oil.
7. Caution: allow excess flours to fall off a fish before dipping it into other ingredients.
8. Also ensure that you do not let the coating peel while you add extra virgin olive oil on top of the fishes.
9. Fix the baking sheet in the middle of the oven and allow it to cook for 13 min. By then, the fishes should be golden brown and you can collect them from the oven, and you can serve immediately. Top it with your lemon zest, parsley and fresh lemon juice.

NUTRITIONS

- 119 Cal,
- 3.4g of fat,
- 293.1mg of sodium,
- 9.3g of carbs,
- 13.5g of protein.

72. SAUCED SHELLFISH IN WHITE WINE

PREPARATION	COOKING	SERVES
10 MIN	10 MIN	2

INGREDIENTS

- 2-lbs fresh cuttlefish
- ½-cup olive oil
- 1-pc large onion, finely chopped
- 1-cup of Robola white wine
- ¼-cup lukewarm water
- 1-pc bay leaf
- ½-bunch parsley, chopped
- 4-pcs tomatoes, grated
- Salt and pepper

DIRECTIONS

1. Take out the hard centerpiece of cartilage (cuttlebone), the bag of ink, and the intestines from the cuttlefish.
2. Wash the cleaned cuttlefish with running water. Slice it into small pieces, and drain excess water.
3. Heat the oil in a saucepan placed over medium-high heat and sauté the onion for 3 minutes until tender.
4. Add the sliced cuttlefish and pour in the white wine. Cook for 5 minutes until it simmers.
5. Pour in the water, and add the tomatoes, bay leaf, parsley, tomatoes, salt, and pepper. Simmer the mixture over low heat until the cuttlefish slices are tender and left with their thick sauce. Serve them warm with rice.
6. Be careful not to overcook the cuttlefish as its texture becomes very hard. A safe rule of thumb is grilling the cuttlefish over a ragingly hot fire for 3 minutes before using it in any recipe.

NUTRITIONS

- Calories: 308,
- Fats: 18.1g,
- Dietary Fiber: 1.5g,
- Carbohydrates: 8g,
- Protein: 25.6g

73. PISTACHIO SOLE FISH

PREPARATION	COOKING	SERVES
5 MIN	10 MIN	2

INGREDIENTS

- 4 (5 ounces) boneless sole fillets
- ½ cup pistachios, finely chopped
- Juice of 1 lemon
- teaspoon extra virgin olive oil

DIRECTIONS

1. Pre-heat your oven to 350 degrees Fahrenheit
2. Wrap baking sheet using parchment paper and keep it on the side
3. Pat fish dry with kitchen towels and lightly season with salt and pepper
4. Take a small bowl and stir in pistachios
5. Place sol on the prepped sheet and press 2 tablespoons of pistachio mixture on top of each fillet
6. Rub the fish with lemon juice and olive oil
7. Bake for 10 minutes until the top is golden and fish flakes with a fork

NUTRITIONS

- *166 Calories*
- *6g Fat*
- *2g Carbohydrates*

74. SPEEDY TILAPIA WITH RED ONION AND AVOCADO

PREPARATION	COOKING	SERVES
10 MIN	5 MIN	2

INGREDIENTS

- 1 tablespoon extra-virgin olive oil
- 1 tablespoon freshly squeezed orange juice
- ¼ teaspoon kosher or sea salt
- 4 (4-ounces) tilapia fillets, more oblong than square, skin-on or skinned
- ¼ cup chopped red onion (about 1/8 onion)
- 1 avocado, pitted, skinned, and sliced

DIRECTIONS

1. In a 9-inch glass pie dish, use a fork to mix together the oil, orange juice, and salt. Working with one fillet at a time, place each in the pie dish and turn to coat on all sides.
2. Arrange the fillets in a wagon-wheel formation, so that one end of each fillet is in the center of the dish and the other end is temporarily draped over the edge of the dish.
3. Top each fillet with 1 tablespoon of onion, then fold the end of the fillet that's hanging over the edge in half over the onion.
4. When finished, you should have 4 folded-over fillets with the fold against the outer edge of the dish and the ends all in the center.
5. Cover the dish with plastic wrap, leaving a small part open at the edge to vent the steam. Microwave on high for about 3 minutes.
6. The fish is done when it just begins to separate into flakes (chunks) when pressed gently with a fork. Top the fillets with the avocado and serve.

NUTRITIONS

- *4 g carbohydrates,*
- *3 g fiber,*

- *22 g protein*

75. SALMON SKILLET SUPPER

PREPARATION	COOKING	SERVES
15 MIN	15 MIN	2

INGREDIENTS

- 1 tablespoon extra-virgin olive oil
- 2 garlic cloves minced
- 1 teaspoon smoked paprika
- 1-pint grape or cherry tomatoes, quartered
- 1 (12-ounces) jar roasted red peppers
- 1 tablespoon water
- ¼ teaspoon freshly ground black pepper
- ¼ teaspoon kosher or sea salt
- 1-pound salmon fillets, skin removed, cut into 8 pieces
- 1 tablespoon freshly squeezed lemon juice (from ½ medium lemon)

DIRECTIONS

1. In a large skillet over medium heat, heat the oil. Add the garlic and smoked paprika and cook for 1 minute, stirring often.
2. Add the tomatoes, roasted peppers, water, black pepper, and salt. Turn up the heat to medium-high, bring to a simmer, and cook for 3 minutes, stirring occasionally and smashing the tomatoes with a wooden spoon toward the end of the cooking time.
3. Add the salmon to the skillet, and spoon some of the sauce over the top.
4. Cover and cook for 10 to 12 minutes, or until the salmon is cooked through (145°F using a meat thermometer) and just starts to flake.
5. Remove the skillet from the heat, and drizzle lemon juice over the top of the fish. Stir the sauce, then break up the salmon into chunks with a fork. You can serve it straight from the skillet.

NUTRITIONS

- 13 g total fat,
- 2 g fiber,
- 31 g protein

76. TUSCAN TUNA AND ZUCCHINI BURGERS

PREPARATION	COOKING	SERVES
10 MIN	10 MIN	2

INGREDIENTS

- 3 slices whole-wheat sandwich bread, toasted
- 2 (5-ounces) cans tuna in olive oil, drained
- 1 cup shredded zucchini
- 1 large egg, lightly beaten
- ¼ cup diced red bell pepper
- 1 tablespoon dried oregano
- 1 teaspoon lemon zest
- ¼ teaspoon freshly ground black pepper
- ¼ teaspoon kosher or sea salt
- 1 tablespoon extra-virgin olive oil
- Salad greens or 4 whole-wheat rolls, for serving (optional)

DIRECTIONS

1. Crumble the toast into bread crumbs using your fingers (or use a knife to cut into ¼-inch cubes) until you have 1 cup of loosely packed crumbs.
2. Pour the crumbs into a large bowl. Add the tuna, zucchini, egg, bell pepper, oregano, lemon zest, black pepper, and salt.
3. Mix well with a fork. With your hands, form the mixture into four (½-cup-size) patties. Place on a plate, and press each patty flat to about ¾-inch thick.
4. In a large skillet over medium-high heat, heat the oil until it's very hot, about 2 minutes. Add the patties to the hot oil, then turn the heat down to medium.
5. Cook the patties for 5 minutes, flip with a spatula, and cook for an additional 5 minutes. Enjoy as is or serve on salad greens or whole-wheat rolls.

NUTRITIONS

- *191 Calories,*
- *10 g total fat,*
- *2 g fiber.*
- *15 g protein*

77. SICILIAN KALE AND TUNA BOWL

PREPARATION	COOKING	SERVES
15 MIN	15 MIN	2

INGREDIENTS

- 1-pound kale
- 3 tablespoons extra-virgin olive oil
- 1 cup chopped onion
- 3 garlic cloves, minced
- 1 (2.25-ounces) can sliced olives, drained
- ¼ cup capers
- ¼ teaspoon crushed red pepper
- 2 teaspoons sugar
- 2 (6-ounces) cans tuna in olive oil, undrained

- 1 (15-ounces) can cannellini beans or great northern beans
- ¼ teaspoon freshly ground black pepper
- ¼ teaspoon kosher or sea salt

DIRECTIONS

1. Fill large stockpot three-quarters full of water, and bring to a boil.
2. Add the kale and cook for 2 minutes. (This is to make the kale less bitter.) Drain the kale in a colander and set aside.
3. Set the empty pot back on the stove over medium heat, and pour in the oil.
4. Add the onion and cook for 4 minutes, stirring often. Add the garlic and cook for 1 minute, stirring often.
5. Add the olives, capers, and crushed red pepper, and cook for 1 minute, stirring often.
6. Add the partially cooked kale and sugar, stirring until the kale is completely coated with oil.
7. Cover the pot and cook for 8 minutes.
8. Remove the kale from the heat, mix in the tuna, beans, pepper, and salt, and serve.

NUTRITIONS

- *Calories 265,*
- *12 g total fat,*

- *7 g fiber,*
- *16 g protein*

78. MEDITERRANEAN COD STEW

PREPARATION	COOKING	SERVES
10 MIN	20 MIN	2

INGREDIENTS

- 2 tablespoons extra-virgin olive oil
- 2 cups chopped onion
- 2 garlic cloves, minced
- ¾ teaspoon smoked paprika
- 1 (14.5-ounces) can diced tomatoes, undrained
- 1 (12-ounces) jar roasted red peppers
- 1 cup sliced olives, green or black
- 1/3 cup dry red wine
- ¼ teaspoon freshly ground black pepper

- ¼ teaspoon kosher or sea salt
- 1½ pounds cod fillets, cut into 1-inch pieces
- 3 cups sliced mushrooms

DIRECTIONS

1. In a large stockpot over medium heat, heat the oil. Add the onion and cook for 4 minutes, stirring occasionally.
2. Add the garlic and smoked paprika and cook for 1 minute, stirring often.
3. Mix in the tomatoes with their juices, roasted peppers, olives, wine, pepper, and salt, and turn the heat up to medium-high. Bring to a boil.
4. Add the cod and mushrooms, and reduce the heat to medium.
5. Cover and cook for about 10 minutes, stirring a few times, until the cod is cooked through and flakes easily, and serve.

NUTRITIONS

- *Calories 220,*
- *8 g total fat,*
- *3 g fiber,*
- *28 g protein*

79. STEAMED MUSSELS IN WHITE WINE SAUCE

PREPARATION	COOKING	SERVES
5 MIN	10 MIN	2

INGREDIENTS

- 2 pounds small mussels
- 1 tablespoon extra-virgin olive oil
- 1 cup thinly sliced red onion
- 3 garlic cloves, sliced
- 1 cup dry white wine
- 2 (¼-inch-thick) lemon slices
- ¼ teaspoon freshly ground black pepper
- ¼ teaspoon kosher or sea salt
- Fresh lemon wedges, for serving (optional)

DIRECTIONS

1. In a large colander in the sink, run cold water over the mussels (but don't let the mussels sit in standing water).
2. All the shells should be closed tight; discard any shells that are a little bit open or any shells that are cracked. Leave the mussels in the colander until you're ready to use them.
3. In a large skillet over medium-high heat, heat the oil. Add the onion and cook for 4 minutes, stirring occasionally.
4. Add the garlic and cook for 1 minute, stirring constantly. Add the wine, lemon slices, pepper, and salt, and bring to a simmer. Cook for 2 minutes.
5. Add the mussels and cover. Cook for 3 minutes, or until the mussels open their shells. Gently shake the pan two or three times while they are cooking.
6. All the shells should now be wide open. Using a slotted spoon, discard any mussels that are still closed. Spoon the opened mussels into a shallow serving bowl, and pour the broth over the top. Serve with additional fresh lemon slices, if desired.

NUTRITIONS

- *Calories 22,*
- *7 g total fat,*
- *1 g fiber,*
- *18 g protein*

80. ORANGE AND GARLIC SHRIMP

PREPARATION	COOKING	SERVES
20 MIN	10 MIN	2

INGREDIENTS

- 1 large orange
- 3 tablespoons extra-virgin olive oil, divided
- 1 tablespoon chopped fresh Rosemary
- 1 tablespoon chopped fresh thyme
- 3 garlic cloves, minced (about 1½ teaspoons)
- ¼ teaspoon freshly ground black pepper
- ¼ teaspoon kosher or sea salt
- 1½ pounds fresh raw shrimp, shells, and tails removed

DIRECTIONS

1. Zest the entire orange using a citrus grater. In a large zip-top plastic bag, combine the orange zest and 2 tablespoons of oil with the Rosemary, thyme, garlic, pepper, and salt.
2. Add the shrimp, seal the bag, and gently massage the shrimp until all the ingredients are combined and the shrimp is completely covered with the seasonings. Set aside.
3. Heat a grill, grill pan, or a large skillet over medium heat. Brush on or swirl in the remaining 1 tablespoon of oil.
4. Add half the shrimp, and cook for 4 to 6 minutes, or until the shrimp turn pink and white, flipping halfway through if on the grill or stirring every minute if in a pan. Transfer the shrimp to a large serving bowl.
5. Repeat with the remaining shrimp, and add them to the bowl.
6. While the shrimp cook, peel the orange and cut the flesh into bite-size pieces. Add to the serving bowl, and toss with the cooked shrimp. Serve immediately or refrigerate and serve cold.

NUTRITIONS

- *Calories 190,*
- *8 g total fat,*
- *1 g fiber,*
- *24 g protein*

81. ROASTED SHRIMP-GNOCCHI BAKE

PREPARATION	COOKING	SERVES
10 MIN	20 MIN	2

INGREDIENTS

- 1 cup chopped fresh tomato
- 2 tablespoons extra-virgin olive oil
- 2 garlic cloves, minced
- ½ teaspoon freshly ground black pepper
- ¼ teaspoon crushed red pepper
- 1 (12-ounces) jar roasted red peppers
- 1-pound fresh raw shrimp, shells and tails removed
- 1-pound frozen gnocchi (not thawed)
- ½ cup cubed feta cheese
- 1/3 cup fresh torn basil leaves

DIRECTIONS

1. Preheat the oven to 425°F. In a baking dish, mix the tomatoes, oil, garlic, black pepper, and crushed red pepper. Roast in the oven for 10 minutes.
2. Stir in the roasted peppers and shrimp. Roast for 10 more minutes, until the shrimp turn pink and white.
3. While the shrimp cooks, cook the gnocchi on the stovetop according to the package directions.
4. Drain in a colander and keep warm. Remove the dish from the oven. Mix in the cooked gnocchi, feta, and basil, and serve.

NUTRITIONS

- *Calories 227,*
- *7 g total fat,*
- *1 g fiber,*
- *20 g protein*

82. SPICY SHRIMP PUTTANESCA

PREPARATION	COOKING	SERVES
5 MIN	15 MIN	2

INGREDIENTS

- 2 tablespoons extra-virgin olive oil
- 3 anchovy fillets, drained and chopped
- 3 garlic cloves, minced
- ½ teaspoon crushed red pepper
- 1 (14.5-ounces) can low-sodium or no-salt-added diced tomatoes, undrained
- 1 (2.25-ounces) can sliced black olives, drained
- 2 tablespoons capers
- 1 tablespoon chopped fresh oregano
- 1-pound fresh raw shrimp, shells and tails removed

DIRECTIONS

1. In a large skillet over medium heat, heat the oil. Mix in the anchovies, garlic, and crushed red pepper.
2. Cook for 3 minutes, stirring frequently and mashing up the anchovies with a wooden spoon until they have melted into the oil.
3. Stir in the tomatoes with their juices, olives, capers, and oregano. Turn up the heat to medium-high, and bring to a simmer.
4. When the sauce is lightly bubbling, stir in the shrimp. Reduce the heat to medium, and cook the shrimp for 6 to 8 minutes, or until they turn pink and white, stirring occasionally, and serve.

NUTRITIONS

- *Calories 214,*
- *10 g total fat,*
- *2 g fiber,*
- *26 g protein*

83. BAKED COD WITH VEGETABLES

PREPARATION	COOKING	SERVES
15 MIN	25 MIN	2

INGREDIENTS

- 1 pound (454 g) thick cod fillet, cut into 4 even portions
- ¼ teaspoon onion powder (optional)
- ¼ teaspoon paprika
- 3 tablespoons extra-virgin olive oil
- 4 medium scallions
- ½ cup fresh chopped basil, divided
- 3 tablespoons minced garlic (optional)
- 2 teaspoons salt
- 2 teaspoons freshly ground black pepper
- ¼ teaspoon dry marjoram (optional)
- 6 sun-dried tomato slices
- ½ cup dry white wine
- ½ cup crumbled feta cheese
- 1 (15-ounce / 425-g) can oil-packed artichoke hearts, drained
- 1 lemon, sliced
- 1 cup pitted kalamata olives
- 1 teaspoon capers (optional)
- 4 small red potatoes, quartered

DIRECTIONS

1. Set oven to 375°F (190°C).
2. Season the fish with paprika and onion powder (if desired).
3. Heat an ovenproof skillet over medium heat and sear the top side of the cod for about 1 minute until golden. Set aside.
4. Heat the olive oil in the same skillet over medium heat. Add the scallions, ¼ cup of basil, garlic (if desired), salt, pepper, marjoram (if desired), tomato slices, and white wine and stir to combine. Boil then removes from heat.
5. Evenly spread the sauce on the bottom of skillet. Place the cod on top of the tomato basil sauce and scatter with feta cheese. Place the artichokes in the skillet and top with the lemon slices.
6. Scatter with the olives, capers (if desired), and the remaining ¼ cup of basil. Pullout from the heat and transfer to the preheated oven. Bake for 15 to 20 minutes
7. Meanwhile, place the quartered potatoes on a baking sheet or wrapped in aluminum foil. Bake in the oven for 15 minutes.
8. Cool for 5 minutes before serving.

NUTRITIONS

- *Calories 1168,*
- *60g fat,*
- *64g protein*

84. SLOW COOKER SALMON IN FOIL

PREPARATION	COOKING	SERVES
5 MIN	2 HOURS	2

INGREDIENTS

- 2 (6-ounce / 170-g) salmon fillets
- 1 tablespoon olive oil
- 2 cloves garlic, minced
- ½ tablespoon lime juice
- 1 teaspoon finely chopped fresh parsley
- ¼ teaspoon black pepper

DIRECTIONS

1. Spread a length of foil onto a work surface and place the salmon fillets in the middle.
2. Blend olive oil, garlic, lime juice, parsley, and black pepper. Brush the mixture over the fillets. Fold the foil over and crimp the sides to make a packet.
3. Place the packet into the slow cooker, cover, and cook on High for 2 hours
4. Serve hot.

NUTRITIONS

- *Calories 446,*
- *21g fat,*
- *65g protein*

85. DILL CHUTNEY SALMON

PREPARATION	COOKING	SERVES
5 MIN	3 MIN	2

INGREDIENTS

Chutney:
- ¼ cup fresh dill
- ¼ cup extra virgin olive oil
- Juice from ½ lemon
- Sea salt, to taste

Fish:
- 2 cups water
- 2 salmon fillets
- Juice from ½ lemon
- ¼ teaspoon paprika
- Salt and freshly ground pepper to taste

DIRECTIONS

1. Pulse all the chutney ingredients in a food processor until creamy. Set aside.
2. Add the water and steamer basket to the Instant Pot. Place salmon fillets, skin-side down, on the steamer basket. Drizzle the lemon juice over salmon and sprinkle with the paprika.
3. Secure the lid. Select the Manual mode and set the cooking time for 3 minutes at High Pressure.
4. Once cooking is complete, do a quick pressure release. Carefully open the lid.
5. Season the fillets with pepper and salt to taste. Serve topped with the dill chutney.

NUTRITIONS

- *Calories 636,*
- *41g fat,*
- *65g protein*

86. GARLIC-BUTTER PARMESAN SALMON AND ASPARAGUS

PREPARATION	COOKING	SERVES
10 MIN	15 MIN	2

INGREDIENTS

- 2 (6-ounce / 170-g) salmon fillets, skin on and patted dry
- Pink Himalayan salt
- Freshly ground black pepper, to taste
- 1 pound (454 g) fresh asparagus, ends snapped off
- 3 tablespoons almond butter
- 2 garlic cloves, minced
- ¼ cup grated Parmesan cheese

DIRECTIONS

1. Prep oven to 400°F (205°C). Line a baking sheet with aluminum foil.
2. Season both sides of the salmon fillets.
3. Situate salmon in the middle of the baking sheet and arrange the asparagus around the salmon.
4. Heat the almond butter in a small saucepan over medium heat.
5. Cook minced garlic
6. Drizzle the garlic-butter sauce over the salmon and asparagus and scatter the Parmesan cheese on top.
7. Bake in the preheated oven for about 12 minutes. You can switch the oven to broil at the end of cooking time for about 3 minutes to get a nice char on the asparagus.
8. Let cool for 5 minutes before serving.

NUTRITIONS

- *Calories 435,*
- *26g fat,*
- *42g protein*

87. LEMON ROSEMARY ROASTED BRANZINO

PREPARATION	COOKING	SERVES
15 MIN	30 MIN	2

INGREDIENTS

- 4 tablespoons extra-virgin olive oil, divided
- 2 (8-ounce) Branzino fillets
- 1 garlic clove, minced
- 1 bunch scallions
- 10 to 12 small cherry tomatoes, halved
- 1 large carrot, cut into ¼-inch rounds
- ½ cup dry white wine
- 2 tablespoons paprika
- 2 teaspoons kosher salt
- ½ tablespoon ground chili pepper
- 2 rosemary sprigs or 1 tablespoon dried rosemary
- 1 small lemon, thinly sliced
- ½ cup sliced pitted kalamata olives

DIRECTIONS

1. Heat a large ovenproof skillet over high heat until hot, about 2 minutes. Add 1 tablespoon of olive oil and heat
2. Add the Branzino fillets, skin-side up, and sear for 2 minutes. Flip the fillets and cook. Set aside.
3. Swirl 2 tablespoons of olive oil around the skillet to coat evenly.
4. Add the garlic, scallions, tomatoes, and carrot, and sauté for 5 minutes
5. Add the wine, stirring until all ingredients are well combined. Carefully place the fish over the sauce.
6. Preheat the oven to 450°F (235°C).
7. Brush the fillets with the remaining 1 tablespoon of olive oil and season with paprika, salt, and chili pepper. Top each fillet with a rosemary sprig and lemon slices. Scatter the olives over fish and around the skillet.
8. Roast for about 10 minutes until the lemon slices are browned. Serve hot.

NUTRITIONS

- Calories 724,
- 43g fat,
- 57g protein

88. GRILLED LEMON PESTO SALMON

PREPARATION	COOKING	SERVES
5 MIN	10 MIN	2

INGREDIENTS

- 10 ounces (283 g) salmon fillet
- 2 tablespoons prepared pesto sauce
- 1 large fresh lemon, sliced
- Cooking spray

DIRECTIONS

1. Preheat the grill to medium-high heat. Spray the grill grates with cooking spray.
2. Season the salmon well. Spread the pesto sauce on top.
3. Make a bed of fresh lemon slices about the same size as the salmon fillet on the hot grill, and place the salmon on top of the lemon slices. Put any additional lemon slices on top of the salmon.
4. Grill the salmon for 10 minutes.
5. Serve hot.

NUTRITIONS

- *Calories 316,*
- *21g fat,*

- *29g protein*

89. STEAMED TROUT WITH LEMON HERB CRUST

PREPARATION	COOKING	SERVES
10 MIN	15 MIN	2

INGREDIENTS

- 3 tablespoons olive oil
- 3 garlic cloves, chopped
- 2 tablespoons fresh lemon juice
- 1 tablespoon chopped fresh mint
- 1 tablespoon chopped fresh parsley
- ¼ teaspoon dried ground thyme
- 1 teaspoon sea salt
- 1 pound (454 g) fresh trout (2 pieces)
- 2 cups fish stock

DIRECTIONS

1. Blend olive oil, garlic, lemon juice, mint, parsley, thyme, and salt. Brush the marinade onto the fish.
2. Insert a trivet in the Instant Pot. Fill in the fish stock and place the fish on the trivet.
3. Secure the lid. Select the Steam mode and set the cooking time for 15 minutes at High Pressure.
4. Once cooking is complete, do a quick pressure release. Carefully open the lid. Serve warm.

NUTRITIONS

- *Calories 477,*
- *30g fat,*

- *52g protein*

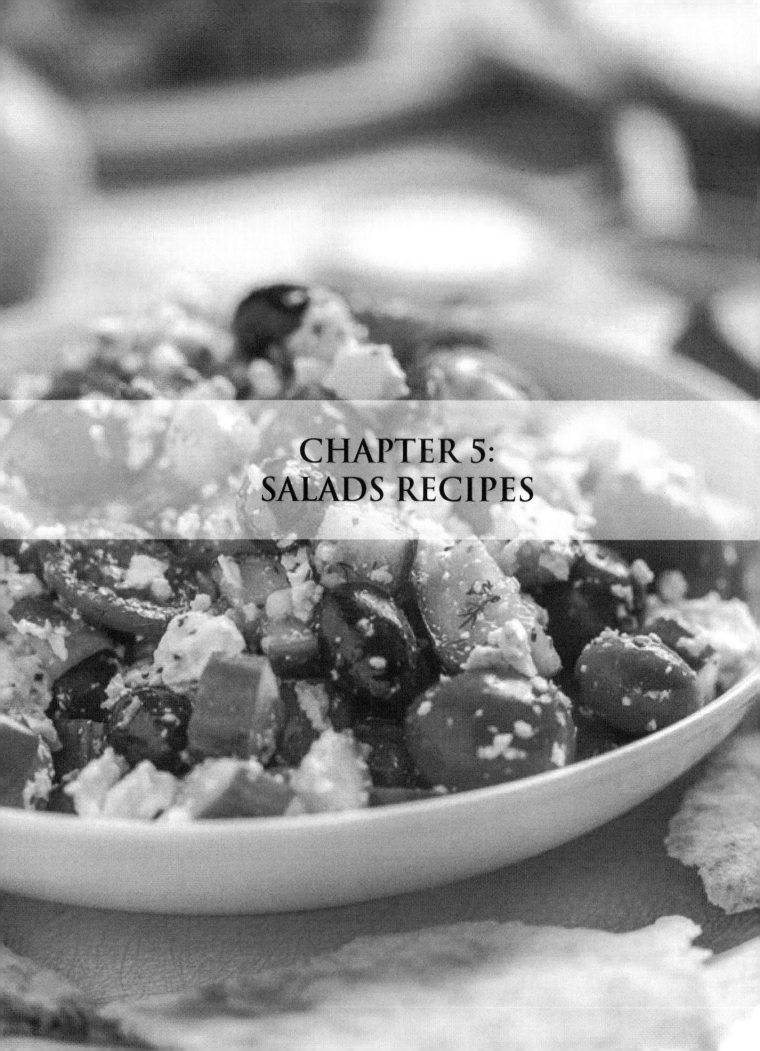

CHAPTER 5:
SALADS RECIPES

90. WASABI TUNA ASIAN SALAD

PREPARATION	COOKING	SERVES
30 MIN	10 MIN	1

INGREDIENTS

- 1 tsp lime juice
- non-stick cooking spray
- pepper/dash of salt
- 1 tsp wasabi paste
- 2 tsp olive oil
- ½ cup chopped or shredded cucumbers
- 1 cup bok choy stalks
- 8 oz raw tuna steak

DIRECTIONS

1. For the fish, preheat your skillet to medium heat. Mix your wasabi and lime juice; coat the tuna steaks. Use a non-stick cooking spray on your skillet for 10 seconds.
2. Put your tuna steaks on the skillet and cook over medium heat until you get the desired doneness.
3. For the salad, slice the cucumber into match-stick tiny sizes. Cut the bok Choy into minute pieces. Toss gently with pepper, salt, and olive oil if you want. Enjoy.

NUTRITIONS

- Calories: 380
- Carbs: 5g
- Fat: 12g
- Protein: 61g

91. LEMON GREEK SALAD

PREPARATION	COOKING	SERVES
15 MIN	5 MIN	1

INGREDIENTS

- 140 oz chicken breast
- 1 cup chopped cucumber
- 1 cup chopped orange/red bell pepper
- 1 cup wedged/sliced/chopped tomatoes
- ¼ cup chopped olives
- 2 tbsp fresh parsley, finely chopped.
- 2 tbsp finely chopped red onion
- 5 tsp lemon juice
- 1 tsp olive oil
- 1 clove minced garlic

DIRECTIONS

1. Preheat your grill to medium heat. Grill the chicken and cook on each side until the chicken is no longer pink or for 5 minutes.
2. Cut the chicken into tiny pieces. In your serving bowl, mix garlic, olives, and parsley. Whisk in olive oil and 4 tsp lemon juice. Add onion, tomatoes, bell pepper, and cucumber.
3. Toss gently. Coat the ingredients with dressing. Add another teaspoon of lemon juice to taste. Divide the salad into two servings and put 6oz chicken on top of each salad. Serve.

NUTRITIONS

- Calories: 380
- Protein: 56g
- Carbs: 14g
- Fat: 12g

92. BROCCOLI SALAD

PREPARATION	COOKING	SERVES
5 MIN	0 MIN	1

INGREDIENTS

- 1/3 tablespoons sherry vinegar
- 1/24 cup olive oil
- 1/3 teaspoons fresh thyme, chopped
- 1/6 teaspoon Dijon mustard
- 1/6 teaspoon honey
- Salt to taste
- 1 1/3 cups broccoli florets
- 1/3 red onions
- 1/12 cup parmesan cheese shaved
- 1/24 cup pecans

DIRECTIONS

1. Mix the sherry vinegar, olive oil, thyme, mustard, honey, and salt in a bowl. In a serving bowl, blend the broccoli florets and onions.
2. Drizzle the dressing on top. Sprinkle with the pecans and parmesan cheese before serving.

NUTRITIONS

- Calories: 199
- Fat: 17.4g
- Carbohydrates: 7.5g
- Fiber: 2.8g
- Protein: 5.2g

93. POTATO CARROT SALAD

PREPARATION	COOKING	SERVES
15 MIN	10 MIN	1

INGREDIENTS

- Water
- 1 potato, sliced into cubes
- 1/2 carrots, cut into cubes
- 1/6 tablespoon milk
- 1/6 tablespoon Dijon mustard
- 1/24 cup mayonnaise
- Pepper to taste
- 1/3 teaspoons fresh thyme, chopped
- 1/6 stalk celery, chopped
- 1/6 scallions, chopped
- 1/6 slice turkey bacon, cooked crispy and crumbled

DIRECTIONS

1. Fill your pot with water. Place it over medium-high heat. Boil the potatoes and carrots for 10 to 12 minutes or until tender. Drain and let cool.
2. In a bowl, mix the milk, mustard, mayonnaise, pepper, and thyme. Stir in the potatoes, carrots, and celery.
3. Coat evenly with the sauce. Cover and refrigerate for 4 hours. Top with the scallions and turkey bacon bits before serving.

NUTRITIONS

- *Calories: 106*
- *Fat: 5.3g*
- *Carbohydrates: 12.6g*
- *Protein: 2g*

94. MARINATED VEGGIE SALAD

PREPARATION	COOKING	SERVES
4H 30 MIN	3 MIN	1

INGREDIENTS

- 1 zucchini, sliced
- 4 tomatoes, sliced into wedges
- ¼ cup red onion, sliced thinly
- 1 green bell pepper, sliced
- 2 tablespoons fresh parsley, chopped
- 2 tablespoons red-wine vinegar
- 2 tablespoons olive oil
- 1 clove garlic, minced
- 1 teaspoon dried basil
- 2 tablespoons water
- Pine nuts, toasted and chopped

DIRECTIONS

1. In a bowl, combine the zucchini, tomatoes, red onion, green bell pepper, and parsley. Pour the vinegar and oil into a glass jar with a lid.
2. Add the garlic, basil, and water. Seal the jar and stir well to combine. Pour the dressing into the vegetable mixture.
3. Cover the bowl, then marinate in the refrigerator for 4 hours. Garnish with the pine nuts before serving.

NUTRITIONS

- *Calories: 65*
- *Fat: 4.7g*
- *Carbohydrates: 5.3g*
- *Protein: 0.9g*

95. MEDITERRANEAN SALAD

PREPARATION	COOKING	SERVES
20 MIN	5 MIN	1

INGREDIENTS

- 1 teaspoon balsamic vinegar
- 1/2 tablespoon basil pesto
- 1/2 cup lettuce
- 1/8 cup broccoli florets, chopped
- 1/8 cup zucchini, chopped
- 1/8 cup tomato, chopped
- 1/8 cup yellow bell pepper, chopped
- 1/2 tablespoons feta cheese, crumbled

DIRECTIONS

1. Arrange the lettuce on a serving platter. Top with the broccoli, zucchini, tomato, and bell pepper. In a bowl, mix the vinegar and pesto. Drizzle the dressing on top. Sprinkle the feta cheese and serve.

NUTRITIONS

- *Calories: 100*
- *Fat: 6g*
- *Carbohydrates: 7g*
- *Protein: 4g*

96. POTATO TUNA SALAD

PREPARATION	COOKING	SERVES
4H 20 MIN	10 MIN	1

INGREDIENTS

- 1 potato, peeled and sliced into cubes
- 1/12 cup plain yogurt
- 1/12 cup mayonnaise
- 1/6 clove garlic, crushed and minced
- 1/6 tablespoon almond milk
- 1/6 tablespoon fresh dill, chopped
- ½ teaspoon lemon zest
- Salt to taste
- 1 cup cucumber, chopped
- ¼ cup scallions, chopped
- ¼ cup radishes, chopped
- (9 oz) canned tuna flakes
- 1/2 hard-boiled eggs, chopped
- 1 cups lettuce, chopped

DIRECTIONS

1. Fill your pot with water. Add the potatoes and boil. Cook for 15 minutes or till slightly tender. Drain and let cool.
2. In a bowl, mix the yogurt, mayo, garlic, almond milk, fresh dill, lemon zest, and salt. Stir in the potatoes, tuna flakes, and eggs. Mix well.
3. Chill in the refrigerator for 4 hours. Stir in the shredded lettuce before serving.

NUTRITIONS

- Calories: 243
- Fat: 9.9g
- Carbohydrates: 22.2g
- Protein: 17.5g

97. HIGH PROTEIN SALAD

PREPARATION	COOKING	SERVES
5 MIN	5 MIN	1

INGREDIENTS

Salad:
- 1(15 oz) can green kidney beans
- 1/4 tablespoon capers
- 1/4 handfuls arugula
- 1(15 oz) can lentils

Dressing:
- 1/1 tablespoon caper brine
- 1/1 tablespoon tamari
- 1/1 tablespoon balsamic vinegar
- 2/2 tablespoon peanut butter
- 2/2 tablespoon hot sauce

- 2/1 tablespoon tahini

DIRECTIONS

1. For the dressing, stir all the ingredients until they come together to form a smooth dressing in a bowl.
2. For the salad, mix the beans, arugula, capers, and lentils. Top with the dressing and serve.

NUTRITIONS

- Calories: 205
- Fat: 2g
- Protein: 13g
- Carbs: 31g

98. RICE AND VEGGIE BOWL

PREPARATION	COOKING	SERVES
5 MIN	15 MIN	1

INGREDIENTS

- 1/3 tablespoon coconut oil
- 1/2 teaspoon ground cumin
- 1/2 teaspoon ground turmeric
- 1/3 teaspoon chili powder
- 1 red bell pepper, chopped
- 1/2 tablespoon tomato paste
- 1 bunch of broccolis, sliced into bite-sized florets with short stems
- 1/2 teaspoon salt, to taste
- 1 large red onion, sliced
- 1/2 garlic cloves, minced
- 1/2 head of cauliflower, sliced into bite-sized florets
- 1/2 cups cooked rice
- ground black pepper to taste

DIRECTIONS

1. Start with warming up the coconut oil over medium-high heat. Stir in the turmeric, cumin, chili powder, salt, and tomato paste.
2. Cook the content for 1 minute. Stir repeatedly until the spices are fragrant. Add the garlic and onion. Fry for 2 to 3 minutes until the onions are softened.
3. Add the broccoli, cauliflower, and bell pepper. Cover, then cook for 3 to 4 minutes and stir occasionally.
4. Add the cooked rice. Stir so it will combine well with the vegetables—Cook for 2 to 3 minutes. Stir until the rice is warm.
5. Check the seasoning and change to taste if desired. Lessen the heat and cook on low for 2 to 3 more minutes so the flavors will meld. Serve with freshly ground black pepper.

NUTRITIONS

- Calories: 260
- Fat: 9g
- Protein: 9g
- Carbs: 36g

99. SQUASH BLACK BEAN BOWL

PREPARATION	COOKING	SERVES
5 MIN	30 MIN	1

INGREDIENTS

- 1 large spaghetti squash, halved,
- 1/3 cup water (or 2 tablespoon olive oil, rubbed on the inside of squash)

Black bean filling:
- 1/2 (15 oz) can of black beans, emptied and rinsed
- 1/2 cup fire-roasted corn (or frozen sweet corn)
- 1/2 cup thinly sliced red cabbage
- 1/2 tablespoon chopped green onion, green and white parts

- ¼ cup chopped fresh coriander
- ½ lime, juiced or to taste
- Pepper and salt, to taste

Avocado mash:
- 1 ripe avocado, mashed
- ½ lime, juiced or to taste
- ¼ teaspoon cumin
- Pepper and pinch of sea salt

DIRECTIONS

1. Warm oven to 400 F. Chop the squash in part and scoop out the seeds with a spoon, like a pumpkin.
2. Fill the roasting pan with 1/3 cup of water. Lay the squash, cut side down, in the pan. Bake for 30 minutes until soft and tender.
3. While this is baking, mix all the ingredients for the black bean filling in a medium-sized bowl. In a small dish, crush the avocado and blend in the ingredients for the avocado mash.
4. Eliminate the squash from the oven and let it cool for 5 minutes. Scrape the squash with a fork so that it looks like spaghetti noodles.
5. Then, fill it with black bean filling and top with avocado mash. Serve and enjoy.

NUTRITIONS

- Calories: 85
- Fat: 0.5g
- Protein: 4g
- Carbs: 6g

100. PEA SALAD

PREPARATION	COOKING	SERVES
40 MIN	0 MIN	1

INGREDIENTS

- 1/2 cup chickpeas, rinsed and drained
- 1/2 cups peas, divided
- Salt to taste
- 1 tablespoon olive oil
- ½ cup buttermilk
- Pepper to taste
- 2 cups pea greens
- 1/2 carrots shaved
- 1/4 cup snow peas, trimmed

DIRECTIONS

1. Add the chickpeas and half of the peas to your food processor. Season with salt. Pulse until smooth. Set aside.
2. In a bowl, toss the remaining peas in oil, milk, salt, and pepper. Transfer the mixture to your food processor. Process until pureed.
3. Transfer this mixture to a bowl. Arrange the pea greens on a serving plate. Top with the shaved carrots and snow peas. Stir in the pea and milk dressing. Serve with the reserved chickpea hummus.

NUTRITIONS

- Calories: 214
- Fat: 8.6g
- Carbohydrates: 27.3g
- Protein: 8g

116

101. SNAP PEA SALAD

PREPARATION	COOKING	SERVES
1 HOUR	0 MIN	1

INGREDIENTS

- 1/2 tablespoons mayonnaise
- ¾ teaspoon celery seed
- ¼ cup cider vinegar
- 1/2 teaspoon yellow mustard
- 1/2 tablespoon sugar
- Salt and pepper to taste
- 1 oz. radishes, sliced thinly
- 2 oz. sugar snap peas, sliced thinly

DIRECTIONS

1. In a bowl, combine the mayonnaise, celery seeds, vinegar, mustard, sugar, salt, and pepper. Stir in the radishes and snap peas. Refrigerate for 30 minutes. Serve.

NUTRITIONS

- *Calories: 69*
- *Fat: 3.7g*
- *Carbohydrates: 7.1g*
- *Protein: 2g*

102. CUCUMBER TOMATO CHOPPED SALAD

PREPARATION	COOKING	SERVES
15 MIN	0 MIN	1

INGREDIENTS

- 1/4 cup light mayonnaise
- 1/2 tablespoon lemon juice
- 1/2 tablespoon fresh dill, chopped
- 1/2 tablespoon chive, chopped
- 1/4 cup feta cheese, crumbled
- Salt and pepper to taste
- 1/2 red onion, chopped
- 1/2 cucumber, diced
- 1/2 radish, diced
- 1 tomato, diced
- Chives, chopped

DIRECTIONS

1. Combine the mayonnaise, lemon juice, fresh dill, chives, feta cheese, salt, and pepper in a bowl. Mix well. Stir in the onion, cucumber, radish, and tomatoes. Coat evenly. Garnish with the chopped chives.

NUTRITIONS

- *Calories: 187*
- *Fat: 16.7g*
- *Carbohydrates: 6.7g*
- *Protein: 3.3g*

103. ZUCCHINI PASTA SALAD

PREPARATION	COOKING	SERVES
4 MIN	0 MIN	1

INGREDIENTS

- 1 tablespoon olive oil
- 1/2 teaspoons Dijon mustard
- 1/3 tablespoons red-wine vinegar
- 1/2 clove garlic, grated
- 2 tablespoons fresh oregano, chopped
- 1/2 shallot, chopped
- ¼ teaspoon red pepper flakes
- 4 oz. zucchini noodles
- ¼ cup Kalamata olives pitted
- 1 cups cherry tomato, sliced in half
- ¾ cup parmesan cheese shaved

DIRECTIONS

1. Mix the olive oil, Dijon mustard, red wine vinegar, garlic, oregano, shallot, and red pepper flakes in a bowl.
2. Stir in the zucchini noodles. Sprinkle on top the olives, tomatoes, and parmesan cheese.

NUTRITIONS

- *Calories: 299*
- *Fat: 24.7g*
- *Carbohydrates: 11.6g*
- *Protein: 7g*

104. EGG AVOCADO SALAD

PREPARATION	COOKING	SERVES
10 MIN	0 MIN	1

INGREDIENTS

- 1/2 avocado
- 1 hard-boiled egg, peeled and chopped
- 1/4 tablespoon mayonnaise
- 1/4 tablespoons freshly squeezed lemon juice
- ¼ cup celery, chopped
- 1/2 tablespoons chives, chopped
- Salt and pepper to taste

DIRECTIONS

1. Add the avocado to a large bowl. Mash the avocado using a fork. Stir in the egg and mash the eggs.
2. Add the mayonnaise, lemon juice, celery, chives, salt, and pepper. Chill in the refrigerator for at least 2o to 30 minutes before serving.

NUTRITIONS

- Calories: 224
- Fat: 18g
- Carbohydrates: 6.1g
- Protein: 10.6g

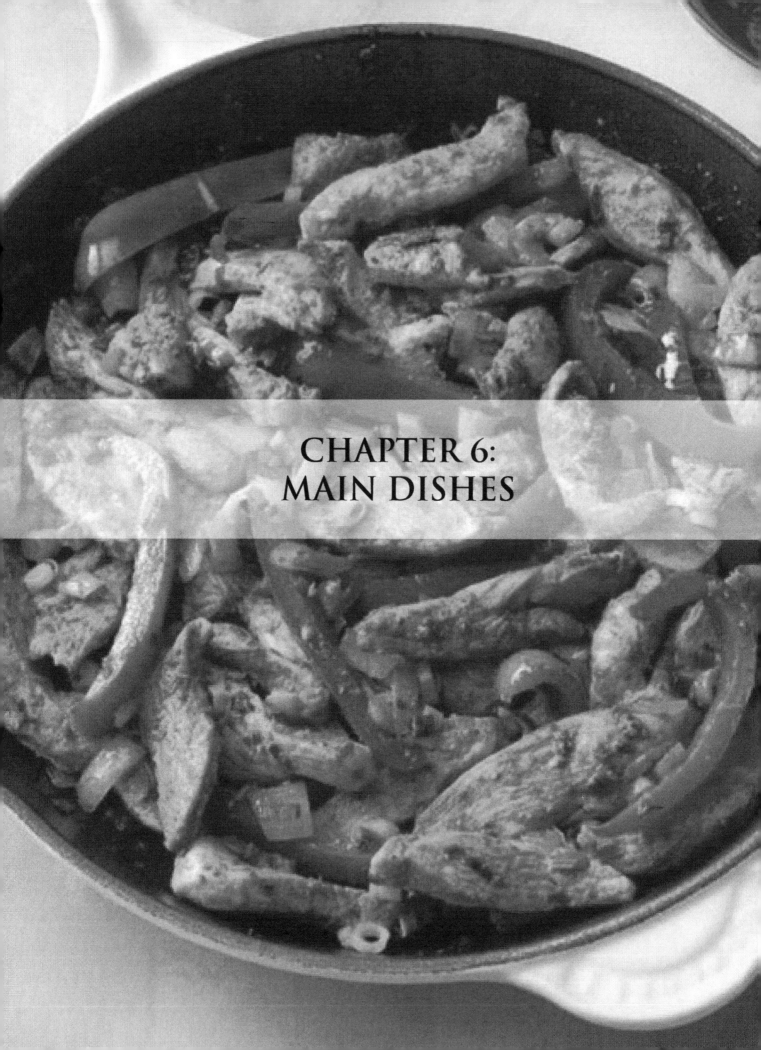

CHAPTER 6:
MAIN DISHES

105. LEAN TURKEY PAPRIKASH

PREPARATION	COOKING	SERVES
15 MIN	15 MIN	4

INGREDIENTS

- Salt and black chili pepper, to taste
- 8 oz. egg noodles
- 2 extra virgin olive oil spoons
- 6 ounces of fat, sliced mushroom
- 1 spoonful of finely chopped onion
- Lean ground turkey, 1 pound
- ½ cup of water
- 1 cubed chicken broth, crumbled
- 1 spoonful of sweet paprika
- 2/3 cup 2% Greek yogurt

DIRECTIONS

1. Pick up a big pot of lightly salted water over high heat to a boil. Cook pasta and drain according to package instructions.
2. Warm-up oil over medium heat in a large skillet, then stir in mushrooms and onion, and cook until tender and lightly brown for a few minutes.
3. Attach turkey to pan, stirring from time to time. Stir in water and bouillon cube until the turkey is fully cooked. Stirring to mix, season with paprika, salt, and pepper.
4. Remove from the heat bath. Stir in yogurt and serve turkey over pasta right away.

NUTRITIONS

- *Calories: 456*
- *Carbs: 45g*
- *Fat: 14g*
- *Protein: 35g*

106. POLLO FAJITAS

PREPARATION	COOKING	SERVES
40 MIN	10 MIN	5

INGREDIENTS

- 1 spoonful of Worcestershire sauce
- 1 spoonful of apple cider vinegar
- 1 tablespoon soy sauce with less sodium
- 1 tablespoon of chili powder
- 1 garlic clove, peeled and chopped
- Dash hot sauce
- 4 (6-ounce) fat-trimmed, skinless chicken breasts sliced into strips
- 1 tablespoon of vegetable oil
- 1 big, thinly sliced onion

- 1 green chili pepper, seeded and sliced
- Salt and ground black chili pepper.
- 8 (6-inch) whole-wheat tortillas
- ½ lemon juice

DIRECTIONS

1. Add Worcestershire sauce, vinegar, soy sauce, chili powder, garlic, and hot sauce in a big Ziploc container.
2. Attach strips of chicken to a Ziploc container. Seal tightly and cover with a shake. Let the chicken marinate within 30 minutes at room temperature (or cool down for many hours), shaking them periodically.
3. Warm oil over high heat in a large skillet, then put strips of chicken and marinade to the saucepan; sauté for 5 to 6 minutes.
4. Add onion plus green pepper to the pan, season with salt and pepper, and sauté until the chicken is thoroughly cooked, within 3 to 4 minutes further.
5. Hot tortillas in a microwave or nonstick pan. Cover tortillas with fajita mixture, and before serving, squeeze with lemon juice.

NUTRITIONS

- *Calories: 210*
- *Carbs: 6g*
- *Fat: 8g*
- *Protein: 28g*

107. CHUNKY CHICKEN QUESADILLA

PREPARATION	COOKING	SERVES
15 MIN	16 MIN	5

INGREDIENTS

- 1 (6-ounce) boneless, skinless breast of chicken, trimmed in fat
- 1 tablespoon low-fat sour cream
- (8-inch) tortillas with whole-wheat
- 1/3 cup salsa
- 1 cup of chopped lettuce
- 1/3 cup shredded cheese with low-fat cheddar

DIRECTIONS

1. Cover a medium nonstick skillet over medium heat with cooking spray and warm. Add the chicken and cook each side for 3 to 5 minutes. Move chicken to a cutting board, once fully cooked.
2. Pour sour cream over 1 tortilla. Slice the chicken breast over sour cream and cover with salsa and lettuce. Sprinkle with cheese, then top with a tortilla.
3. Recoat skillet over low heat with cooking spray and cover—Cook quesadilla, about 3 minutes per side until golden, using a large spatula to flip it. Remove, slice, and serve from skillet.

NUTRITIONS

- *Calories: 190*
- *Carbs: 23g*
- *Fat: 7g*
- *Protein: 9g*

108. CHICKEN FETTUCCINE WITH SHIITAKE MUSHROOMS

PREPARATION	COOKING	SERVES
15 MIN	25 MIN	4

INGREDIENTS

- Salt and black chili pepper, to taste
- 8-ounce whole-wheat fettuccine
- 2 spoonful of extra virgin olive oil
- 6-ounce boneless, skinless breasts of chicken, trimmed with fat and cut into strips
- Roasted garlic cloves and hazelnuts
- 2 ounces of shiitake mushrooms stemmed and sliced (about 1 to 1 ½cups)
- 2 teaspoons lemon zest
- 2 lemon juice teaspoons
- ½ cup Parmesan grated cheese
- 1/2 tablespoon of fresh basil

DIRECTIONS

1. Pick up a big pot of lightly salted water over high heat to a boil. Cook fettuccine as instructed on the box. Drain the sauce, reserving ½ cup of water for the sauce.
2. In the meantime, warm oil over medium heat in a big, nonstick skillet. Attach strips of chicken, then sauté for 3 to 4 minutes.
3. Add mushrooms and garlic. Cook, stirring periodically, for 4 to 5 minutes until the mushrooms are tender. Add lemon zest, lemon juice, salt, and pepper to taste.
4. Add pasta, reserved broth, Parmesan, and basil into the skillet. Nice toss and serve.

NUTRITIONS

- Calories: 444
- Carbs: 43g
- Fat: 13g
- Protein: 33g

109. CHICKEN YAKITORI

PREPARATION	COOKING	SERVES
15 MIN	15 MIN	5

INGREDIENTS

- ½ cup of soy sauce with less sodium
- ½ cup sherry or white wine to prepare
- ½ cup low-sodium chicken broth
- 1/2 teaspoon ginger
- Pinch of garlic powder
- 1/2 cup scallions hacked
- 4 (6-ounce) boneless, skinless, fat-free chicken breasts, sliced into 2-inch cubes

DIRECTIONS

1. When using skewers of bamboo or metal spindles, soak in water for 30 minutes to stop burning the fuel.
2. Put soy sauce, sherry, chicken broth, ginger, garlic powder, and scallions into a small pot. Bring fixings to a boil over medium-high heat, and remove from heat immediately.
3. Preheat the broiler for the oven. Begin threading chicken on skewers. Coat a broiler pan using a cooking spray and placed skewers of chicken on the pan. Brush with sherry sauce to every skewer.
4. Place the saucepan under the broiler until the chicken is browned, 3 minutes. Remove the pan from the oven and turn over each chicken skewer, brushing the chicken sauce repeatedly.
5. Return the saucepan to the broiler until the chicken is well browned and cooked through. Serve.

NUTRITIONS

- Calories: 160
- Carbs: 8g
- Fat: 7g
- Protein: 16g

110. MUSCLE MEATBALLS

PREPARATION	COOKING	SERVES
15 MIN	20 MIN	16 MEATBALLS

INGREDIENTS

- 1 ½ pound 93 percent ground turkey
- 2 egg whites or 6 spoonful of liquid egg white replace
- ½ cup rubbed wheat germ
- 1/4 cup fast-cooking oats:
- 1 tablespoon of whole flaxseeds
- 1 tablespoon Parmesan cheese
- 1/2 teaspoon seasoning for all-use
- 1/4 teaspoon black chili pepper

DIRECTIONS

1. Preheat the oven to 400°F. Cover a baking dish of 9" by 13" with cooking spray. Put all the fixings in a large bowl, and mix gently together to combine.
2. Shape the mixture into 16 meatballs and put it in the baking platter. Bake for 7 minutes, then flip each meatball with a spatula.
3. Return to the oven and cook for around 8 to 13 minutes, until the meatballs are no longer pink in the middle. Serve.

NUTRITIONS

- *Calories: 266*
- *Carbs: 11g*
- *Fat: 5g*
- *Protein: 46g*

111. ORANGE AND HONEY-GLAZED CHICKEN

PREPARATION	COOKING	SERVES
15 MIN	10 MIN	5

INGREDIENTS

- 4 (6-ounce) boneless, skinless breasts of chicken trimmed in fat
- 2 tablespoons of orange juice
- 2 tablespoons of honey
- 1 tablespoon of lemon juice.
- 1/8 tablespoon salt

DIRECTIONS

1. Preheat to 375°F on the burner. Cover with cooking spray a 9-inch by 13-inch baking dish, and add chicken.
2. Combine orange juice, sugar, lemon juice, and salt in a small bowl. Baste the orange juice mixture on every piece of chicken.
3. Put foil over the dish and bake for 10 minutes. Remove the chicken foil, and turn it. Bake chicken for another ten to fifteen minutes until fried and the juices run free.

NUTRITIONS

- Calories: 200
- Carbs: 14g
- Fat: 6g
- Protein: 24g

112. THAI BASIL CHICKEN

PREPARATION	COOKING	SERVES
15 MIN	10 MIN	4

INGREDIENTS

- 4 (6-ounce) boneless, skinless breasts of chicken trimmed in fat
- 3 garlic cloves, peeled and chopped
- 2 jalapeño chilies, hairy
- 1 tablespoon fish sauce
- 1 tablespoon granulated sugar
- ¼ cup of fresh basil
- 1 tablespoon fresh mint
- 1 spoonful of unsalted, dry-roasted peanuts

DIRECTIONS

1. Break each breast into approximately 8 strips. Placed on aside. Cover a big, nonstick skillet over medium-high heat with cooking spray and warm. Also, add the garlic and jalapeños. Stir continuously, stirring until garlic is only golden.
2. Add chicken strips and cook, frequently stirring, for about 8 to 10 minutes until chicken is thoroughly cooked. Add sugar and fish sauce, cook for 30 seconds. Until eating, garnish with the basil, mint, and peanuts.

NUTRITIONS

- *Calories: 170*
- *Carbs: 15g*
- *Fat: 1g*
- *Protein: 29g*

113. CHICKEN CURRY

PREPARATION	COOKING	SERVES
15 MIN	27 MIN	5

INGREDIENTS

- 1 small chopped onion
- 1 clove of garlic, minced and peeled
- 3 spoonful of curry powder
- 1 tablespoon of sweet paprika
- 1 bay leaf
- 1 teaspoon cinnamon
- ½ teaspoon peeled and rubbed fresh ginger
- Salt and black ground pepper to taste
- 4 (6-ounce) boneless, skinless, fat-cut chicken breasts, cut into 1-inch cubes
- 1 tablespoon of tomato paste
- ½ cup of water
- ½ citrus
- ½ teaspoon chili Indian powder
- 1 cup 2% Greek yogurt

DIRECTIONS

1. Cover a large skillet over medium heat with cooking spray and hold. Sauté the onion for about 5 minutes, until translucent.
2. Add garlic, curry powder, paprika, bay leaf, cinnamon, ginger, salt, and pepper into the skillet; stir for 2 minutes.
3. Add the chicken and the tomato paste and water to the saucepan; whisk to mix. Bring liquid to a boil, lower heat to low, and cook for 10 minutes.
4. Stir in chili powder and lemon juice. Simmer within 5 minutes until the chicken is cooked through. Take off the heat and take off the bay leaf and remove it. Add yogurt and serve.

NUTRITIONS

- Calories: 306
- Carbs: 50g
- Fat: 5g
- Protein: 16g

114. ITALIAN PARMESAN CHICKEN

PREPARATION	COOKING	SERVES
15 MIN	25 MIN	4

INGREDIENTS

- 2 spoonful of extra virgin olive oil
- 2 teaspoons of chopped garlic
- Breadcrumbs with 1/4 cup seasoning
- ¼ cup Parmesan grated cheese
- 4 (6-ounce) boneless, skinless breasts of chicken, trimmed in fat

DIRECTIONS

1. Preheat the oven to 425°F. Put the olive oil plus garlic in a medium heat-proof dish. Warm-up for 30 to 60 seconds in the microwave to mix flavors. Combine breadcrumbs and cheese in a small, medium dish.
2. Coat the chicken breast in the oil mixture and let the excess wash away. Then, cover the mix with breadcrumbs and put it in a shallow baking dish. Repeat until you bread all the chicken breasts.
3. Put the chicken in the oven for 10 minutes, then flip over and the juices run clear, around 10 to 15 minutes more. Take off the oven, and eat.

NUTRITIONS

- *Calories: 363*
- *Carbs: 10g*
- *Fat: 7g*
- *Protein: 54g*

115. CHICKEN AND BROCCOLI STIR-FRY

PREPARATION	COOKING	SERVES
15 MIN	10 MIN	5

INGREDIENTS

- 2 tablespoons of red wine
- 1 tablespoon soy sauce with less sodium
- ½ tablespoon of cornstarch
- 1 tablespoon of granulated sugar
- 1 tsp salt
- Broccoli
- 1 red bell pepper, chopped and seeded
- 1/2 sliced onion
- 4 (6-ounce) boneless, skinless, fat-free chicken breasts, trimmed into thin stripes

DIRECTIONS

1. Combine the red wine, soy sauce, cornstarch, sugar, and salt in a small cup. Whisk well with a fork until cornstarch dissolves.
2. Cover a big, nonstick skillet over medium-high heat with cooking spray and warm. Stir in broccoli, pepper bell, and onion until tender. Add chicken and stir-fry for around 2 to 3 minutes until browned.
3. Pour soy sauce mixture over vegetables and chicken. Stir-fry until sauce thickens, within 2 to 4 minutes. Take off heat and serve.

NUTRITIONS

- *Calories: 377*
- *Carbs: 10g*
- *Fat: 13g*
- *Protein: 17g*

116. GREEK PITA PIZZA

PREPARATION	COOKING	SERVES
15 MIN	10 MIN	5

INGREDIENTS

- 1 (6-ounce) boneless, skinless breast of chicken, trimmed in fat
- Whole-wheat pita bread
- ½ tablespoon extra-virgin olive oil
- 2 Sliced olives
- 1 tsp vinegar with red wine
- 1/2 clove of garlic, minced and peeled
- 1/4 teaspoon of dried oregano
- 1/4 teaspoon of dried basil
- Salt and black chili pepper, to taste

- ¼ cup fresh spinach
- Low-fat cheese crumbled
- ½ tomatoes, seeded, chopped

DIRECTIONS

1. Preheat the broiler to high on the burner. Cover a small skillet over medium heat with cooking spray and hold. Put the chicken in the skillet and cook for 3 to 5 minutes.
2. When juices run clear, remove chicken from the heat; set aside. Let the chicken breast cool, and then chop into small bits.
3. In the meantime, put pita bread on a baking sheet, and brush with oil lightly. Broil up for 2 minutes 4 inches from the sun.
4. Put olives, vinegar, garlic, oregano, basil, salt, chili pepper, and any remaining oil in a small cup. Healthy balance to blend.
5. Layer a mixture of olives over the pita. Then put the spinach, feta, onion, and chicken. Broil until the feta gets warm and softened, about 3 minutes more.

NUTRITIONS

- Calories: 200
- Carbs: 33g

- Fat: 5g
- Protein: 6g

117. BOW-TIE PASTA SALAD WITH CHICKEN AND CHICKPEAS

PREPARATION	COOKING	SERVES
15 MIN	0 MIN	5

INGREDIENTS

- Salt, just to taste
- Whole-wheat bow-tie pasta 8 ounces
- 3 (6-ounce) fat-cut chicken breasts, fried, shredded
- ½ (15 ounces) of chickpeas can be drained and rinsed
- 1 canned sliced black olive (2.25-ounce), drained
- Celery stalks, shredded
- 2 cucumbers, split
- ½ cup shredded carrots
- ½ yellow, finely chopped onion
- Sliced Parmesan cheese

- 1 tbsp of extra virgin olive oil
- 1/3 cup red vinegar
- ½ teaspoon Worcestershire sauce
- ½ tablespoon of spicy brown mustard
- ½ clove of garlic, minced and peeled
- 1 tbsp basil chopped or 1 teaspoon dried basil
- ¼ teaspoon black chili pepper
-

DIRECTIONS

1. Pick up a big pot of lightly salted water over high heat to a boil. Cook the pasta, as stated in the instructions box. Drain and run the pasta for about 30 seconds under cold water, or until it is fully cool.
2. Move pasta to a big bowl and add the ingredients leftover. To blend, use tongs to mix thoroughly. Cover the bowl and cool for at least ½ hours or till night. Throw in the salad before serving.

NUTRITIONS

- Calories: 317
- Carbs: 44g

- Fat: 12g
- Protein: 8g

118. GREEK STYLE QUESADILLAS

PREPARATION	COOKING	SERVES
10 MIN	10 MIN	4

INGREDIENTS

- 4 whole-wheat tortillas
- 1 cup Mozzarella cheese, shredded
- 1 cup fresh spinach, chopped
- 2 tablespoon Greek yogurt
- 1 egg, beaten
- ¼ cup green olives, sliced
- 1 tablespoon olive oil
- 1/3 cup fresh cilantro, chopped

DIRECTIONS

1. In the bowl, combine mozzarella cheese, spinach, yogurt, egg, olives, and cilantro. Then pour olive oil into the skillet.
2. In the skillet, place one tortilla and spread it with a mozzarella mixture. Top it with the second tortilla and spread it with cheese mixture again.
3. Then place the third tortilla and spread it with all remaining cheese mixture. Cover it with the last tortilla and fry it for 5 minutes from each side over medium heat.

NUTRITIONS

- *Calories: 193*
- *Fat: 7.7g*
- *Carbs: 23.6g*
- *Protein: 8.3g*

119. LIGHT PAPRIKA MOUSSAKA

PREPARATION	COOKING	SERVES
15 MIN	45 MIN	3

INGREDIENTS

- 1 eggplant, trimmed
- 1 cup ground chicken
- 1/3 cup white onion, diced
- 3 oz. Cheddar cheese, shredded
- 1 potato, sliced
- 1 teaspoon olive oil
- 1 teaspoon salt
- ½ cup milk
- 1 tablespoon butter
- 1 tablespoon ground paprika
- 1 tablespoon Italian seasoning
- 1 teaspoon tomato paste

DIRECTIONS

1. Slice the eggplant in length and sprinkle with salt. In the skillet, pour olive oil and add sliced potato. Roast potato for 2 minutes from each side. Then transfer it to the plate.
2. Put eggplant in the skillet and roast it for 2 minutes from each side too. In the pan, pour milk and bring it to a boil, then put the tomato paste, Italian seasoning, paprika, butter, and cheddar cheese.
3. Then mix up together onion with ground chicken. Arrange the sliced potato in the casserole in one layer. Then add ½ part of all sliced eggplants.
4. Spread the eggplants with ½ part of the chicken mixture. Then add the remaining eggplants. Pour the milk mixture over the eggplants—Bake moussaka for 30 minutes at 355F. Serve.

NUTRITIONS

- *Calories: 387*
- *Fat: 21.2g*
- *Carbs: 26.3g*
- *Protein: 25.4g*

120. CUCUMBER BOWL WITH SPICES AND GREEK YOGURT

PREPARATION	COOKING	SERVES
10 MIN	20 MIN	3

INGREDIENTS

- 4 cucumbers
- ½ teaspoon chili pepper
- ¼ cup fresh parsley, chopped
- ¾ cup fresh dill, chopped
- 2 tablespoons lemon juice
- ½ teaspoon salt
- ½ teaspoon ground black pepper
- ¼ teaspoon sage
- ½ teaspoon dried oregano
- 1/3 cup Greek yogurt

DIRECTIONS

1. Make the cucumber dressing: blend the dill and parsley until you get green mash. Then combine green mash with lemon juice, salt, ground black pepper, sage, dried oregano, Greek yogurt, and chili pepper. Churn the mixture well.
2. Chop the cucumbers roughly and combine them with cucumber dressing. Mix up well. Refrigerate the cucumber for 20 minutes. Serve.

NUTRITIONS

- *Calories: 114*
- *Fat: 1.6g*
- *Carbs: 23.2g*
- *Protein: 7.6g*

121. SWEET POTATO BACON MASH

PREPARATION	COOKING	SERVES
10 MIN	20 MIN	4

INGREDIENTS

- 3 sweet potatoes, peeled
- 4 oz. bacon, chopped
- 1 cup chicken stock
- 1 tablespoon butter
- 1 teaspoon salt
- 2 oz. Parmesan, grated

DIRECTIONS

1. Dice sweet potato and put it in the pan. Add chicken stock and close the lid. Boil the vegetables until they are soft. After this, drain the chicken stock.
2. Mash the sweet potato with the help of the potato masher. Add grated cheese and butter. Mix up together salt and chopped bacon. Fry the mixture until it is crunchy (10-15 minutes).
3. Add cooked bacon to the mashed sweet potato and mix up with the help of the spoon. It is recommended to serve the meal warm or hot.

NUTRITIONS

- *Calories: 304*
- *Fat: 18.1*
- *Carbs: 18.8*
- *Protein: 17*

122. PROSCIUTTO WRAPPED MOZZARELLA BALLS

PREPARATION	COOKING	SERVES
10 MIN	10 MIN	4

INGREDIENTS

- 8 Mozzarella balls, cherry size
- 4 oz. bacon, sliced
- ¼ teaspoon ground black pepper
- ¾ teaspoon dried rosemary
- 1 teaspoon butter

DIRECTIONS

1. Sprinkle the sliced bacon with ground black pepper and dried rosemary. Wrap every mozzarella ball in the sliced bacon and secure them with toothpicks. Melt butter.
2. Brush wrapped mozzarella balls with butter. Line the baking tray with the parchment and arrange mozzarella balls in it. Bake the meal for 10 minutes at 365F. Serve.

NUTRITIONS

- Calories: 323
- Fat: 26.8 g
- Carbs: 0.6 g
- Protein: 20.6 g

123. MEDITERRANEAN BURRITO

PREPARATION	COOKING	SERVES
10 MIN	0 MIN	2

INGREDIENTS

- 2 wheat tortillas
- 2 oz. red kidney beans, canned, drained
- 2 tablespoons hummus
- 2 teaspoons tahini sauce
- 1 cucumber
- 2 lettuce leaves
- 1 tablespoon lime juice
- 1 teaspoon olive oil
- ½ teaspoon dried oregano

DIRECTIONS

1. Mash the red kidney beans until you get a puree. Then spread the wheat tortillas with beans mash from one side. Add hummus and tahini sauce.
2. Cut the cucumber into the wedges and place them over tahini sauce. Then add lettuce leaves. Make the dressing: mix up together olive oil, dried oregano, and lime juice.
3. Drizzle the lettuce leaves with the dressing and wrap the wheat tortillas in the shape of burritos.

NUTRITIONS

- *Calories: 288*
- *Fat: 10.2 g*
- *Carbs: 38.2 g*
- *Protein: 12.5 g*

CHAPTER 7:
MEAT RECIPES

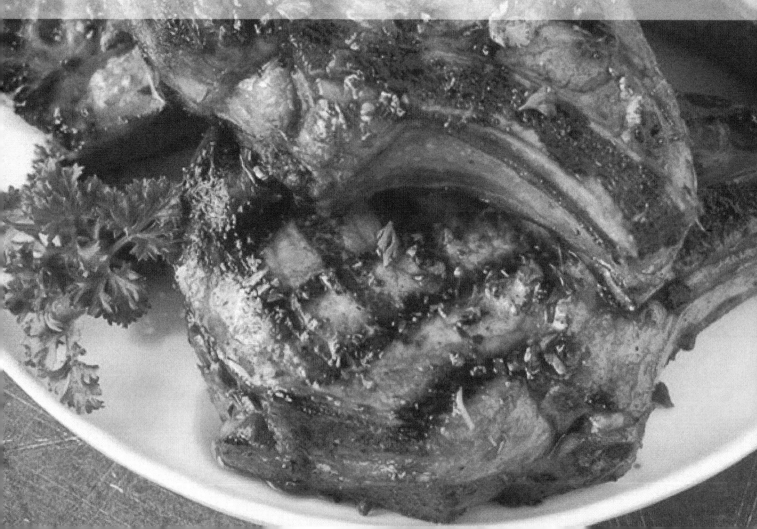

124. TENDER LAMB CHOPS

PREPARATION	COOKING	SERVES
10 MIN	6 HOURS	8

INGREDIENTS

- 8 lamb chops
- ½ teaspoon dried thyme
- 1 onion, sliced
- 1 teaspoon dried oregano
- 2 garlic cloves, minced
- Pepper and salt

DIRECTIONS

1. Add sliced onion into the slow cooker. Combine thyme, oregano, pepper, and salt. Rub over lamb chops.
2. Place lamb chops in the slow cooker and top with garlic. Pour ¼ cup water around the lamb chops. Cover and cook on low heat within 6 hours. Serve and enjoy.

NUTRITIONS

- Calories: 40
- Fat: 1.9 g
- Carbohydrates: 2.3 g
- Protein: 3.4 g

125. SMOKY PORK & CABBAGE

PREPARATION	COOKING	SERVES
10 MIN	8 HOURS	6

INGREDIENTS

- 3 lb. pork roast
- 1/2 cabbage head, chopped
- 1 cup of water
- 1/3 cup liquid smoke
- 1 tablespoon kosher salt

DIRECTIONS

1. Rub pork with kosher salt and place into the pot. Pour liquid smoke over the pork. Add water. Cook on low within 7 hours.
2. Remove pork from the crockpot and add cabbage to the bottom of the pot. Place pork on top of the cabbage. Cook again within 1 more hour. Shred pork with a fork and serves.

NUTRITIONS

- *Calories: 484*
- *Fat: 21.5 g*
- *Carbohydrates: 4 g*
- *Protein: 66 g*

126. SEASONED PORK CHOPS

PREPARATION	COOKING	SERVES
10 MIN	4 HOURS	4

INGREDIENTS

- 4 pork chops
- 2 garlic cloves, minced
- 1 cup chicken broth
- 1 tablespoon poultry seasoning
- 1/4 cup olive oil
- Pepper and salt

DIRECTIONS

1. In a bowl, whisk together olive oil, poultry seasoning, garlic, broth, pepper, and salt. Pour olive oil mixture into the slow cooker, then place pork chops in the pot. Cook on high within 4 hours. Serve and enjoy.

NUTRITIONS

- *Calories: 386*
- *Fat: 32.9 g*
- *Carbohydrates: 3 g*
- *Protein: 20 g*

127. BEEF STROGANOFF

PREPARATION	COOKING	SERVES
10 MIN	8 HOURS	2

INGREDIENTS

- 1/2 lb. beef stew meat
- 10 oz mushroom soup, homemade
- 1 medium onion, chopped
- 1/2 cup sour cream
- 2 1/2 oz mushrooms, sliced
- Pepper and salt

DIRECTIONS

1. Add all ingredients except sour cream into the crockpot and mix well. Cook on low within 8 hours. Add sour cream and stir well. Serve and enjoy.

NUTRITIONS

- *Calories 470*
- *Fat 25 g*
- *Carbohydrates 8.6 g*
- *Protein 49 g*

128. LEMON BEEF

PREPARATION	COOKING	SERVES
10 MIN	6 HOURS	4

INGREDIENTS

- 1 lb. beef chuck roast
- 1 fresh lime juice
- 1 garlic clove, crushed
- 1 teaspoon chili powder
- 2 cups lemon-lime soda
- 1/2 teaspoon salt

DIRECTIONS

1. Place beef chuck roast into the slow cooker. Season roast with garlic, chili powder, and salt. Pour lemon-lime soda over the roast.
2. Cook on low within 6 hours. Shred the meat using a fork. Add lime juice over shredded roast and serve.

NUTRITIONS

- *Calories: 355*
- *Fat: 16.8 g*
- *Carbohydrates: 14 g*
- *Protein 35.5: g*

129. HERB PORK ROAST

PREPARATION	COOKING	SERVES
10 MIN	14 MIN	10

INGREDIENTS

- 5 lb. pork roast, boneless or bone-in
- 1 tablespoon dry herb mix
- 4 garlic cloves, cut into slivers
- 1 tablespoon salt

DIRECTIONS

1. Using a knife, make small slices all over the meat, then insert garlic slivers into the cuts. In a small bowl, mix Italian herb mix and salt and rub all over pork roast.
2. Place pork roast in the pot. Cook on low within 14 hours. Extract meat from pot and shred using a fork. Serve and enjoy.

NUTRITIONS

- Calories: 327
- Fat: 8 g
- Carbohydrates: 0.5 g
- Protein: 59 g

130. GREEK BEEF ROAST

PREPARATION	COOKING	SERVES
10 MIN	8 HOURS	6

INGREDIENTS

- 2 lb. lean top round beef roast
- 1 tablespoon Italian seasoning
- 6 garlic cloves, minced
- 1 onion, sliced
- 2 cups beef broth
- ½ cup red wine
- 1 teaspoon red pepper flakes
- Pepper
- Salt

DIRECTIONS

1. Season meat with pepper and salt and place into the pot. Pour remaining ingredients over meat. Cook on low within 8 hours. Shred the meat using a fork. Serve and enjoy.

NUTRITIONS

- *Calories: 231*
- *Fat: 6 g*
- *Carbohydrates: 4 g*
- *Protein: 35 g*

131. TOMATO PORK CHOPS

PREPARATION	COOKING	SERVES
10 MIN	6 HOURS	4

INGREDIENTS

- 4 pork chops, bone-in
- 1 tablespoon garlic, minced
- ½ small onion, chopped
- 6 oz can tomato paste
- 1 bell pepper, chopped
- ¼ teaspoon red pepper flakes
- 1 teaspoon Worcestershire sauce
- 1 tablespoon dried Italian seasoning
- 14 1/2 oz can tomato, diced
- 2 teaspoon olive oil
- ¼ teaspoon pepper
- 1 teaspoon kosher salt

DIRECTIONS

1. Heat-up oil in a pan over medium heat. Season pork chops with pepper and salt. Sear pork chops in the pan until brown from both sides.
2. Transfer pork chops into the pot. Add remaining ingredients over pork chops. Cook on low heat within 6 hours. Serve and enjoy.

NUTRITIONS

- Calories: 325
- Fat: 23.4 g
- Carbohydrates: 10 g
- Protein: 20 g

132. GREEK PORK CHOPS

PREPARATION	COOKING	SERVES
10 MIN	6 MIN	8

INGREDIENTS

- 8 pork chops, boneless
- 4 teaspoon dried oregano
- 2 tablespoon Worcestershire sauce
- 3 tablespoon fresh lemon juice
- ¼ cup olive oil
- 1 teaspoon ground mustard
- 2 teaspoon garlic powder
- 2 teaspoon onion powder
- Pepper
- Salt

DIRECTIONS

1. Whisk together oil, garlic powder, onion powder, oregano, Worcestershire sauce, lemon juice, mustard, pepper, and salt.
2. Place pork chops in a dish, then pour marinade over pork chops and coat well. Place in refrigerator overnight—Preheat the grill.
3. Put pork chops on the grill and cook within 3-4 minutes on each side. Serve and enjoy.

NUTRITIONS

- Calories: 324
- Fat: 26.5 g
- Carbohydrates: 2.5 g
- Protein: 18 g

133. PORK CACCIATORE

PREPARATION	COOKING	SERVES
10 MIN	6 HOURS	6

INGREDIENTS

- 1 ½ lb. pork chops
- 1 teaspoon dried oregano
- 1 cup beef broth
- 3 tablespoon tomato paste
- 14 oz can tomato, diced
- 2 cups mushrooms, sliced
- 1 small onion, diced
- 1 garlic clove, minced
- 2 tablespoon olive oil
- ¼ teaspoon pepper
- ½ teaspoon salt

DIRECTIONS

1. Warm-up oil in your pan over medium heat. Add pork chops to the pan and cook until brown on both sides. Transfer pork chops into the pot.
2. Pour remaining ingredients over the pork chops. Cook on low heat within 6 hours. Serve and enjoy.

NUTRITIONS

- Calories: 440
- Fat: 33 g
- Carbohydrates: 6 g
- Protein: 28 g

134. PORK WITH TOMATO & OLIVES

PREPARATION	COOKING	SERVES
10 MIN	30 MIN	6

INGREDIENTS

- 6 pork chops, boneless and cut into thick slices
- 1/8 teaspoon ground cinnamon
- 1/2 cup olives, pitted and sliced
- 8 oz can tomato, crushed
- 1/4 cup beef broth
- 2 garlic cloves, chopped
- 1 large onion, sliced
- 1 tablespoon olive oil

DIRECTIONS

1. Warm-up olive oil in a pan over medium heat. Place pork chops in a pan and cook until lightly brown and set aside.
2. Cook onion plus garlic in the same pan over medium heat, until onion is softened. Add broth and bring to boil over high heat.
3. Return pork to pan and stir in crushed tomatoes and remaining ingredients. Cover and simmer for 20 minutes. Serve and enjoy.

NUTRITIONS

- Calories: 321
- Fat: 23 g
- Carbohydrates: 7 g
- Protein: 19 g

135. PORK ROAST

PREPARATION	COOKING	SERVES
10 MIN	1H 35 MIN	6

INGREDIENTS

- 3 lb. pork roast, boneless
- 1 cup of water
- 1 onion, chopped
- 3 garlic cloves, chopped
- 1 tablespoon black pepper
- 1 rosemary sprig
- 2 fresh oregano sprigs
- 2 fresh thyme sprigs
- 1 tablespoon olive oil
- 1 tablespoon kosher salt

DIRECTIONS

1. Warm oven to 350 F. Season pork roast with pepper and salt. Heat olive oil in a stockpot and sear pork roast on each side, about 4 minutes.
2. Add onion and garlic. Pour in the water, oregano, and thyme and bring to boil for a minute—cover pot and roast within 1 1/2 hours. Serve and enjoy.

NUTRITIONS

- Calories: 502
- Fat: 23.8 g
- Carbohydrates: 3 g
- Protein: 65 g

136. EASY BEEF KOFTA

PREPARATION	COOKING	SERVES
10 MIN	10 MIN	8

INGREDIENTS

- 2 lb. ground beef
- 4 garlic cloves, minced
- 1 onion, minced
- 2 teaspoon cumin
- 1 cup fresh parsley, chopped
- ¼ teaspoon pepper
- 1 teaspoon salt

DIRECTIONS

1. Add all the listed ingredients into the mixing bowl and mix until combined. Roll meat mixture into the kabab shapes and cook in a hot pan for 4-6 minutes on each side or until cooked. Serve and enjoy.

NUTRITIONS

- *Calories: 223*
- *Fat: 7.3 g*
- *Carbohydrates: 2.5 g*
- *Protein: 35 g*

137. LEMON PEPPER PORK TENDERLOIN

PREPARATION	COOKING	SERVES
10 MIN	25 MIN	4

INGREDIENTS

- 1 lb. pork tenderloin
- 3/4 teaspoon lemon pepper
- 2 teaspoon dried oregano
- 1 tablespoon olive oil
- 3 tablespoon feta cheese, crumbled
- 3 tablespoon olive tapenades

DIRECTIONS

1. Add pork, oil, lemon pepper, and oregano in a zip-lock bag and rub well and place in a refrigerator for 2 hours.
2. Remove pork from zip-lock bag. Make a lengthwise slice through the center of the tenderloin using a sharp knife. Spread olive tapenade on half tenderloin and sprinkle with feta cheese.
3. Fold another half of the meat over to the original shape of the tenderloin. Tie close pork tenderloin with twine at 2-inch intervals—Grill pork tenderloin for 20 minutes. Cut into slices and serve.

NUTRITIONS

- Calories: 215
- Fat: 9.1 g
- Carbohydrates: 1 g
- Protein: 30.8 g

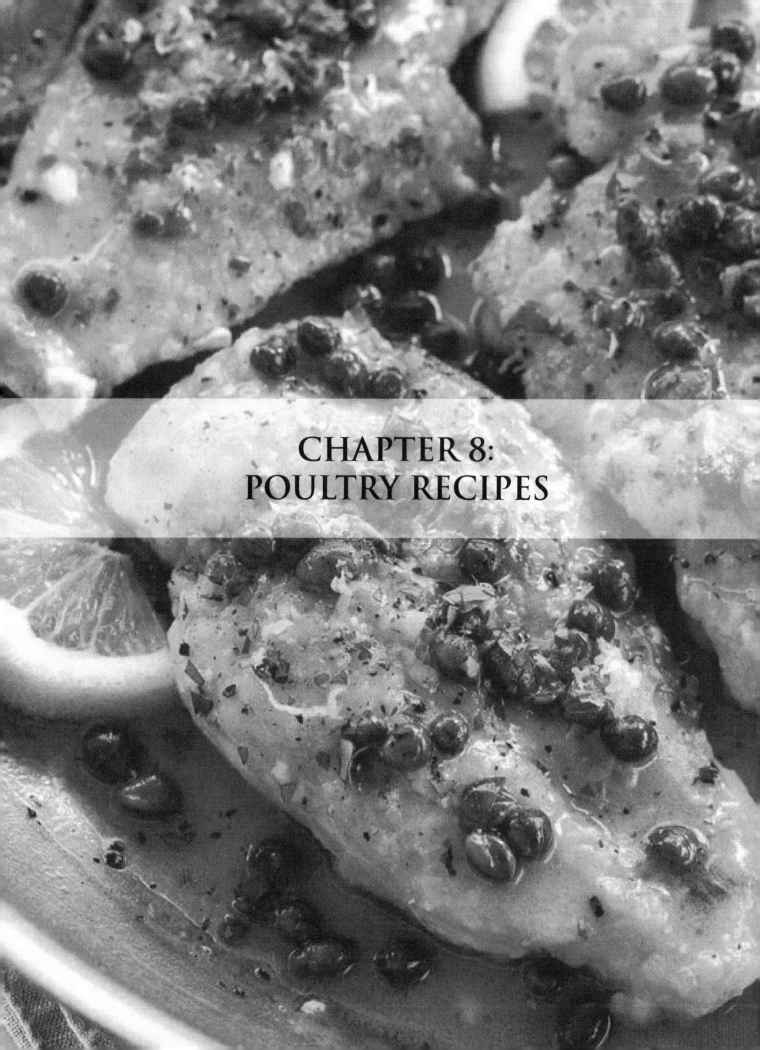

CHAPTER 8:
POULTRY RECIPES

138. CHICKEN CAPER

PREPARATION	COOKING	SERVES
5 MIN	25 MIN	4

INGREDIENTS

- 2 pounds boneless chicken tenderloins, skinless, and excess fat removed
- 1 tbsp garlic gusto seasoning
- ½ cup chicken broth (low sodium)
- 2 tbsp fresh lemon juice
- 4 tbsp capers
- 2 tbsp butter (not margarine)
- ground pepper and natural sea salt - to taste

DIRECTIONS

1. In a single layer, place the chicken on the bottom of your pot. Add the broth, lemon juice, and garlic seasoning to a bowl and whisk.
2. Pour the mixture over the chicken and sprinkle over with the capers—cook on high for 10 minutes. Remove chicken and set it aside. Set to sauté and bring the liquid to a boil.
3. Add the butter and whisk together. Allow the sauce to cook until the liquid reduces to half. Spread the sauce over the chicken—season with pepper and salt. Serve.

NUTRITIONS

- *Calories: 262*
- *Fat: 5.9g*
- *Carbohydrates: 0.6g*
- *Protein: 48.3g*

139. TURKEY SAUSAGE SPAGHETTI

PREPARATION	COOKING	SERVES
10 MIN	15 MIN	4

INGREDIENTS

- 4 cups Zucchini, spiraled
- 1 ½ pound Lean turkey sausage
- 1 tbsp Tuscan seasoning
- 2 cups Tomato sauce (no added sugar)
- 8 tbsp fresh parmesan cheese (grated)

DIRECTIONS

1. Cut the turkey sausage into ½-inch chunks. Place the chunks in a pan and cook over medium-high heat for about 8 minutes, or until it turns brown. Stir occasionally.
2. Add the Tuscan seasoning and tomato sauce to the pan. Stir thoroughly to coat completely. Adjust heat to high and bring the batter to a boil, about 4 min.
3. Add the noodles and toss well—Cook for extra 2 minutes, or until the noodles become soft and the chicken fully cooked.
4. Transfer to your serving plates and sprinkle over with the parmesan cheese. Serve.

NUTRITIONS

- Calories: 179
- Fat: 8.5g
- Carbohydrates: 8.5g
- Protein: 19.3g

140. SPICY TURKEY AND CAULIFLOWER

PREPARATION	COOKING	SERVES
10 MIN	20 MIN	4

INGREDIENTS

- 1 tbsp Roasted garlic oil (or another oil, with fresh garlic)
- 1 ½ pound Boneless turkey meat, skinless and cut into thin slices
- 1 tbsp Curry powder
- 4 cups Cauliflower florets
- 1 ½ cup Light coconut milk
- Ground pepper and natural sea salt - to taste

DIRECTIONS

1. Slice the turkey and set it aside. Chop the cauliflower into ½-inch florets. Add the garlic oil to your pan and heat on high.
2. Once the oil gets heated, add the turkey and sprinkle it over with curry. Stir thoroughly and cook for about 10 minutes.
3. Add the coconut milk and cauliflower. Cook until the turkey is fully cooked with cauliflower tender, about 10 minutes. Season with pepper and salt. Serve.

NUTRITIONS

- *Calories: 231*
- *Fat: 5.4g*
- *Carbohydrates: 6.3g*
- *Protein: 38g*

141. SPINACH-CHICKEN NOODLES

PREPARATION	COOKING	SERVES
15 MIN	15 MIN	3

INGREDIENTS

- 1 ½ lb. boneless chicken breasts, skinless
- 1 tbsp olive oil
- 1 cup plain Greek yogurt (low-fat)
- ½ cup chicken broth
- ½ tsp garlic powder
- ½ tsp Italian seasoning
- ¼ cup parmesan cheese
- 1 cup spinach, chopped
- 3-6 slices sun-dried tomatoes
- 1 tbsp garlic, chopped
- 1 ½ cup zucchini noodles

DIRECTIONS

1. For the chicken, heat-up oil over medium heat with your pan. Pat-dry the chicken breasts using a paper towel, and season with pepper and chicken.
2. Place in the pan and cook each side for about 5 minutes, or until it turns brown. Transfer the chicken from the pan to your plate.
3. Add the broth, yogurt, Italian seasoning, garlic powder, and parmesan cheese to the pan. Whisk and cook until it becomes slightly thick.
4. Add the tomatoes and spinach, and simmer until the spinach becomes wilted. Return the chicken and toss to coat well, then serve over the zoodles.
5. For the zoodles, preheat your oven to 350 degrees. Cut the zucchini into tiny spirals—place parchment paper on a baking sheet.
6. Spread the zucchini noodles on the sheet. Sprinkle sea salt and toss. Bake the zoodles for about 15 minutes or more, depending on how soft you want it. Serve.

NUTRITIONS

- *Calories: 414*
- *Fat: 15g*
- *Carbohydrates: 8g*
- *Protein: 60g*

142. DIJON CHICKEN VEGGIES

PREPARATION	COOKING	SERVES
5 MIN	25 MIN	4

INGREDIENTS

- 1 ½ pounds boneless chicken thighs (skinless)
- 1 tbsp Tuscan seasoning
- 4 tbsp balsamic
- 1 tbsp Dijon mustard
- 2 cups cherry/grape tomatoes (halved)
- 2 cups zucchini (sliced into 3/8-inch slices)
- 1/3 cup water

DIRECTIONS

1. Add the mustard, balsamic, and seasoning to a bowl and whisk together. Put the chicken in your bowl, then toss thoroughly.
2. Put it in your refrigerator to marinade, about 20 min to 8 hours. Preheat your oven to 425, then place your cast-iron skillet over medium-high heat.
3. Shake off any excess marinade and place the chicken in the skillet. Cook for about 5 min, or until seared. Do the same for the other side of the chicken.
4. Meanwhile, prepare the veggies. Add water to the marinade that remains in the bowl and whisk thoroughly to combine well.
5. Sprinkle the veggies around the skillet and season with a pinch of salt and pepper. Pour the marinade on the veggies and toss to combine everything.
6. Transfer to the oven and cook for extra 15 minutes. Remove from heat and serve.

NUTRITIONS

- Calories: 280
- Fat: 9.9g
- Carbohydrates: 7.5g
- Protein: 38.7g

143. SESAME GINGER CHICKEN

PREPARATION	COOKING	SERVES
10 MIN	15 MIN	4

INGREDIENTS

- 4 tsp Orange oil
- 1 ½ lb. Boneless chicken breast (skinless)
- 1 tbsp Toasted sesame ginger seasoning

DIRECTIONS

1. Put the chicken breast on a cutting board and flatten it to 3/8-inch-thick with your meat mallet. Sprinkle over with seasoning.
2. Add the orange oil to a nonstick pan and heat over medium-high heat. Add the chicken and cook each side for about 8 minutes, or until the chick is well cooked. Serve.

NUTRITIONS

- Calories: 247
- Fat: 9.9g
- Carbohydrates: 0.5g
- Protein: 36.5g

144. CREAMY GARLIC SAUCE TURKEY

PREPARATION	COOKING	SERVES
15 MIN	28 MIN	4

INGREDIENTS

- 1 ½ lb. Boneless turkey meat, skinless and cut into thin slices
- 2 tbsp Roasted garlic oil
- 1 medium onion, diced
- 1 tbsp Garlic and spring onion seasoning
- ½ cup Vegetable broth
- 1-2 tbsp Grass-fed butter

DIRECTIONS

1. Put the oil in your pan, then heat over medium-high heat. Add the onions to the pan and cook for 2 minutes. Add the turkey and cook for about 5 minutes. Stir occasionally.
2. Add the seasoning and cook for extra 20 minutes, or until the turkey is fully cooked. Add the broth and simmer for 1 more minute. Serve.

NUTRITIONS

- *Calories: 441*
- *Carbs: 6g*
- *Fat: 46g*
- *Protein: 3g*

145. TOMATO ROTISSERIE

PREPARATION	COOKING	SERVES
15 MIN	4 MIN	3

INGREDIENTS

- 3 lb. Rotisserie chicken
- 15 Petite tomatoes, diced
- 9 Tortillas
- 1 cup shredded cheese
- ½ cup Plain Greek yogurt
- 1 Avocado
- 1 Lime

DIRECTIONS

1. Shred your chicken, then put it in a microwave-safe bowl. Add tomatoes and the seasoning to the bowl and mix.
2. Microwave for 4 minutes on high. Fill the tortillas with the chicken. Top with the remaining ingredients and spritz of lime.

NUTRITIONS

- *Calories: 170*
- *Carbs: 1g*
- *Fat: 11g*
- *Protein: 15g*

146. BALSAMIC STRAWBERRY CHICKEN

PREPARATION	COOKING	SERVES
15 MIN	20 MIN	4

INGREDIENTS

- 1 ½ lb. boneless chicken breast, skinless
- 1 tbsp seasoning
- 1 cup fresh strawberries
- 1 tbsp balsamic mosto Cotto
- ½ tsp peppercorn
- 1 pinch sea salt
- 4 tbsp lemon oil

DIRECTIONS

1. Preheat your grill to medium-high heat. Season, the chicken with the seasoning. Place on the grill and cook each side for about 10 minutes. Remove from heat and set it aside.
2. For the dressing, add other ingredients to your food processor and puree until the mixture becomes smooth. Slice the chicken diagonally and drizzle the dressing over it. Serve.

NUTRITIONS

- Calories: 367
- Carbs: 17g
- Fat: 11g
- Protein: 45g

147. CAULIFLOWER TOMATO SHAKSHUKA

PREPARATION	COOKING	SERVES
5 MIN	20 MIN	2

INGREDIENTS

- 1-pound Riced cauliflower
- 4 tsp extra virgin olive oil
- 4 tbsp Chopped onion
- 1 tbsp India seasoning
- 1 can diced tomatoes (with no added sugar)
- 1 can Pureed tomatoes (with no added sugar)
- 4 Fresh eggs

DIRECTIONS

1. Cook the cauliflower following the instructions on the package. Put the oil in your skillet and heat it over medium-high heat.
2. Stir in the onions and sauté for about 2 minutes, or until the onions become translucent. Sprinkle over the mixture with the spices and sauté for an extra 1 minute.
3. Now add the cooked cauliflower to the skillet and stir thoroughly. Add a pinch of natural salt. (optional)
4. Stir in the tomatoes and mix thoroughly. Boil the mixture in your skillet. Then simmer for an additional 5 minutes.
5. Open the pot and crack the eggs over the mixture—season with pepper and salt. Close the skillet and cook for 3 minutes to poach the egg. You can cook for about 6-7 for a hard-cooked egg. Turn off heat and serve.

NUTRITIONS

- Calories: 228
- Fat: 14.5g
- Carbohydrates: 10.3g
- Protein: 15.3g

148. TURKEY SHRIMP

PREPARATION	COOKING	SERVES
15 MIN	30 MIN	4

INGREDIENTS

- 2 tbsp roasted garlic oil
- 1 medium onion, diced
- 1 tbsp garlic gusto seasoning
- 1 lb. boneless turkey meat, skinless and cut into thin slices
- ½ lb. medium-size shrimp, precooked, peeled, with tails removed
- 3 scallions, chopped
- ¾ cup frank's red-hot seasoning
- lemon juice - splash

DIRECTIONS

1. Put the oil in your skillet and heat over medium-high heat. Add the onion and sauté until it becomes translucent, about 2 minutes.
2. Add the turkey and cook for about 10 minutes. Stir occasionally. Add the garlic seasoning and cook until the turkey is fully cooked about 12 minutes.
3. Add other ingredients and cook for about 5 minutes, or until the sauce begins to bubble. Serve.

NUTRITIONS

- Calories: 361
- Carbs: 0g
- Fat: 8g
- Protein: 22g

149. BROCCOLI CHICKEN THIGHS

PREPARATION	COOKING	SERVES
5 MIN	20 MIN	4

INGREDIENTS

- 4 boneless chicken thighs, skinless
- 2 tsp seasoning, or use a mixture of garlic, salt, onion, pepper, and parsley
- 4 tbsp balsamic mosto cotto or use a balsamic reduction
- ¼ cup chicken broth, low sodium
- 4 cups steamed broccoli florets, crisp-tender

DIRECTIONS

1. Season the chicken thighs. Grease your pan with nonstick cooking spray. Place over high heat. Once it starts to shimmer, add the chicken.
2. Reduce the heat to medium and cook each side for about 7 min, or until it is well cooked. Remove the chicken and set it aside.
3. Add the broth and balsamic to the pan. Scrape all brown bits at the bottom of the pan. Once the sauce reduces by half, add the broccoli and chicken back to the pan. Toss to coat thoroughly. Serve immediately.

NUTRITIONS

- Calories: 314
- Fat: 10.8g
- Carbohydrates: 8.8g
- Protein: 43.6g

150. BELL PEPPER CASHEW CHICKEN

PREPARATION	COOKING	SERVES
10 MIN	20 MIN	4

INGREDIENTS

- 4 tsp lemon or roasted garlic oil or any other oil of choice
- 1 ½ lb. boneless chicken breast, skinless and sliced into thin strips
- 1 tbsp. Thai seasoning
- 2 cups of green bell pepper, thin strips
- 2 cups of red bell pepper, thin strips
- 3 scallions, sliced - put the greens and whites separate
- 24 cashews, chopped

DIRECTIONS

1. Over medium-high heat, heat the oil with your pan. Put the chicken strips to the pan and cook each side for about 5 min, or until it turns opaque.
2. Add the white scallions and peppers to the pan. Sprinkle seasoning over the mixture and stir thoroughly to combine.
3. Close the lid and cook for an extra 7 min over high heat until the chicken is well cooked. Stir occasionally.
4. Remove and sprinkle the scallion greens and nuts over. Serve hot. It can be served over riced cauliflower.

NUTRITIONS

- Calories: 323
- Fat: 13.1g
- Carbohydrates: 12.3g
- Protein: 38.7g

151. TOMATO PUTTANESCA

PREPARATION	COOKING	SERVES
15 MIN	0 MIN	4

INGREDIENTS

- 4 tsp roasted garlic oil
- 1 ½ lb. boneless turkey meat, skinless and cut into thin slices
- 1 cup diced tomatoes
- 1 tsp Italian seasoning
- 1 tbsp garlic & spring onion seasoning
- 2 cups bell pepper, sliced
- 2 tbsp capers, drained

DIRECTIONS

1. Heat the oil in your pan until it starts to sizzle. Add the turkey and cook for about 5 minutes. Add other ingredients and reduce the heat to medium. Close the pan and sauté for 12 minutes or until the turkey is fully cooked. Serve.

NUTRITIONS

- *Calories: 70*
- *Carbs: 8g*
- *Fat: 3g*
- *Protein: 2g*

152. HERBED LEMON CHICKEN

PREPARATION	COOKING	SERVES
10 MIN	30 MIN	4

INGREDIENTS

- 1 ½ lb. Boneless chicken breasts, skinless
- 4 tsp Lemon oil or use oil with lemon juice and zest
- 1 tbsp Seasoning or use salt and pepper
- 2-3 tbsp Herbs (fresh chopped tarragon, parsley, rosemary, thyme, chives, etc., or combo)

DIRECTIONS

1. Preheat your grill to 350. Toss all the fixings in a bowl. Grill each side of the chicken within 9-11 minutes, or until the chicken is well cooked. Serve.

NUTRITIONS

- Calories: 234
- Fat: 8.8g
- Carbohydrates: 0g
- Protein: 36.1g

153. PHOENIX CHICKEN SOUP

PREPARATION	COOKING	SERVES
15 MIN	20 MIN	6

INGREDIENTS

- 4 tsp roasted garlic oil
- 1 ½ lb. boneless chicken breasts (skinless, sliced into thin strips)
- 4 minced scallions whites, and chopped greens
- 1 tbsp phoenix sunrise seasoning
- 1 tbsp garlic gusto seasoning
- 8 cups chicken broth
- ½ cup Roma or grape tomatoes, chopped
- 1/3 cup fresh chopped cilantro
- 1 lime, juiced
- 1 medium avocado, diced

DIRECTIONS

1. Put the oil in a pot and heat over medium-high heat. Add the scallions and chicken. Sauté for about 2 minutes. Add the broth, seasonings, and tomatoes. Stir and bring to a boil.
2. Lower the heat to medium. Simmer for about 15 minutes. Meanwhile, prepare the lime, cilantro, and avocado.
3. Add the lime juice and cilantro to the pot and stir. Add the avocado to the serving bowls. Scoop the soup onto the avocado and serve.

NUTRITIONS

- Calories: 423
- Carbs: 58g
- Fat: 15g
- Protein: 12g

154. BELL PEPPER TURKEY SONOMA

PREPARATION	COOKING	SERVES
15 MIN	30 MIN	4

INGREDIENTS

- 4 tsp roasted garlic oil or used any oil of your choice
- 1 cup scallions
- 1 cup red bell pepper, sliced thin
- 1 cup yellow bell pepper, sliced thin
- 20 oz boneless turkey meat, skinless and cut into thin slices
- 1 tbsp phoenix sunrise seasoning

DIRECTIONS

1. Heat the oil over medium-high heat with your pan. Add the scallions and cook for about 5 minutes. Add pepper and stir. Cook for 7 minutes.
2. Once done, transfer to your dish and keep it warm. Return the pan and add the sliced turkey. Sprinkle the seasoning over and cook for about 15-20 minutes. Stir often. Once the turkey is well cooked, add the pepper and stir well. Serve.

NUTRITIONS

- *Calories: 425*
- *Carbs: 31g*
- *Fat: 12g*
- *Protein: 25g*

155. GRILLED CHICKEN

PREPARATION	COOKING	SERVES
15 MIN	0 MIN	3

INGREDIENTS

- 2 lb. boneless chicken breasts, skinless
- 1 ½ tbsp flavor quake seasoning
- 4 tsp roasted garlic oil

DIRECTIONS

1. Season the chicken in a bowl and allow it to sit for about 15 minutes or more in your refrigerator. Preheat your grill to 325 degrees.
2. Put the chicken on the preheated grill, cook each side for about 5 minutes, or until the chicken is fully cooked. Remove and let it cool, then serve.

NUTRITIONS

- *Calories: 110*
- *Carbs: 0g*
- *Fat: 3g*
- *Protein: 22g*

156. CREAMY CHICKEN ASPARAGUS

PREPARATION	COOKING	SERVES
10 MIN	15 MIN	4

INGREDIENTS

- 4 tsp Roasted garlic oil
- 1 ¾ lb. Boneless chicken breast, skinless, and chopped into 1-inch chunks
- ½ cup Chicken broth, low sodium
- 1 tbsp Garlic Gusto seasoning
- 8 tbsp Light cream cheese
- 4 cups fresh asparagus, chopped into 2-inch pieces
- Seasoning (salt, garlic, and pepper)

DIRECTIONS

1. Put the oil in your pan and heat it over medium-high heat. Stir in the chicken breast and cook for about 10 min, or until the chicken becomes slightly brown. Stir occasionally.
2. Put the chicken broth in the pan and scrape all the brown bits from the pan's bottom. Add the garlic seasoning, asparagus, and cream cheese.
3. Adjust to high and cook until the cream cheese completely melts. Stir frequently. Bring mixture to a boil.
4. Simmer until the sauce becomes thick. Equally, divide into 4 portions and sprinkle over with the seasoning. Serve hot.

NUTRITIONS

- Calories: 302
- Fat: 12.8g
- Carbohydrates: 7.1g
- Protein: 39g

157. TACO TOMATO SEASONED TURKEY

PREPARATION	COOKING	SERVES
5 MIN	10 MIN	4

INGREDIENTS

- 1 ½ pound Boneless turkey meat, skinless and cut into thin slices
- 1 tbsp Low salt tex-mex seasoning
- ½ cup Fresh tomatoes, chopped
- 1 tsp Seasoning (optional)
- Favorite taco condiments

DIRECTIONS

1. In a single layer, place the turkey in the bottom of your pot. Sprinkle the seasonings over the turkey. Spread the tomatoes over the turkey.
2. Cook on high for 10 minutes. Remove the chicken and shred it with your forks. Pour the sauce over and serve.

NUTRITIONS

- Calories: 198
- Fat: 4.3g
- Carbohydrates: 0.9g
- Protein: 36.3g

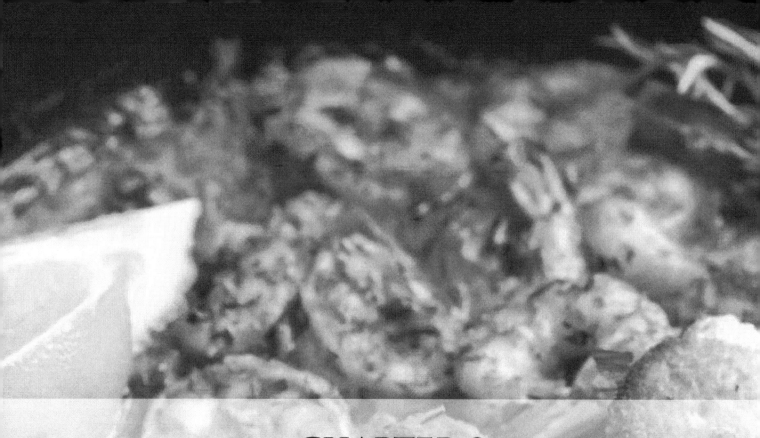

CHAPTER 9:
SEAFOOD RECIPES

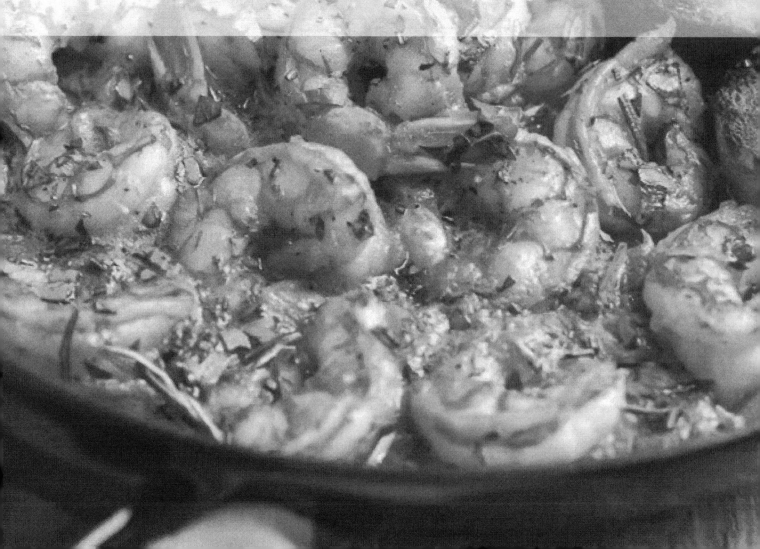

158. SHRIMP WITH GARLIC

PREPARATION	COOKING	SERVES
10 MIN	25 MIN	2

INGREDIENTS

- 1 lb. shrimp
- ¼ teaspoon baking soda
- 2 tablespoons oil
- 2 teaspoon minced garlic
- ¼ cup vermouth
- 2 tablespoons unsalted butter
- 1 teaspoon parsley

DIRECTIONS

1. In a bowl, toss shrimp with baking soda and salt, let it stand for a couple of minutes. In a skillet, heat olive oil and add shrimp
2. Add garlic, red pepper flakes and cook for 1-2 minutes. Add vermouth and cook within 4-5 minutes. When ready, remove from heat and serve

NUTRITIONS

- *Calories: 289*
- *Carbohydrate: 2 g*
- *Fat: 17 g*
- *Protein: 7 g*

159. SABICH SANDWICH

PREPARATION	COOKING	SERVES
5 MIN	15 MIN	2

INGREDIENTS

- 2 tomatoes
- Olive oil
- ½ lb. eggplant
- ¼ cucumber
- 1 tablespoon lemon
- 1 tablespoon parsley
- ¼ head cabbage
- 2 tablespoons wine vinegar
- 2 pita bread
- ½ cup hummus
- ¼ tahini sauce

- 2 hard-boiled eggs

DIRECTIONS

1. In a skillet, fry eggplant slices until tender. In a bowl, add tomatoes, cucumber, parsley, lemon juice, and season salad.
2. In another bowl, toss cabbage with vinegar. In each pita pocket, add hummus, eggplant, and drizzle tahini sauce. Top with eggs and tahini sauce. Serve.

NUTRITIONS

- *Calories: 269*
- *Carbohydrate: 2 g*
- *Fat: 14 g*
- *Protein: 7 g*

160. SALMON WITH VEGETABLES

PREPARATION	COOKING	SERVES
10 MIN	15 MIN	4

INGREDIENTS

- 2 tablespoons olive oil
- 2 carrots
- 1 head fennel
- 2 squash
- ¼ onion
- 1-inch ginger
- 1 cup white wine
- 2 cups of water
- 2 parsley sprigs
- 2 tarragon sprigs
- 6 oz. salmon fillets
- 1 cup cherry tomatoes
- 1 scallion

DIRECTIONS

1. In a skillet, heat olive oil, add fennel, squash, onion, ginger, carrot, and cook until vegetables are soft. Add wine, water, parsley and cook for another 4-5 minutes
2. Season salmon fillets and place them in the pan. Cook within 5 minutes per side or until it is ready. Transfer salmon to a bowl, spoon tomatoes and scallion around salmon and serve.

NUTRITIONS

- *Calories: 301*
- *Carbohydrate: 2 g*
- *Fat: 17 g*
- *Protein: 8 g*

161. CRISPY FISH

PREPARATION	COOKING	SERVES
5 MIN	15 MIN	4

INGREDIENTS

- Thick fish fillets
- ¼ cup all-purpose flour
- 1 egg
- 1 cup bread crumbs
- 2 tablespoons vegetables
- Lemon wedge

DIRECTIONS

1. In a dish, add flour, egg, breadcrumbs in different dishes and set aside. Dip each fish fillet into the flour, egg, and then bread crumbs bowl.
2. Place each fish fillet in a heated skillet and cook for 4-5 minutes per side. Serve with lemon wedges.

NUTRITIONS

- *Calories: 189*
- *Carbohydrate: 2 g*
- *Fat: 17 g*
- *Protein: 7 g*

162. MOULES MARINIERES

PREPARATION	COOKING	SERVES
10 MIN	30 MIN	4

INGREDIENTS

- 2 tablespoons unsalted butter
- 1 leek
- 1 shallot
- 2 cloves garlic
- 2 bay leaves
- 1 cup white wine
- 2 lb. mussels
- 2 tablespoons mayonnaise
- 1 tablespoon lemon zest
- 2 tablespoons parsley
- 1 sourdough bread

DIRECTIONS

1. In a saucepan, melt butter, add leeks, garlic, bay leaves, shallot, and cook until vegetables are soft. Boil, add mussels and cook for 1-2 minutes.
2. Transfer mussels to a bowl and cover. Whisk in remaining butter with mayonnaise and return mussels to the pot. Add lemon juice, parsley lemon zest, and stir to combine.

NUTRITIONS

- Calories: 321
- Carbohydrate: 2 g
- Fat: 17 g
- Protein: 9 g

163. STEAMED MUSSELS WITH COCONUT-CURRY

PREPARATION	COOKING	SERVES
15 MIN	20 MIN	4

INGREDIENTS

- 6 sprigs cilantro
- 2 cloves garlic
- 2 shallots
- ¼ teaspoon coriander seeds
- ¼ teaspoon red chili flakes
- 1 teaspoon zest
- 1 can coconut milk
- 1 tablespoon vegetable oil
- 1 tablespoon curry paste
- 1 tablespoon brown sugar
- 1 tablespoon fish sauce

- 2 lb. mussels

DIRECTIONS

1. In a bowl, combine lime zest, cilantro stems, shallot, garlic, coriander seed, chili, and salt. In a saucepan, heat oil adds garlic, shallots, pounded paste, and curry paste.
2. Cook for 3-4 minutes; add coconut milk, sugar, and fish sauce. Bring to a simmer and add mussels. Stir in lime juice, cilantro leaves and cook for a couple of more minutes. When ready, remove from heat and serve.

NUTRITIONS

- *Calories: 209*
- *Carbohydrate: 6 g*
- *Fat: 7 g*
- *Protein: 17 g*

164. TUNA NOODLE CASSEROLE

PREPARATION	COOKING	SERVES
15 MIN	20 MIN	4

INGREDIENTS

- 2 oz. egg noodles
- 4 oz. fraiche
- 1 egg
- 1 teaspoon cornstarch
- 1 tablespoon juice from 1 lemon
- 1 can tuna
- 1 cup peas
- ¼ cup parsley

DIRECTIONS

1. Place noodles in a saucepan with water and bring to a boil. In a bowl, combine egg, crème Fraiche and lemon juice; whisk well.
2. When noodles are cooked, add crème Fraiche mixture to the skillet and mix well. Add tuna, peas, parsley lemon juice and mix well. When ready, remove from heat and serve.

NUTRITIONS

- *Calories: 214*
- *Carbohydrate: 2 g*
- *Fat: 7 g*
- *Protein: 19 g*

165. SEARED SCALLOPS

PREPARATION	COOKING	SERVES
15 MIN	20 MIN	4

INGREDIENTS

- 1 lb. sea scallops
- 1 tablespoon canola oil

DIRECTIONS

1. Season scallops and refrigerates for a couple of minutes. In a skillet, heat oil, add scallops, and cook for 1-2 minutes per side. When ready, remove from heat and serve.

NUTRITIONS

- Calories: 283
- Carbohydrate: 10 g
- Fat: 8 g
- Protein: 9 g

166. BLACK COD

PREPARATION	COOKING	SERVES
15 MIN	20 MIN	4

INGREDIENTS

- ¼ cup miso paste
- ¼ cup sake
- 1 tablespoon mirin
- 1 teaspoon soy sauce
- 1 tablespoon olive oil
- 4 black cod fillets

DIRECTIONS

1. In a bowl, combine miso, soy sauce, oil, and sake. Rub mixture over cod fillets and let it marinate for 20-30 minutes. Adjust broiler and broil cod filets for 10-12 minutes. When fish is cook, remove, and serve.

NUTRITIONS

- *Calories: 231*
- *Carbohydrate: 2 g*
- *Fat: 15 g*
- *Protein: 8 g*

167. MISO-GLAZED SALMON

PREPARATION	COOKING	SERVES
10 MIN	40 MIN	4

INGREDIENTS

- ¼ cup red miso
- ¼ cup sake
- 1 tablespoon soy sauce
- 1 tablespoon vegetable oil
- 4 salmon fillets

DIRECTIONS

1. In a bowl, combine sake, oil, soy sauce, and miso. Rub mixture over salmon fillets and marinate for 20-30 minutes. Preheat a broiler. Broil salmon for 5-10 minutes. When ready, remove, and serve.

NUTRITIONS

- *Calories: 198*
- *Carbohydrate: 5 g*
- *Fat: 10 g*
- *Protein: 6 g*

168. ARUGULA AND SWEET POTATO SALAD

PREPARATION	COOKING	SERVES
10 MIN	20 MIN	4

INGREDIENTS

- 1 lb. sweet potatoes
- 1 cup walnuts
- 1 tablespoon olive oil
- 1 cup of water
- 1 tablespoon soy sauce
- 3 cups arugula

DIRECTIONS

1. Bake potatoes at 400 F until tender, remove and set aside. In a bowl, drizzle walnuts with olive oil and microwave for 2-3 minutes or until toasted. In a bowl, mix all salad fixings and mix well. Pour over the soy sauce and serve.

NUTRITIONS

- *Calories: 189*
- *Carbohydrate: 2 g*
- *Fat: 7 g*
- *Protein: 10 g*

169. NICOISE SALAD

PREPARATION	COOKING	SERVES
15 MIN	10 MIN	4

INGREDIENTS

- 1 oz. red potatoes
- 1 package of green beans
- 2 eggs
- ½ cup tomatoes
- 2 tablespoons wine vinegar
- ¼ teaspoon salt
- ½ teaspoon pepper
- ½ teaspoon thyme
- ¼ cup olive oil
- 6 oz. tuna
- ¼ cup Kalamata olives

DIRECTIONS

1. In a bowl, combine all ingredients. Add salad dressing and serve.

NUTRITIONS

- *Calories: 189*
- *Carbohydrate: 2 g*
- *Fat: 7 g*
- *Protein: 15 g*

170. SHRIMP CURRY

PREPARATION	COOKING	SERVES
15 MIN	20 MIN	4

INGREDIENTS

- 2 tablespoons peanut oil
- ¼ onion
- 2 cloves garlic
- 1 teaspoon ginger
- 1 teaspoon cumin
- 1 teaspoon turmeric
- 1 teaspoon paprika
- ¼ red chili powder
- 1 can tomatoes
- 1 can coconut milk
- 1 lb. peeled shrimp

- 1 tablespoon cilantro

DIRECTIONS

1. In a skillet, add onion and cook for 4-5 minutes. Add ginger, cumin, garlic, chili, paprika and cook on low heat. Pour the tomatoes, coconut milk, and simmer for 10-12 minutes.
2. Stir in shrimp, cilantro, and cook for 2-3 minutes. When ready, remove, and serve.

NUTRITIONS

- Calories: 178
- Carbohydrate: 3 g
- Fat: 17 g
- Protein: 9 g

171. SALMON PASTA

PREPARATION	COOKING	SERVES
10 MIN	25 MIN	2

INGREDIENTS

- 5 tablespoons butter
- ¼ onion
- 1 tablespoon all-purpose flour
- 1 teaspoon garlic powder
- 2 cups skim milk
- ¼ cup Romano cheese
- 1 cup green peas
- ¼ cup canned mushrooms
- 8 oz. salmon
- 1 package penne pasta

DIRECTIONS

1. Bring a pot with water to a boil. Add pasta and cook for 10-12 minutes. In a skillet, melt butter, add onion and sauté until tender. Stir in garlic powder, flour, milk, and cheese.
2. Add mushrooms, peas and cook on low heat for 4-5 minutes. Toss in salmon and cook for another 2-3 minutes when ready, serve with cooked pasta.

NUTRITIONS

- *Calories: 211*
- *Carbohydrate: 7 g*
- *Fat: 18 g*
- *Protein: 17 g*

172. CRAB LEGS

PREPARATION	COOKING	SERVES
5 MIN	20 MIN	3

INGREDIENTS

- 3 lb. crab legs
- ¼ cup salted butter, melted and divided
- ½ lemon, juiced
- ¼ tsp. garlic powder

DIRECTIONS

1. In a bowl, toss the crab legs and two tablespoons of the melted butter together. Place the crab legs in the basket of the fryer.
2. Cook at 400 F for fifteen minutes, giving the basket a shake halfway through. Combine the remaining butter with the lemon juice and garlic powder.
3. Crack open the cooked crab legs and remove the meat. Serve with the butter dip on the side, and enjoy!

NUTRITIONS

- Calories: 392
- Fat: 10g
- Protein: 18g
- Carbs: 8g

173. CRUSTY PESTO SALMON

PREPARATION	COOKING	SERVES
5 MIN	15 MIN	2

INGREDIENTS

- ¼ cup s, roughly chopped
- ¼ cup pesto
- 2 x 4-oz. salmon fillets
- 2 tbsp. unsalted butter, melted

DIRECTIONS

1. Mix the s and pesto. Place the salmon fillets in a round baking dish, roughly six inches in diameter.
2. Brush the fillets with butter, followed by the pesto mixture, ensuring to coat both the top and bottom. Put the baking dish inside the fryer. Cook for 12 minutes at 390 F. Serves warm.

NUTRITIONS

- Calories: 290
- Fat: 11g
- Protein: 20g
- Carbs: 9g

174. BUTTERY COD

PREPARATION	COOKING	SERVES
10 MIN	12 MIN	2

INGREDIENTS

- 2 x 4-oz. cod fillets
- 2 tbsp. salted butter, melted
- 1 tsp. Old Bay seasoning
- ½ medium lemon, sliced

DIRECTIONS

1. Place the cod fillets in a skillet. Brush with melted butter, season with Old Bay, and top with a few lemon wedges.
2. Cover the fish in aluminum foil, then place it in your deep fryer. Cook for eight minutes at 350 F. The cod is done when it is easily peeled. Serve hot

NUTRITIONS

- *Calories: 394*
- *Fat: 5g*
- *Protein: 12g*
- *Carbs: 4g*

175. SESAME TUNA STEAK

PREPARATION	COOKING	SERVES
5 MIN	12 MIN	2

INGREDIENTS

- 1 tbsp. coconut oil, melted
- 2 x 6-oz. tuna steaks
- ½ tsp. garlic powder
- 2 tsp. black sesame seeds
- 2 tsp. white sesame seeds

DIRECTIONS

1. Apply the coconut oil to the tuna steaks with a brunch, then season with garlic powder. Combine the black and white sesame seeds. Embed them in the tuna steaks, covering the fish all over.
2. Place the tuna into your air fryer. Cook within 8 minutes at 400 F, turning the fish halfway through. The tuna steaks are ready when they have reached a temperature of 145 F. Serve straightaway.

NUTRITIONS

- *Calories: 160*
- *Fat: 6g*
- *Protein: 26g*
- *Carbs: 7g*

176. LEMON GARLIC SHRIMP

PREPARATION	COOKING	SERVES
10 MIN	15 MIN	2

INGREDIENTS

- 1 medium lemon, zest & juice
- ½ lb. medium shrimp, shelled and deveined
- ½ tsp. Old Bay seasoning
- 2 tbsp unsalted butter, melted
- ½ tsp. minced garlic

DIRECTIONS

1. Put the grated zest and juice lemon over the same bowl. Toss in the shrimp, Old Bay, and butter, mixing everything to make sure the shrimp is completely covered.
2. Transfer to a round baking dish roughly six inches wide, then place this dish in your fryer—Cook at 400 F for 6 minutes. Serve hot, drizzling any leftover sauce over the shrimp.

NUTRITIONS

- *Calories: 490*
- *Fat: 9g*
- *Protein: 12g*
- *Carbs: 11g*

177. FOIL PACKET SALMON

PREPARATION	COOKING	SERVES
5 MIN	15 MIN	2

INGREDIENTS

- 2 x 4-oz. skinless salmon fillets
- 2 tbsp unsalted butter, melted
- ½ tsp. garlic powder
- 1 medium lemon
- ½ tsp. dried dill

DIRECTIONS

1. Cut the sheets of aluminum foil into two squares measuring roughly 5" x 5". Lay each of the salmon fillets at the center of each piece.
2. Brush both fillets with a tablespoon of bullets and season with a quarter-teaspoon of garlic powder. Halve the lemon and grate the skin of one half over the fish.
3. Cut four half-slices of lemon, using two to top each fillet. Season each fillet with a quarter-teaspoon of dill.
4. Fold the tops and sides of the aluminum foil over the fish to create a kind of packet. Place each one in the fryer—Cook for 12 minutes at 400°F. Serve hot.

NUTRITIONS

- Calories: 240
- Fat: 13g
- Protein: 21g
- Carbs: 9g

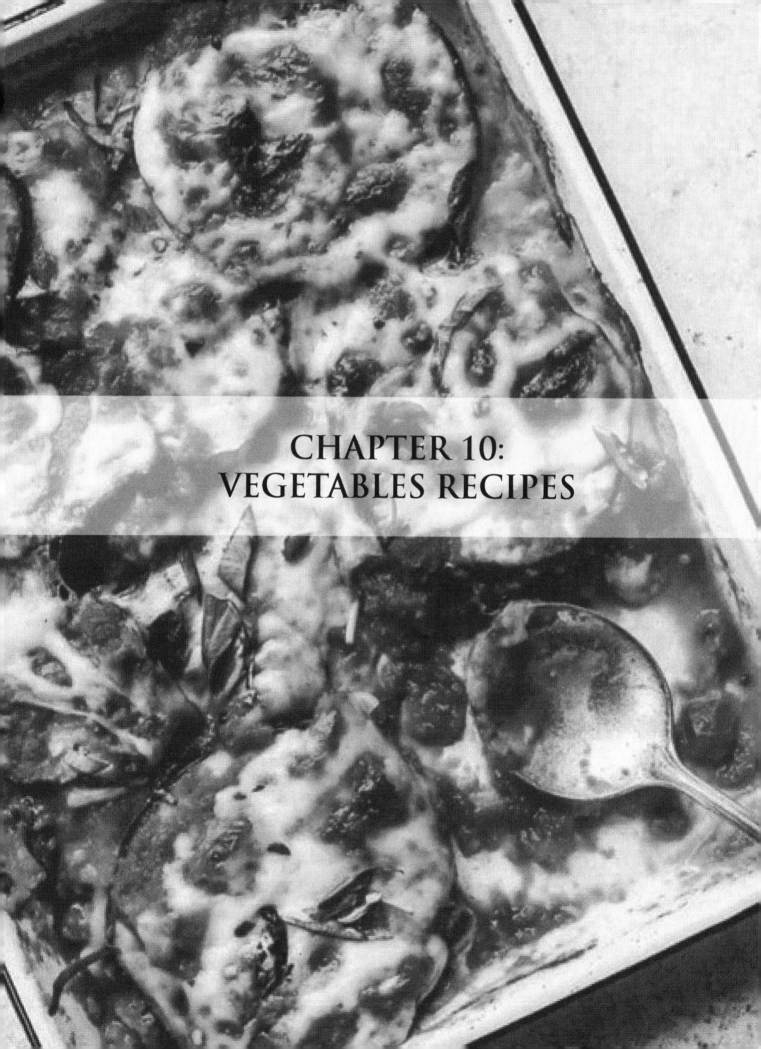

CHAPTER 10:
VEGETABLES RECIPES

178. BABY CORN IN CHILI-TURMERIC SPICE

PREPARATION	COOKING	SERVES
5 MIN	8 MIN	5

INGREDIENTS

- ¼ cup of water
- ¼ teaspoon baking soda
- ¼ teaspoon salt
- ¼ teaspoon turmeric powder
- ½ teaspoon curry powder
- ½ teaspoon red chili powder
- 1 cup chickpea flour or besan
- 10 pieces' baby corn, blanched

DIRECTIONS

1. Preheat the air fryer to 4000F. Position the air fryer basket with aluminum foil and brush with oil. In a mixing bowl, mix all ingredients except for the corn.
2. Whisk until well combined. Dip the corn in the batter and place it inside the air fryer. Cook for 8 minutes until golden brown.

NUTRITIONS

- *Calories: 89*
- *Carbohydrates: 14.35g*
- *Protein: 4.75g*
- *Fat: 1.54g*

179. BAKED CHEESY EGGPLANT WITH MARINARA

PREPARATION	COOKING	SERVES
20 MIN	45 MIN	3

INGREDIENTS

- 1 clove garlic, sliced
- 1 large eggplant
- 1 tablespoon olive oil
- 1 tablespoon olive oil
- 1/2 pinch salt, or as needed
- 1/4 cup & 2 tbsp bread crumbs
- 1/2 cup and 2 tablespoons ricotta cheese
- 1/4 cup grated Parmesan cheese
- 1/4 cup grated Parmesan cheese
- 1/4 cup water, + more as needed
- 1/4 teaspoon red pepper flakes
- 1-1/2 cups prepared marinara sauce
- 1-1/2 teaspoons olive oil
- 2 tablespoons shredded pepper jack cheese
- salt
- ground black pepper

DIRECTIONS

1. Cut the eggplant crosswise into 5 pieces. Peel a pumpkin, grate it and cut it into two cubes. Lightly turn skillet with 1 tbsp olive oil. Heat the oil at 390 ° F for 5 minutes. Add half of the aubergines and cook 2 minutes on each side. Transfer to a plate.
2. Add 1 tablespoon of olive oil and add garlic—Cook for one minute. Add the chopped aubergines—season with pepper flakes and salt.
3. Cook for 4 minutes. Lower the heat to 330oF and continue cooking the eggplants until soft, about 8 more minutes.
4. Stir in water and marinara sauce. Cook for 7 minutes until heated through. Stirring now and then. Transfer to a bowl.
5. In a bowl, whisk well pepper, salt, pepper jack cheese, Parmesan cheese, and ricotta. Evenly spread cheeses over eggplant strips and then fold in half.
6. Lay folded eggplant in baking pan. Pour the marinara sauce on top. Mix olive oil and breadcrumbs in a small bowl. Sprinkle all over the sauce.
7. Cook for 15 minutes at 390F until tops are lightly browned. Serve and enjoy.

NUTRITIONS

- Calories: 405
- Carbs: 41.1g
- Protein: 12.7g
- Fat: 21.4g

180. BAKED POLENTA WITH CHILI-CHEESE

PREPARATION	COOKING	SERVES
5 MIN	10 MIN	3

INGREDIENTS

- 1 commercial polenta roll, sliced
- 1 cup cheddar cheese sauce
- 1 tablespoon chili powder

DIRECTIONS

1. Place the baking dish accessory in the air fryer. Set the polenta slices in the baking dish. Add the chili powder and cheddar cheese sauce. Conceal the air fryer and cook for 10 minutes at 3900F. Serve.

NUTRITIONS

- Calories: 206
- Carbs: 25.3g
- Protein: 3.2g
- Fat: 4.2g

181. BAKED PORTOBELLO PASTA 'N CHEESE

PREPARATION	COOKING	SERVES
10 MIN	30 MIN	4

INGREDIENTS

- 1 cup milk
- 1 cup shredded mozzarella cheese
- 1 large clove garlic, minced
- 1 tablespoon vegetable oil
- 1/4 cup margarine
- 1/4 teaspoon dried basil
- 1/4-pound portobello mushrooms, thinly sliced
- 2 tablespoons all-purpose flour
- 2 tablespoons soy sauce
- 4-ounce penne pasta, cooked

according to manufacturer's Directions for Cooking
- 5-ounce frozen chopped spinach, thawed

DIRECTIONS

1. Lightly grease the baking pan of the air fryer with oil. For 2 minutes, heat on 360oF. Add mushrooms and cook for a minute. Transfer to a plate.
2. In the same pan, melt margarine for a minute. Stir in basil, garlic, and flour—Cook for 3 minutes. Stir and cook for another 2 minutes.
3. Stir in half of the milk slowly while whisking continuously. Cook for another 2 minutes. Mix well. Cook for another 2 minutes. Stir in remaining milk and cook for another 3 minutes.
4. Add cheese and mix well. Stir in soy sauce, spinach, mushrooms, and pasta. Mix well. Top with remaining cheese. Cook for 15 minutes at 390 F until tops are lightly browned. Serve and enjoy.

NUTRITIONS

- *Calories: 482*
- *Carbs: 32.1g*
- *Protein: 16.0g*
- *Fat: 32.1g*

182. BAKED POTATO TOPPED WITH CREAM CHEESE' N OLIVES

PREPARATION	COOKING	SERVES
15 MIN	40 MIN	1

INGREDIENTS

- ¼ teaspoon onion powder
- 1 medium russet potato, scrubbed and peeled
- 1 tablespoon chives, chopped
- 1 tablespoon Kalamata olives
- 1 teaspoon olive oil
- 1/8 teaspoon salt
- a dollop of vegan butter
- a dollop of vegan cream cheese

DIRECTIONS

1. Place inside the air fryer basket and cook for 40 minutes. Be sure to turn the potatoes once halfway. Position the potatoes in a mixing container and pour olive oil, onion powder, salt, and vegan butter.
2. Preheat the air fryer to 400 F. Serve the potatoes with vegan cream cheese, Kalamata olives, chives, and other vegan toppings that you want.

NUTRITIONS

- *Carbohydrates: 68.34g*
- *Calories: 504*
- *Protein: 9.31g*
- *Fat: 21.53g*

183. MEXICAN BAKED ZUCCHINI

PREPARATION	COOKING	SERVES
10 MIN	30 MIN	4

INGREDIENTS

- 1 tablespoon olive oil
- 1-1/2 pounds' zucchini, cubed
- 1/2 cup chopped onion
- 1/2 teaspoon garlic salt
- 1/2 teaspoon paprika
- 1/2 teaspoon dried oregano
- 1/2 teaspoon cayenne pepper, or to taste
- 1/2 cup cooked long-grain rice
- 1/2 cup cooked pinto beans
- 1-1/4 cups salsa
- 3/4 cup shredded Cheddar cheese

DIRECTIONS

1. Lightly grease the baking pan of the air fryer with olive oil. Add onions and zucchini and for 10 minutes, cook at 360 F. Halfway through cooking time, stir.
2. Season with cayenne, oregano, paprika, and garlic salt. Mix well. Stir in salsa, beans, and rice—Cook for 5 minutes. Stir in cheddar cheese and mix well.
3. Cover pan with foil. Cook for 15 minutes at 390 F until bubbly. Serve and enjoy.

NUTRITIONS

- *Calories: 263*
- *Carbs: 24.6g*
- *Protein: 12.5g*
- *Fat: 12.7g*

184. BANANA PEPPER STUFFED WITH TOFU' N SPICES

PREPARATION	COOKING	SERVES
5 MIN	10 MIN	8

INGREDIENTS

- ½ teaspoon red chili powder
- ½ teaspoon turmeric powder
- 1 onion, finely chopped
- 1 package firm tofu, crumbled
- 1 teaspoon coriander powder
- 3 tablespoons coconut oil
- 8 banana peppers, top-end sliced and seeded
- Salt to taste

DIRECTIONS

1. Preheat the air fryer for 5 minutes. In a mixing bowl, combine the tofu, onion, coconut oil, turmeric powder, red chili powder, coriander powder, and salt. Mix until well combined.
2. Scoop the tofu mixture into the hollows of the banana peppers. Place the stuffed peppers in the air fryer. Close and cook for 10 minutes at 3250F. Serve.

NUTRITIONS

- *Calories: 72*
- *Carbohydrates: 4.1g*
- *Protein: 1.2g*
- *Fat: 5.6g*

185. BELL PEPPER-CORN WRAPPED IN TORTILLA

PREPARATION	COOKING	SERVES
5 MIN	15 MIN	4

INGREDIENTS

- 1 small red bell pepper, chopped
- 1 small yellow onion, diced
- 1 tablespoon water
- 2 cobs grilled corn kernels
- 4 large tortillas
- 4 pieces' commercial vegan nuggets, chopped
- mixed greens for garnish

DIRECTIONS

1. Preheat the air fryer to 400F. In a skillet heated over medium heat, water sautés the vegan nuggets together with the onions, bell peppers, and corn kernels. Set aside.
2. Place filling inside the corn tortillas. Fold the tortillas and place them inside the air fryer and cook for 15 minutes until the tortilla wraps are crispy. Serve with mixed greens on top.

NUTRITIONS

- Calories: 548
- Carbohydrates: 43.54g
- Protein: 46.73g
- Fat: 20.76g

186. BLACK BEAN BURGER WITH GARLIC-CHIPOTLE

PREPARATION	COOKING	SERVES
10 MIN	20 MIN	3

INGREDIENTS

- ½ cup corn kernels
- ½ teaspoon chipotle powder
- ½ teaspoon garlic powder
- ¾ cup of salsa
- 1 ¼ teaspoon chili powder
- 1 ½ cup rolled oats
- 1 can black beans, rinsed and drained
- 1 tablespoon soy sauce

DIRECTIONS

1. In a mixing container, mix all components and mix using your hands. Form small patties using your hands and set aside. Brush patties with oil if desired.
2. Place the grill pan in the air fryer and place the patties on the grill pan accessory. Conceal the lid and cook for twenty minutes on each side at 330F.

NUTRITIONS

- Calories: 395
- Carbs: 52.2g
- Protein: 24.3g
- Fat: 5.8g

187. BROWN RICE, SPINACH 'N TOFU FRITTATA

PREPARATION	COOKING	SERVES
20 MIN	55 MIN	4

INGREDIENTS

- ½ cup baby spinach, chopped
- ½ cup kale, chopped
- ½ onion, chopped
- ½ teaspoon turmeric
- 1 ¾ cups brown rice, cooked
- 1 flax egg, 1 tbsp flaxseed meal plus 3 tablespoons cold water
- 1 package firm tofu
- 1 tablespoon olive oil
- 1 yellow pepper, chopped
- 2 tablespoons soy sauce

- 2 teaspoons arrowroot powder
- 2 teaspoons Dijon mustard
- 2/3 cup almond milk
- 3 big mushrooms, chopped
- 3 tablespoons nutritional yeast
- 4 cloves garlic, crushed
- 4 spring onions, chopped
- a handful of basil leaves, chopped

DIRECTIONS

1. Preheat the air fryer to 3750F. Grease your pan that will fit inside the air fryer. Prepare the frittata crust by mixing the brown rice and flax egg.
2. Press the rice onto the baking dish until you form a crust. Brush with a little oil and cook for 10 minutes. Meanwhile, heat olive oil in a skillet over medium flame and sauté the garlic and onions for 2 minutes.
3. Add the pepper and mushroom and continue stirring for 3 minutes. Stir in the kale, spinach, spring onions, and basil. Remove from the pan and set aside.
4. In a food processor, pulse the tofu, mustard, turmeric, soy sauce, nutritional yeast, vegan milk, and arrowroot powder. Pour in a mixing bowl and stir in the sautéed vegetables.
5. Pour the vegan frittata mixture over the rice crust and cook in the air fryer for 40 minutes.

NUTRITIONS

- *Calories: 226*
- *Carbohydrates: 30.44g*
- *Protein: 10.69g*
- *Fat: 8.05g*

188. BRUSSELS SPROUTS WITH BALSAMIC OIL

PREPARATION	COOKING	SERVES
5 MIN	15 MIN	4

INGREDIENTS

- ¼ teaspoon salt
- 1 tablespoon balsamic vinegar
- 2 cups Brussels sprouts, halved
- 2 tablespoons olive oil

DIRECTIONS

1. Preheat the air fryer for 5 minutes. Combine all components in a bowl until the zucchini fries are well coated. Place in the air fryer basket. Close and cook for 15 minutes at 350F. Serve.

NUTRITIONS

- *Calories: 82*
- *Carbohydrates: 4.6g*
- *Protein: 1.5g*
- *Fat: 6.8g*

189. BUTTERED CARROT-ZUCCHINI WITH MAYO

PREPARATION	COOKING	SERVES
15 MIN	25 MIN	4

INGREDIENTS

- 1 tablespoon grated onion
- 2 tablespoons butter, melted
- 1/2-pound carrots, sliced
- 1-1/2 zucchinis, sliced
- 1/4 cup water
- 1/4 cup mayonnaise
- 1/4 teaspoon prepared horseradish
- 1/4 teaspoon salt
- 1/4 teaspoon ground black pepper
- 1/4 cup Italian bread crumbs

DIRECTIONS

1. Lighten skillet with cooking spray. Add the carrots. Cook for 360 minutes at 360oF. Put the zucchini and continue cooking for another five minutes.
2. Meanwhile, in a bowl, whisk together the pepper, salt, horseradish, onion, mayonnaise, and water. Pour into a vegetable skillet. Pull well over the coat.
3. In a small container, mix the melted butter and breadcrumbs. Sprinkle over the vegetables. Cook for 10 minutes at 390 F until tops are lightly browned. Serve and enjoy.

NUTRITIONS

- Calories: 223
- Carbs: 13.8g
- Protein: 2.7g
- Fat: 17.4g

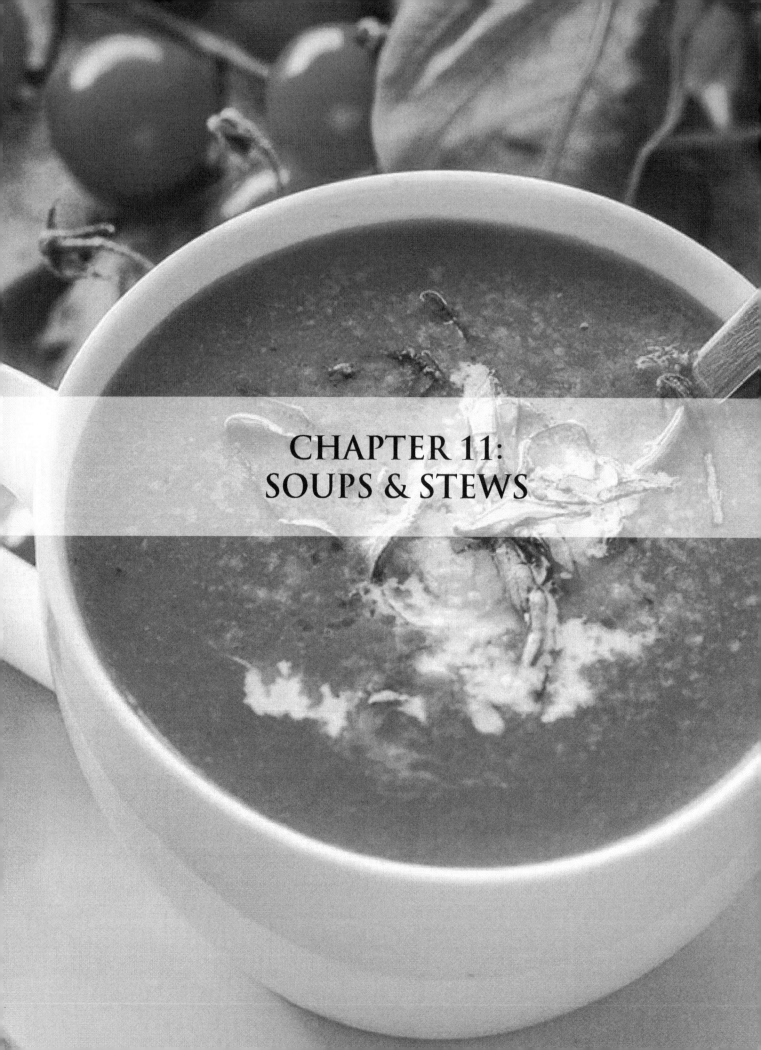

CHAPTER 11:
SOUPS & STEWS

190. ROASTED TOMATO SOUP

PREPARATION	COOKING	SERVES
20 MIN	50 MIN	6

INGREDIENTS

- 3 pounds of tomatoes in a halved manner
- 6 garlic(smashed)
- 2 onions (cut)
- 4 teaspoons of cooking oil or virgin oil
- Salt to taste
- Freshly ground pepper
- 1/4 cup of heavy cream(optional)
- Sliced fresh basil leaves for garnish

DIRECTIONS

1. Preheat the oven to medium heat of about 427°F. In your mixing bowl, mix the halved tomatoes, garlic, olive oil, onions, salt, and pepper.
2. Spread the tomato mixture on the already prepared baking sheet. For a process of 20- 28 minutes, roast and stir.
3. Then remove it from the oven, and the roasted vegetables should now be transferred to a soup pot. Stir in the basil leaves. Blend in small portions in a blender, then serve immediately.

NUTRITIONS

- *Calories: 200*
- *Carbs: 15g*
- *Fat: 8g*
- *Protein: 5g*

191. CHEESEBURGER SOUP

PREPARATION	COOKING	SERVES
15 MIN	45 MIN	4

INGREDIENTS

- 1/4 cup of chopped onion
- 1 can (14.5 oz.) diced tomato
- 1 lb. of 90% lean ground beef
- 3/4 cup of chopped celery
- 2 teaspoon of Worcestershire sauce
- 3 cups of low sodium chicken broth
- 1/4 teaspoon of salt
- 1 teaspoon of dried parsley
- 7 cups of baby spinach
- 1/4 teaspoon of ground pepper
- 4 oz. of reduced-fat shredded cheddar cheese

DIRECTIONS

1. Get a large soup pot and cook the beef until it becomes brown. Add the celery, onion, and sauté until it becomes tender.
2. Remove and drain excess liquid. Stir in the broth, tomatoes, parsley, Worcestershire sauce, pepper, and salt.
3. Simmer on low heat within 20 minutes. Add spinach and leave it to cook until it becomes wilted in about 1-3 minutes. Top each of your servings with 1 ounce of cheese.

NUTRITIONS

- Calories: 400
- Carbohydrates: 11 g
- Protein: 44 g
- Fat: 20 g

192. QUICK LENTIL CHILI

PREPARATION	COOKING	SERVES
15 MIN	1H 20 MIN	10

INGREDIENTS

- 1 1/2 cups of seeded or diced pepper
- 1 1/2 cups of coarsely chopped onions
- 5 cups of vegetable broth, low-sodium
- 1 tablespoon of garlic
- 1/4 teaspoon of freshly ground pepper
- 1 cup of red lentils
- 3 filled teaspoons of chili powder
- 1 tablespoon of grounded cumin

DIRECTIONS

1. Place your pot over medium heat. Combine your onions, red peppers, low sodium vegetable broth, garlic, salt, and pepper.
2. Cook and always stir until the onions are more translucent and all the liquid evaporated. It will take about 10 minutes.
3. Add the remaining broth, lime juice, chili powder, lentils, cumin, and boil. Reduce heat at this point, cover it for about 15 minutes to simmer until the lentils are appropriately cooked.
4. Put a little water if the batter seems to be thick. The chili will be appropriately done when most of the water is absorbed. Serve and enjoy.

NUTRITIONS

- Calories: 196
- Carbs: 35g
- Fat: 1g
- Protein: 11g

193. CREAMY CAULIFLOWER SOUP

PREPARATION	COOKING	SERVES
15 MIN	30 MIN	6

INGREDIENTS

- 5 cups cauliflower rice
- 8 oz. cheddar cheese, grated
- 2 cups unsweetened almond milk
- 2 cups vegetable stock
- 2 tbsp water
- 1 small onion, chopped
- 2 garlic cloves, minced
- 1 tbsp olive oil
- Pepper
- Salt

DIRECTIONS

1. Heat-up olive oil in a large stockpot over medium heat. Add onion and garlic and cook for 1-2 minutes. Add cauliflower rice and water.
2. Cover and cook for 5-7 minutes. Now add vegetable stock and almond milk and stir well. Bring to boil. Turn heat to low and simmer for 5 minutes.
3. Turn off the heat. Slowly add cheddar cheese and stir until smooth—season soup with pepper and salt. Stir well and serve hot.

NUTRITIONS

- Calories: 214
- Fat: 16.5 g
- Carbohydrates: 7.3 g
- Protein: 11.6 g

194. CRACKPOT CHICKEN TACO SOUP

PREPARATION	COOKING	SERVES
15 MIN	6 HOURS	6

INGREDIENTS

- 2 frozen boneless chicken breasts
- 2 cans of white beans or black beans
- 1 can of diced tomatoes
- Green chili's
- 1/2 onion chopped
- 1/2 packet of taco seasoning
- 1/2 teaspoon of Garlic salt
- 1 cup of chicken broth
- Salt and pepper to taste
- Tortilla chips, cheese, sour cream, and cilantro as toppings, as well as chili pepper (this is optional).

DIRECTIONS

1. Put your frozen chicken into the crockpot and place the other ingredients into the pot too. Cook for about 6-8 hours.
2. Take out the chicken and shred it to the size you want. Finally, place the shredded chicken into the crockpot and put it on a slow cooker. Stir and allow cooking.
3. You can add more beans and tomatoes also to help stretch the meat and make it tastier.

NUTRITIONS

- Calories: 136
- Carbs: 25g
- Fat: 0g
- Protein: 8g

195. THYME TOMATO SOUP

PREPARATION	COOKING	SERVES
5 MIN	20 MIN	6

INGREDIENTS

- 2 tbsp ghee
- 2 large red onions, diced
- 1/2 cup raw cashew nuts, diced
- 2 (28 oz.) cans tomatoes
- 1 tsp. fresh thyme leaves + extra to garnish
- 1 1/2 cups water
- Salt and black pepper to taste

DIRECTIONS

1. Dissolve ghee in a pot over medium heat and sauté the onions for 4 minutes until softened. Stir in the tomatoes, thyme, water, cashews, and season with salt and black pepper.
2. Cover and bring to simmer for 10 minutes until thoroughly cooked. Open, turn the heat off, and puree the ingredients with an immersion blender.
3. Adjust to taste and stir in the heavy cream. Spoon into soup bowls and serve.

NUTRITIONS

- *Calories: 310*
- *Fats: 27 g*
- *Carbohydrates: 3g*
- *Protein: 11g*

196. MUSHROOM & JALAPEÑO STEW

PREPARATION	COOKING	SERVES
20 MIN	50 MIN	4

INGREDIENTS

- 2 tsp. olive oil
- 1 cup leeks, chopped
- 1 garlic clove, minced
- 1/2 cup celery stalks, chopped
- 1/2 cup carrots, chopped
- 1 green bell pepper, chopped
- 1 jalapeño pepper, chopped
- 2 1/2 cups mushrooms, sliced
- 1 1/2 cups vegetable stock
- 2 tomatoes, chopped
- 2 thyme sprigs, chopped

- 1 rosemary sprig, chopped
- 2 bay leaves
- 1/2 tsp. salt
- 1/4 tsp. ground black pepper
- 2 tbsp vinegar

DIRECTIONS

1. Set a pot over medium heat and warm oil. Add in garlic and leeks and sauté until soft and translucent.
2. Add in the black pepper, celery, mushrooms, and carrots. Cook as you stir for 12 minutes; stir in a splash of vegetable stock to ensure there is no sticking.
3. Stir in the rest of the ingredients. Set heat to medium; allow to simmer for 25 to 35 minutes or until cooked through. Divide into individual bowls and serve warm.

NUTRITIONS

- *Calories: 65*
- *Fats: 2.7 g*

- *Carbohydrates: 9 g*
- *Protein: 2.7 g*

197. LIME-MINT SOUP

PREPARATION	COOKING	SERVES
5 MIN	20 MIN	4

INGREDIENTS

- 4 cups vegetable broth
- 1/4 cup of mint leaves, chopped
- 1/4 cup chopped scallions, white and green parts
- 3 garlic cloves, minced
- 3 tablespoons freshly squeezed lime juice

DIRECTIONS

1. In a large stockpot, combine the broth, mint, scallions, garlic, and lime juice. Bring to a boil over medium-high heat. Adjust the heat to low, simmer for 15 minutes, and serve.

NUTRITIONS

- *Calories: 360*
- *Fat: 2 g*
- *Carbohydrates: 5 g*
- *Protein: 5 g*

198. SAVORY SPLIT PEA SOUP

PREPARATION	COOKING	SERVES
5 MIN	50 MIN	6

INGREDIENTS

- 1 (16-ounce) package dried green split peas, soaked overnight
- 5 cups vegetable broth or water
- 2 teaspoons garlic powder
- 2 teaspoons onion powder
- 1 teaspoon dried oregano
- 1 teaspoon dried thyme
- 1/4 teaspoon freshly ground black pepper

DIRECTIONS

1. Mix the split peas, broth, garlic powder, onion powder, oregano, thyme, and pepper in a large stockpot. Bring to a boil over medium-high heat.
2. Adjust to medium-low, and simmer for 45 minutes, stirring every 5 to 10 minutes. Serve warm.

NUTRITIONS

- *Calories: 160*
- *Carbs: 27g*
- *Fat: 2g*
- *Protein: 10g*

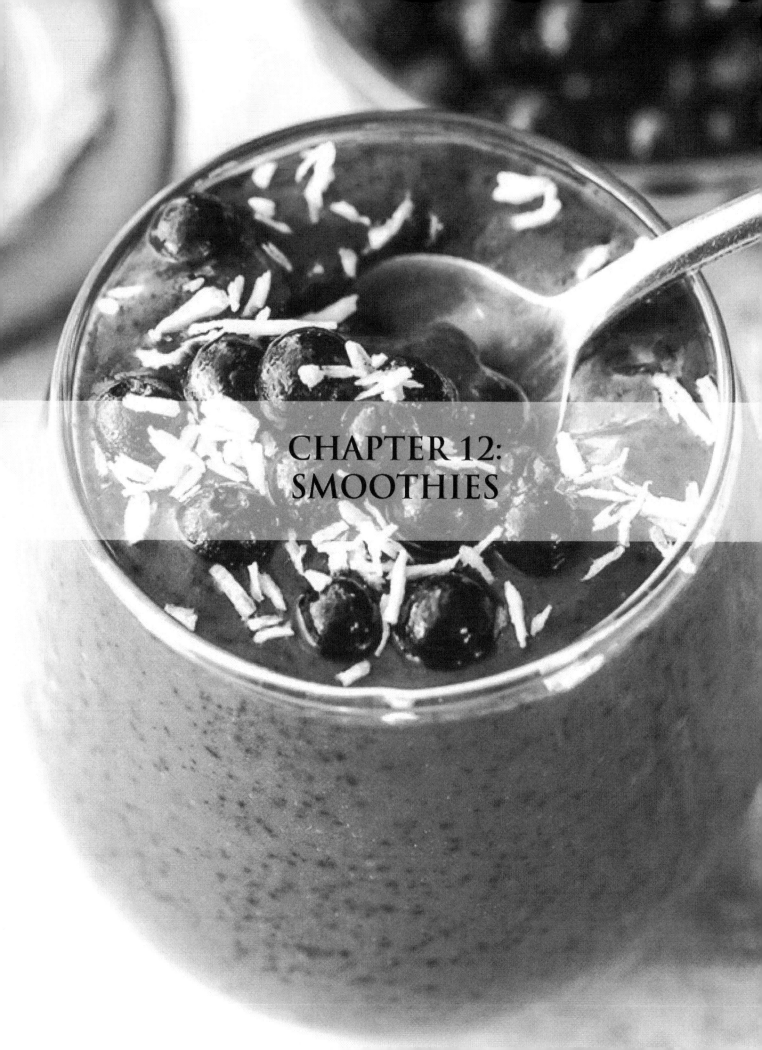

CHAPTER 12: SMOOTHIES

199. AVOCADO BLUEBERRY SMOOTHIE

PREPARATION	COOKING	SERVES
5 MIN	0 MIN	1

INGREDIENTS

- 1 tsp chia seeds
- ½ cup unsweetened coconut milk
- 1 avocado
- ½ cup blueberries

DIRECTIONS

1. Add all the listed fixings to the blender and blend until smooth and creamy. Serve immediately and enjoy.

NUTRITIONS

- *Calories: 389*
- *Fat: 34.6g*
- *Carbs: 20.7g*
- *Protein: 4.8g*

200. VEGAN BLUEBERRY SMOOTHIE

PREPARATION	COOKING	SERVES
5 MIN	0 MIN	2

INGREDIENTS

- 2 cups blueberries
- 1 tbsp hemp seeds
- 1 tbsp chia seeds
- 1 tbsp flax meal
- 1/8 tsp orange zest, grated
- 1 cup fresh orange juice
- 1 cup unsweetened coconut milk

DIRECTIONS

1. Toss all your ingredients into your blender, then process till smooth and creamy. Serve immediately and enjoy.

NUTRITIONS

- Calories: 212
- Fat: 6.6g
- Carbs: 36.9g
- Protein: 5.2g

201. BERRY PEACH SMOOTHIE

PREPARATION	COOKING	SERVES
5 MIN	0 MIN	2

INGREDIENTS

- 1 cup of coconut water
- 1 tbsp hemp seeds
- 1 tbsp agave
- ½ cup strawberries
- ½ cup blueberries
- ½ cup cherries
- ½ cup peaches

DIRECTIONS

1. Toss all your ingredients into your blender, then process till smooth and creamy. Serve immediately and enjoy.

NUTRITIONS

- Calories: 117
- Fat: 2.5g
- Carbs: 22.5g
- Protein: 3.5g

202. CANTALOUPE BLACKBERRY SMOOTHIE

PREPARATION	COOKING	SERVES
5 MIN	0 MIN	2

INGREDIENTS

- 1 cup coconut milk yogurt
- ½ cup blackberries
- 2 cups fresh cantaloupe
- 1 banana

DIRECTIONS

1. Toss all your ingredients into your blender, then process till smooth. Serve and enjoy.

NUTRITIONS

- Calories: 160
- Fat: 4.5g
- Carbs: 33.7g
- Protein: 1.8g

203. CANTALOUPE KALE SMOOTHIE

PREPARATION	COOKING	SERVES
5 MIN	5 MIN	2

INGREDIENTS

- 8 oz. water
- 1 orange, peeled
- 3 cups kale, chopped
- 1 banana, peeled
- 2 cups cantaloupe, chopped
- 1 zucchini, chopped

DIRECTIONS

1. Toss all your ingredients into your blender, then process till smooth and creamy. Serve immediately and enjoy.

NUTRITIONS

- *Calories: 203*
- *Fat: 0.5g*
- *Carbs: 49.2g*
- *Protein: 5.6g*

204. MIX BERRY CANTALOUPE SMOOTHIE

PREPARATION	COOKING	SERVES
5 MIN	0 MIN	2

INGREDIENTS

- 1 cup alkaline water
- 2 fresh Seville orange juices
- ¼ cup fresh mint leaves
- 1 ½ cups mixed berries
- 2 cups cantaloupe

DIRECTIONS

1. Toss all your ingredients into your blender, then process till smooth. Serve immediately and enjoy.

NUTRITIONS

- *Calories: 122*
- *Fat: 1g*
- *Carbs: 26.1g*
- *Protein: 2.4g*

205. AVOCADO KALE SMOOTHIE

PREPARATION	COOKING	SERVES
5 MIN	0 MIN	3

INGREDIENTS

- 1 cup of water
- ½ Seville orange, peeled
- 1 avocado
- 1 cucumber, peeled
- 1 cup kale
- 1 cup of ice cubes

DIRECTIONS

1. Toss all your ingredients into your blender, then process till smooth and creamy. Serve immediately and enjoy.

NUTRITIONS

- Calories: 160
- Fat: 13.3g
- Carbs: 11.6g
- Protein: 2.4g

206. APPLE KALE CUCUMBER SMOOTHIE

PREPARATION	COOKING	SERVES
5 MIN	5 MIN	1

INGREDIENTS

- ¾ cup of water
- ½ green apple, diced
- ¾ cup kale
- ½ cucumber

DIRECTIONS

1. Toss all your ingredients into your blender, then process till smooth and creamy. Serve immediately and enjoy.

NUTRITIONS

- Calories: 86
- Fat: 0.5g
- Carbs: 21.7g
- Protein: 1.9g

207. CUCUMBER SMOOTHIE

PREPARATION	COOKING	SERVES
5 MIN	0 MIN	2

INGREDIENTS

- 1 cup of ice cubes
- 20 drops liquid stevia
- 2 fresh lime, peeled and halved
- 1 tsp lime zest, grated
- 1 cucumber, chopped
- 1 avocado, pitted and peeled
- 2 cups kale
- 1 tbsp creamed coconut
- ¾ cup of coconut water

DIRECTIONS

1. Toss all your ingredients into your blender, then process till smooth and creamy. Serve immediately and enjoy.

NUTRITIONS

- *Calories: 313*
- *Fat: 25.1g*
- *Carbs: 24.7g*
- *Protein: 4.9g*

208. CAULIFLOWER VEGGIE SMOOTHIE

PREPARATION	COOKING	SERVES
5 MIN	0 MIN	4

INGREDIENTS

- 1 zucchini, peeled and chopped
- 1 Seville orange, peeled
- 1 apple, diced
- 1 banana
- 1 cup kale
- ½ cup cauliflower

DIRECTIONS

1. Toss all your ingredients into your blender, then process till smooth and creamy. Serve immediately and enjoy.

NUTRITIONS

- Calories: 71
- Fat: 0.3g
- Carbs: 18.3g
- Protein: 1.3g

209. SOURSOP SMOOTHIE

PREPARATION	COOKING	SERVES
5 MIN	5 MIN	2

INGREDIENTS

- 3 quartered frozen Burro Bananas
- 1-1/2 cups of Homemade Coconut Milk
- 1/4 cup of Walnuts
- 1 teaspoon of Sea Moss Gel
- 1 teaspoon of Ground Ginger
- 1 teaspoon of Soursop Leaf Powder
- 1 handful of kale

DIRECTIONS

1. Prepare and put all ingredients in a blender or a food processor. Blend it well until you reach a smooth consistency. Serve and enjoy your Soursop Smoothie!

NUTRITIONS

- *Calories: 213*
- *Fat: 3.1g*
- *Carbs: 6g*
- *Protein: 8g*

210. CUCUMBER-GINGER WATER

PREPARATION	COOKING	SERVES
5 MIN	0 MIN	2

INGREDIENTS

- 1 sliced Cucumber
- 1 smashed thumb of Ginger Root
- 2 cups of Spring Water

DIRECTIONS

1. Prepare and put all ingredients in a jar with a lid. Let the water infuse overnight. Store it in the refrigerator. Serve and enjoy your Cucumber-Ginger Water throughout the day!

NUTRITIONS

- *Calories: 117*
- *Fat: 2g*
- *Carbs: 6g*
- *Protein: 9.7g*

211. STRAWBERRY MILKSHAKE

PREPARATION	COOKING	SERVES
5 MIN	0 MIN	2

INGREDIENTS

- 2 cups of Homemade Hempseed Milk
- 1 cup of frozen Strawberries
- Agave Syrup, to taste

DIRECTIONS

1. Prepare and put all ingredients in a blender or a food processor. Blend it well until you reach a smooth consistency. Serve and enjoy your Strawberry Milkshake!

NUTRITIONS

- *Calories: 222*
- *Fat: 4g*
- *Carbs: 3g*
- *Protein: 6g*

212. CACTUS SMOOTHIE

PREPARATION	COOKING	SERVES
5 MIN	10 MIN	2

INGREDIENTS

- 1 medium Cactus
- 2 cups of Homemade Coconut Milk
- 2 frozen Baby Bananas
- 1/2 cup of Walnuts
- 1 Date
- 2 teaspoons of Hemp Seeds

DIRECTIONS

1. Take the Cactus, remove all pricks, wash it, and cut into medium pieces. Put all the listed fixings in a blender or a food processor.
2. Blend it well until you reach a smooth consistency. Serve and enjoy your Cactus Smoothie!

NUTRITIONS

- *Calories: 123*
- *Fat: 3g*
- *Carbs: 6g*
- *Protein: 2.5g*

213. PRICKLY PEAR JUICE

PREPARATION	COOKING	SERVES
5 MIN	10 MIN	2

INGREDIENTS

- 6 Prickly Pears
- 1/3 cup of Lime Juice
- 1/3 cup of Agave
- 1-1/2 cups of Spring Water

DIRECTIONS

1. Take prickly pear, cut off the ends, slice off the skin, and put in a blender. Do the same with the other pears. Add lime juice with agave to the blender and blend well for 30–40 seconds.
2. Strain the prepared mixture through a nut milk bag or cheesecloth and pour it back into the blender. Pour spring water in and blend it repeatedly. Serve and enjoy your Prickly Pear Juice!

NUTRITIONS

- *Calories: 312*
- *Fat: 6g*
- *Carbs: 11g*
- *Protein: 8g*

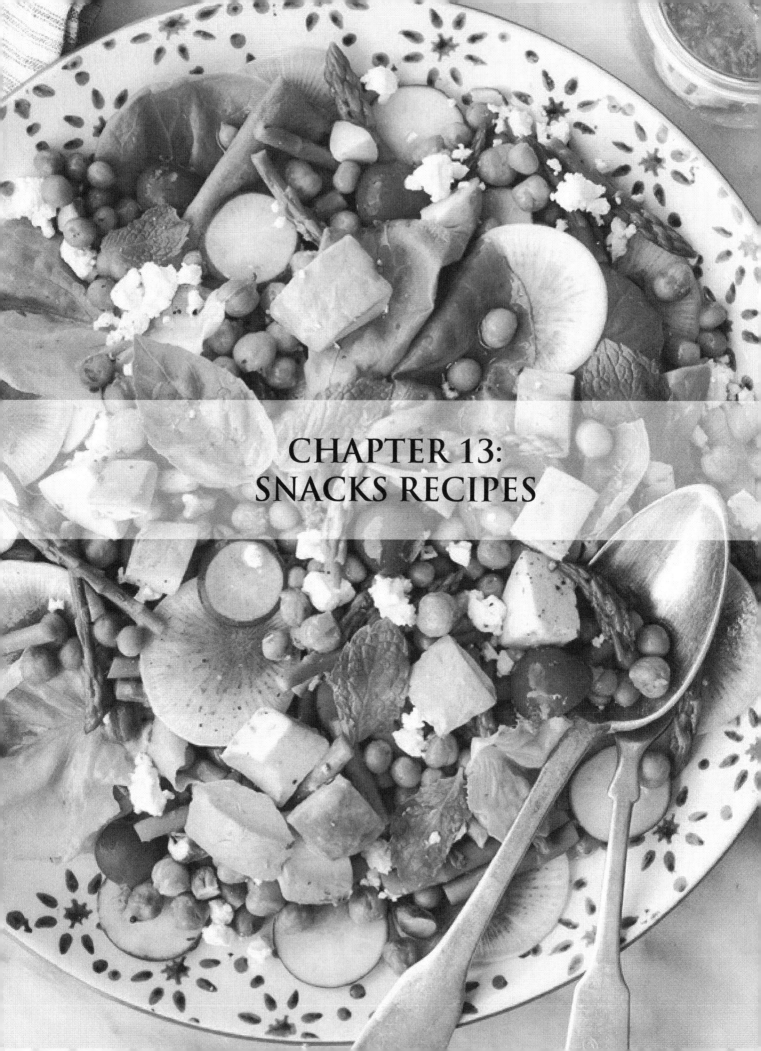

CHAPTER 13:
SNACKS RECIPES

214. EASY SALMON BURGER

PREPARATION	COOKING	SERVES
5 MIN	15 MIN	6

INGREDIENTS

- 16 ounces pink salmon, minced
- 1 cup prepared mashed potatoes
- 1 medium onion, chopped
- 1 stalk celery, finely chopped
- 1 large egg, lightly beaten
- 2 tablespoons fresh cilantro, chopped
- 1 cup breadcrumbs
- Vegetable oil, for deep frying
- Salt and freshly ground black pepper

DIRECTIONS

1. Combine the salmon, mashed potatoes, onion, celery, egg, and cilantro in a mixing bowl. Season to taste and mix thoroughly.
2. Spoon about 2 tablespoon mixture, roll in breadcrumbs, and then form into small patties.
3. Heat oil in a non-stick frying pan. Cook your salmon patties for 5 minutes on each side or until golden brown and crispy. Serve in burger buns and with coleslaw on the side if desired.

NUTRITIONS

- *Calories 230*
- *Fat 7.9 g*
- *Carbs 20.9 g*
- *Protein 18.9 g*

215. SALMON SANDWICH WITH AVOCADO AND EGG

PREPARATION	COOKING	SERVES
15 MIN	10 MIN	4

INGREDIENTS

- 8 ounces smoked salmon, thinly sliced
- 1 medium ripe avocado, thinly sliced
- 4 large poached eggs
- 4 slices whole-wheat bread
- 2 cups arugula or baby rocket
- Salt and freshly ground black pepper

DIRECTIONS

1. Place 1 bread slice on a plate top with arugula, avocado, salmon, and poached egg. Season with salt and pepper. Repeat the procedure for the remaining ingredients. Serve and enjoy.

NUTRITIONS

- Calories: 310
- Fat: 18.2 g
- Carbohydrates: 16.4 g
- Protein: 21.3 g

216. SALMON SPINACH AND COTTAGE CHEESE SANDWICH

PREPARATION	COOKING	SERVES
15 MIN	10 MIN	4

INGREDIENTS

- 4 ounces of cottage cheese
- 1/4 cup chives, chopped
- 1 teaspoon capers
- 1/2 teaspoon grated lemon rind
- 4 smoked salmon
- 2 cups loose baby spinach
- 1 medium red onion, sliced thinly
- 8 slices rye bread
- Kosher salt and freshly ground black pepper

DIRECTIONS

1. Preheat your griddle or Panini press. Mix cottage cheese, chives, capers, and lemon rind in a small bowl.
2. Spread and divide the cheese mixture on 4 bread slices. Top with spinach, onion slices, and smoked salmon.
3. Cover with remaining bread slices. Grill the sandwiches until golden and grill marks form on both sides. Transfer to a serving dish. Serve and enjoy.

NUTRITIONS

- *Calories: 261*
- *Fat 9.9 g*
- *Carbohydrates 22.9 g*
- *Protein 19.9 g*

217. SALMON FETA AND PESTO WRAP

PREPARATION	COOKING	SERVES
15 MIN	10 MIN	4

INGREDIENTS

- 8 ounces smoked salmon fillet, thinly sliced
- 1 cup feta cheese
- 8 Romaine lettuce leaves
- 4 pita bread
- 1/4 cup basil pesto sauce

DIRECTIONS

1. Place 1 pita bread on a plate. Top with lettuce, salmon, feta cheese, and pesto sauce. Fold or roll to enclose filling. Repeat the procedure for the remaining ingredients. Serve and enjoy.

NUTRITIONS

- Calories: 379
- Fat 17.7 g
- Carbohydrates: 36.6 g
- Protein: 18.4 g

218. SALMON CREAM CHEESE AND ONION ON BAGEL

PREPARATION	COOKING	SERVES
15 MIN	10 MIN	4

INGREDIENTS

- 8 ounces smoked salmon fillet, thinly sliced
- 1/2 cup cream cheese
- 1 medium onion, thinly sliced
- 4 bagels (about 80g each), split
- 2 tablespoons fresh parsley, chopped
- Freshly ground black pepper, to taste

DIRECTIONS

1. Spread the cream cheese on each bottom's half of bagels. Top with salmon and onion, season with pepper, sprinkle with parsley, and then cover with bagel tops. Serve and enjoy.

NUTRITIONS

- Calories: 309
- Fat 14.1 g
- Carbohydrates 32.0 g
- Protein 14.7 g

219. GREEK BAKLAVA

PREPARATION	COOKING	SERVES
20 MIN	20 MIN	18

INGREDIENTS

- 1 package phyllo dough
- 1 lb. chopped nuts
- 1 cup butter
- 1 teaspoon ground cinnamon
- 1 cup of water
- 1 cup white sugar
- 1 teaspoon. vanilla extract
- 1/2 cup honey

DIRECTIONS

1. Warm oven to 175°C or 350°Fahrenheit. Spread butter on the sides and bottom of a 9-in by the 13-in pan.
2. Chop the nuts, then mix with cinnamon; set it aside. Unfurl the phyllo dough, then halve the whole stack to fit the pan. Use a damp cloth to cover the phyllo to prevent drying as you proceed.
3. Put two phyllo sheets in the pan, then butter well. Repeat to make eight layered phyllo sheets. Scatter 2-3 tablespoons of the nut mixture over the sheets
4. Place two more phyllo sheets on top; butter, then sprinkle with nuts. Layer as you go. The final layer should be six to eight phyllo sheets deep.
5. Make square or diamond shapes with a sharp knife up to the bottom of the pan. You can slice into four long rows for diagonal shapes. Bake until crisp and golden for 50 minutes.
6. Meanwhile, boil water and sugar until the sugar melts to make the sauce; mix in honey and vanilla. Let it simmer for 20 minutes.
7. Take the baklava out of the oven, then drizzle with sauce right away; cool. Serve the baklava in cupcake papers. You can also freeze them without cover. The baklava will turn soggy when wrapped.

NUTRITIONS

- Calories: 393
- Carbohydrate: 37.5 g
- Fat: 25.9 g
- Protein: 6.1 g

220. GLAZED BANANAS IN PHYLLO NUT CUPS

PREPARATION	COOKING	SERVES
30 MIN	45 MIN	6

INGREDIENTS

- 3/4 cup shelled pistachios
- 1/2 cup sugar
- 1 teaspoon. ground cinnamon
- 4 sheets phyllo dough (14 inches x 9 inches)
- 1/4 cup butter, melted

Sauce:
- 3/4 cup butter, cubed
- 3/4 cup packed brown sugar
- 3 medium firm bananas, sliced
- 1/4 teaspoon. ground cinnamon
- 3 to 4 cups of vanilla ice cream

DIRECTIONS

1. Finely chop sugar and pistachios in a food processor; move to a bowl, then mix in cinnamon. Slice each phyllo sheet into 6 four-inch squares, get rid of the trimmings. Pile the squares, then use plastic wrap to cover.
2. Slather melted butter on each square one at a time, then scatter a heaping tablespoonful of pistachio mixture. Pile 3 squares, flip each at an angle to misalign the corners.
3. Force each stack on the sides and bottom of an oiled eight-oz. Custard cup. Bake for 15-20 minutes in a 350 degrees F oven until golden; cool for 5 minutes. Move to a wire rack to cool completely.
4. Melt and boil brown sugar and butter in a saucepan to make the sauce; lower heat. Mix in cinnamon and bananas gently; heat thoroughly.
5. Put ice cream in the phyllo cups until full, then put banana sauce on top. Serve right away.

NUTRITIONS

- *Calories: 735*
- *Carbohydrate: 82 g*
- *Fat: 45 g*
- *Protein: 7 g*

221. SALMON APPLE SALAD SANDWICH

PREPARATION	COOKING	SERVES
15 MIN	10 MIN	4

INGREDIENTS

- 4 ounces canned pink salmon, drained and flaked
- 1 medium red apple, cored and diced
- 1 celery stalk, chopped
- 1 shallot, finely chopped
- 1/3 cup light mayonnaise
- 8 slices whole-grain bread, toasted
- 8 Romaine lettuce leaves
- Salt and freshly ground black pepper

DIRECTIONS

1. Combine the salmon, apple, celery, shallot, and mayonnaise in a mixing bowl. Season with salt and pepper.
2. Put 1 slice of bread on your plate, top with lettuce and salmon salad, and then covers with another piece of bread—repeat the procedure for the remaining ingredients. Serve and enjoy.

NUTRITIONS

- *Calories: 315*
- *Fat 11.3 g*
- *Carbohydrates 40.4 g*
- *Protein 15.1 g*

222. SMOKED SALMON AND CHEESE ON RYE BREAD

PREPARATION	COOKING	SERVES
15 MIN	10 MIN	4

INGREDIENTS

- 8 ounces smoked salmon, thinly sliced
- 1/3 cup mayonnaise
- 2 tablespoons lemon juice
- 1 tablespoon Dijon mustard
- 1 teaspoon garlic, minced
- 4 slices cheddar cheese
- 8 slices rye bread
- 8 Romaine lettuce leaves
- Salt and freshly ground black pepper

DIRECTIONS

1. Mix the mayonnaise, lemon juice, mustard, and garlic in a small bowl. Flavor with salt plus pepper and set aside.
2. Spread dressing on 4 bread slices. Top with lettuce, salmon, and cheese. Cover with remaining rye bread slices. Serve and enjoy.

NUTRITIONS

- *Calories: 365*
- *Fat: 16.6 g*
- *Carbohydrates: 31.6 g*
- *Protein: 18.8 g*

223. BULGUR LAMB MEATBALLS

PREPARATION	COOKING	SERVES
10 MIN	15 MIN	6

INGREDIENTS

- 1 and ½ cups Greek yogurt
- ½ teaspoon cumin, ground
- 1 cup cucumber, shredded
- ½ teaspoon garlic, minced
- A pinch of salt and black pepper
- 1 cup bulgur
- 2 cups of water
- 1-pound lamb, ground
- ¼ cup parsley, chopped
- ¼ cup shallots, chopped
- ½ teaspoon allspice, ground
- ½ teaspoon cinnamon powder
- 1 tablespoon olive oil

DIRECTIONS

1. In a bowl, mix the bulgur with the water, cover the bowl, leave aside for 10 minutes, drain and transfer to a bowl.
2. Add the meat, the yogurt, and the rest of the ingredients except the oil, stir well and shape medium meatballs out of this mix.
3. Heat-up a pan with the oil over medium-high heat, add the meatballs, cook them for 7 minutes on each side, arrange them all on a platter and serve as an appetizer.

NUTRITIONS

- *Calories 300*
- *Fat 9.6 g*
- *Carbs 22.6 g*
- *Protein 6.6 g*

224. CUCUMBER BITES

PREPARATION	COOKING	SERVES
10 MIN	0 MIN	12

INGREDIENTS

- 1 English cucumber, sliced into 32 rounds
- 10 ounces hummus
- 16 cherry tomatoes, halved
- 1 tablespoon parsley, chopped
- 1-ounce feta cheese, crumbled

DIRECTIONS

1. Spread the hummus on each cucumber round, divide the tomato halves on each. Sprinkle the cheese and parsley on to, and serve.

NUTRITIONS

- *Calories 162*
- *Fat 3.4 g*
- *Fiber 2 g*
- *Carbs 6.4 g*
- *Protein 2.4 g*

225. STUFFED AVOCADO

PREPARATION	COOKING	SERVES
10 MIN	0 MIN	2

INGREDIENTS

- 1 avocado, halved and pitted
- 10 ounces of canned tuna, drained
- 2 tablespoons sun-dried tomatoes, chopped
- 1 and ½ tablespoon basil pesto
- 2 tablespoons black olives, pitted and chopped
- Salt and black pepper to the taste
- 2 teaspoons pine nuts, toasted and chopped
- 1 tablespoon basil, chopped

DIRECTIONS

1. In a bowl, mix the tuna plus sun-dried tomatoes and the rest of the ingredients except the avocado and stir. Stuff the avocado halves with the tuna mix and serve as an appetizer.

NUTRITIONS

- *Calories 233*
- *Fat 9 g*
- *Carbs 11.4 g*
- *Protein 5.6 g*

226. HUMMUS WITH GROUND LAMB

PREPARATION	COOKING	SERVES
10 MIN	15 MIN	8

INGREDIENTS

- 10 ounces hummus
- 12 ounces lamb meat, ground
- ½ cup pomegranate seeds
- ¼ cup parsley, chopped
- 1 tablespoon olive oil
- Pita chips for serving

DIRECTIONS

1. Heat-up pan with the oil over medium-high heat, add the meat, and brown for 15 minutes, stirring often.
2. Spread the hummus on a platter, spread the ground lamb all over, also spread the pomegranate seeds and the parsley, and serve with pita chips as a snack.

NUTRITIONS

- *Calories 133*
- *Fat 9.7 g*
- *Carbs 6.4 g*
- *Protein 5 g*

227. WRAPPED PLUMS

PREPARATION	COOKING	SERVES
5 MIN	0 MIN	8

INGREDIENTS

- 2 ounces prosciutto, cut into 16 pieces
- 4 plums, quartered
- 1 tablespoon chives, chopped
- A pinch of red pepper flakes, crushed

DIRECTIONS

1. Wrap each plum quarter in a prosciutto slice, arrange them all on a platter, sprinkle the chives and pepper flakes all over, and serve.

NUTRITIONS

- *Calories 30*
- *Fat 1 g*
- *Carbs 4 g*
- *Protein 2 g*

228. VEGGIE FRITTERS

PREPARATION	COOKING	SERVES
10 MIN	10 MIN	4

INGREDIENTS

- 2 garlic cloves, minced
- 2 yellow onions, chopped
- 4 scallions, chopped
- 2 carrots, grated
- 2 teaspoons cumin, ground
- ½ teaspoon turmeric powder
- Salt and black pepper to the taste
- ¼ teaspoon coriander, ground
- 2 tablespoons parsley, chopped
- ¼ teaspoon lemon juice
- ½ cup almond flour
- 2 beets, peeled and grated
- 2 eggs, whisked
- ¼ cup tapioca flour
- 3 tablespoons olive oil

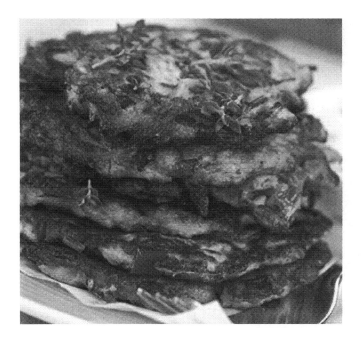

DIRECTIONS

1. In a bowl, combine the garlic, onions, scallions, and the rest of the ingredients except the oil, stir well and shape medium fritters out of this mix.
2. Heat oil in a pan over medium-high heat, add the fritters, cook for 5 minutes on each side, arrange on a platter and serve.

NUTRITIONS

- *Calories 209*
- *Fat 11.2 g*
- *Carbs 4.4 g*
- *Protein 4.8 g*

229. WHITE BEAN DIP

PREPARATION	COOKING	SERVES
10 MIN	0 MIN	4

INGREDIENTS

- 15 oz white beans, drained & rinsed
- 6 ounces canned artichoke hearts, drained and quartered
- 4 garlic cloves, minced
- 1 tablespoon basil, chopped
- 2 tablespoons olive oil
- Juice of ½ lemon
- Zest of ½ lemon, grated
- Salt and black pepper to the taste

DIRECTIONS

1. In your food processor, combine the beans, artichokes, and the rest of the ingredients except the oil and pulse well. Add the oil gradually, pulse the mix again, divide into cups, and serve as a party dip.

NUTRITIONS

- *Calories 274*
- *Fat 11.7 g*
- *Carbs 18.5 g*
- *Protein 16.5 g*

230. EGGPLANT DIP

PREPARATION	COOKING	SERVES
10 MIN	40 MIN	4

INGREDIENTS

- 1 eggplant, poked with a fork
- 2 tablespoons tahini paste
- 2 tablespoons lemon juice
- 2 garlic cloves, minced
- 1 tablespoon olive oil
- Salt and black pepper to the taste
- 1 tablespoon parsley, chopped

DIRECTIONS

1. Put the eggplant in a roasting pan, bake at 400° F for 40 minutes, cool down, peel and transfer to your food processor.
2. Add the remaining ingredients except for the parsley, pulse well, divide into small bowls and serve as an appetizer with the parsley sprinkled on top.

NUTRITIONS

- *Calories 121*
- *Fat 4.3 g*
- *Carbs 1.4 g*
- *Protein 4.3 g*

231. CUCUMBER ROLLS

PREPARATION	COOKING	SERVES
5 MIN	0 MIN	6

INGREDIENTS

- 1 big cucumber, sliced lengthwise
- 1 tablespoon parsley, chopped
- 8 ounces canned tuna, drained and mashed
- Salt and black pepper to the taste
- 1 teaspoon lime juice

DIRECTIONS

1. Arrange cucumber slices on a working surface, divide the rest of the ingredients, and roll. Arrange all the rolls on a surface and serve.

NUTRITIONS

- *Calories 200*
- *Fat 6 g*
- *Carbs 7.6 g*
- *Protein 3.5 g*

232. OLIVES AND CHEESE STUFFED TOMATOES

PREPARATION	COOKING	SERVES
10 MIN	0 MIN	24

INGREDIENTS

- 24 cherry tomatoes, top cut off, and insides scooped out
- 2 tablespoons olive oil
- ¼ teaspoon red pepper flakes
- ½ cup feta cheese, crumbled
- 2 tablespoons black olive paste
- ¼ cup mint, torn

DIRECTIONS

1. In a bowl, mix the olives paste with the rest of the ingredients except the cherry tomatoes and whisk. Stuff the cherry tomatoes with this mix, arrange them all on a platter, and serve.

NUTRITIONS

- *Calories 136*
- *Fat 8.6 g*
- *Carbs 5.6 g*
- *Protein 5.1 g*

233. TOMATO SALSA

PREPARATION	COOKING	SERVES
5 MIN	0 MIN	6

INGREDIENTS

- 1 garlic clove, minced
- 4 tablespoons olive oil
- 5 tomatoes, cubed
- 1 tablespoon balsamic vinegar
- ¼ cup basil, chopped
- 1 tablespoon parsley, chopped
- 1 tablespoon chives, chopped
- Salt and black pepper to the taste
- Pita chips for serving

DIRECTIONS

1. Mix the tomatoes plus garlic in a bowl, and the rest of the ingredients except the pita chips, stir, divide into small cups and serve with the pita chips on the side.

NUTRITIONS

- *Calories 160*
- *Fat 13.7 g*
- *Carbs 10.1 g*
- *Protein 2.2*

234. CHILI MANGO AND WATERMELON SALSA

PREPARATION	COOKING	SERVES
5 MIN	0 MIN	12

INGREDIENTS

- 1 red tomato, chopped
- Salt and black pepper to the taste
- 1 cup watermelon, seedless, peeled and cubed
- 1 red onion, chopped
- 2 mangos, peeled and chopped
- 2 chili peppers, chopped
- ¼ cup cilantro, chopped
- 3 tablespoons lime juice
- Pita chips for serving

DIRECTIONS

1. In a bowl, mix the tomato, watermelon, onion, and the rest of the ingredients except the pita chips and toss well. Divide the mix into small cups and serve with pita chips on the side.

NUTRITIONS

- *Calories 62*
- *Fat g*
- *Carbs 3.9 g*
- *Protein 2.3 g*

235. CREAMY SPINACH AND SHALLOTS DIP

PREPARATION	COOKING	SERVES
10 MIN	0 MIN	4

INGREDIENTS

- 1-pound spinach, roughly chopped
- 2 shallots, chopped
- 2 tablespoons mint, chopped
- ¾ cup cream cheese, soft
- Salt and black pepper to the taste

DIRECTIONS

1. Combine the spinach with the shallots and the rest of the ingredients in a blender and pulse. Divide into small bowls and serve.

NUTRITIONS

- Calories 204
- Fat 11.5 g
- Carbs 4.2 g
- Protein 5.9 g

236. FETA ARTICHOKE DIP

PREPARATION	COOKING	SERVES
10 MIN	30 MIN	8

INGREDIENTS

- 8 ounces artichoke hearts, drained and quartered
- ¾ cup basil, chopped
- ¾ cup green olives, pitted and chopped
- 1 cup parmesan cheese, grated
- 5 ounces feta cheese, crumbled

DIRECTIONS

1. In your food processor, mix the artichokes with the basil and the rest of the ingredients, pulse well, and transfer to a baking dish. Introduce in the oven, bake at 375° F for 30 minutes and serve.

NUTRITIONS

- *Calories 186*
- *Fat 12.4 g*
- *Carbs 2.6 g*
- *Protein 1.5 g*

237. AVOCADO DIP

PREPARATION	COOKING	SERVES
5 MIN	0 MIN	8

INGREDIENTS

- ½ cup heavy cream
- 1 green chili pepper, chopped
- Salt and pepper to the taste
- 4 avocados, pitted, peeled, and chopped
- 1 cup cilantro, chopped
- ¼ cup lime juice

DIRECTIONS

1. Pour the cream with the avocados and the rest of the ingredients in a blender, and pulse well. Divide the mix into bowls and serve cold.

NUTRITIONS

- Calories 200
- Fat 14.5 g
- Carbs 8.1 g
- Protein 7.6 g

238. GOAT CHEESE AND CHIVES SPREAD

PREPARATION	COOKING	SERVES
10 MIN	0 MIN	4

INGREDIENTS

- 2 ounces goat cheese, crumbled
- ¾ cup sour cream
- 2 tablespoons chives, chopped
- 1 tablespoon lemon juice
- Salt and black pepper to the taste
- 2 tablespoons extra virgin olive oil

DIRECTIONS

1. Mix the goat cheese with the cream and the rest of the ingredients in a bowl, and whisk well. Keep in the fridge for 10 minutes and serve.

NUTRITIONS

- *Calories 220*
- *Fat 11.5 g*
- *Carbs 8.9 g*
- *Protein 5.6 g*

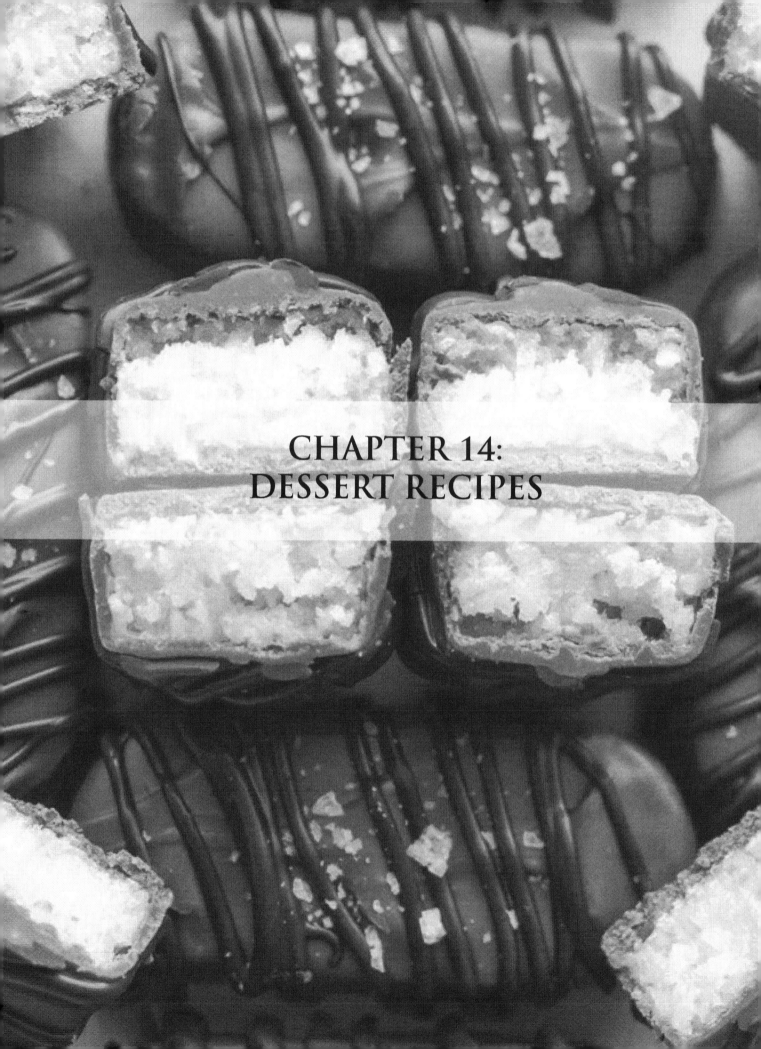

CHAPTER 14:
DESSERT RECIPES

239. BOUNTY BARS

PREPARATION	COOKING	SERVES
20 MIN	0 MIN	12

INGREDIENTS

- 1 cup coconut cream
- 3 cups shredded unsweetened coconut
- 1/4 cup extra virgin coconut oil
- 1/2 teaspoon vanilla powder
- 1/4 cup powdered erythritol
- 1 1/2 oz. cocoa butter
- 5 oz. dark chocolate

DIRECTIONS

1. Heat the oven at 350 °F and toast the coconut in it for 5-6 minutes. Remove from the oven once toasted and set aside to cool.
2. Take a medium-sized bowl and add coconut oil, coconut cream, vanilla, erythritol, and toasted coconut. Mix the ingredients well to prepare a smooth mixture.
3. Make 12 bars of equal size with your hands from the prepared mixture and adjust in the tray lined with parchment paper.
4. Place the tray in the fridge within 1 hour. In the meantime, put the cocoa butter and dark chocolate in a glass bowl.
5. Simmer a cup of water in a saucepan over medium heat and place the bowl over it to melt the cocoa butter and the dark chocolate.
6. Remove from the heat once appropriately melted, mix well until blended, and set aside to cool.
7. Take the coconut bars and coat them with dark chocolate mixture one by one using a wooden stick. Adjust on the tray lined with parchment paper and drizzle the remaining mixture over them.
8. Refrigerate for around one hour before you serve the delicious bounty bars.

NUTRITIONS

- Calories: 230
- Fat: 25 g
- Carbohydrates: 5 g
- Protein: 32 g

240. SHAKE CAKE

PREPARATION	COOKING	SERVES
15 MIN	15 MIN	1

INGREDIENTS

- 1 shake packet
- ¼ teaspoon baking powder
- 2 tablespoons egg beaters
- 2 tablespoons water
- 1 tablespoon reduced-fat cream cheese
- ½ packet Splenda

DIRECTIONS

1. Preheat the oven to 3500F. Mix all ingredients in a bowl. Pour in a muffin cup and bake for 15 minutes. Allow cooling.

NUTRITIONS

- *Calories: 271*
- *Protein: 8.7g*
- *Carbs: 19.4g*
- *Fat: 7.9g*

241. AVOCADO KALE BOWL

PREPARATION	COOKING	SERVES
10 MIN	0 MIN	2

INGREDIENTS

- ½ avocado, sliced
- 1 cup kale leaves
- 1 banana, sliced
- ½ cup raspberries
- 1 cup almond milk
- 1 kiwi, sliced
- 2 drops stevia
- ½ cup ice
- 1 tsp chia seeds

DIRECTIONS

1. Place avocado, kale, stevia, banana, almond milk, and ice in a blender. Process until smooth and creamy.
2. Transfer to a bowl. Serve and decorate the bowl by placing chia seeds, kiwi, and raspberries

NUTRITIONS

- *Calories: 230*
- *Fat: 1 g*
- *Carbohydrates: 12 g*
- *Protein: 15 g*

242. HOMEMADE COCONUT ICE CREAM

PREPARATION	COOKING	SERVES
10 MIN	10 MIN	4

INGREDIENTS

- 2 cups evaporated low-fat milk
- 1/3 cup low-fat condensed milk
- 1 cup low-fat coconut milk
- 1 cup stevia/xylitol/bacon syrup
- 2 scoops whey protein concentrate
- 2 tsp. sugar-free coconut extract
- 1 tsp. dried coconut

DIRECTIONS

1. Put all of the fixings in a mixing bowl and combine well. Heat the mixture over medium heat until it starts to bubble.
2. Remove from heat and allow the mixture to cool down. Chill mixture for about an hour then freezes in ice cream maker as outlined by the manufacturer's directions.

NUTRITIONS

- Calories: 182
- Fat: 2 g
- Carbohydrates: 20 g
- Protein: 22 g

243. BERRIES WITH COCONUT CREAM

PREPARATION	COOKING	SERVES
5 MIN	0 MIN	2

INGREDIENTS

- 1 cup fat-free cream cheese
- ¼ cup coconut chunks
- ½ tsp. sugar-free coconut extract
- ½ cup mixed berries
- 3 tsp. stevia/xylitol/yacon syrup

DIRECTIONS

1. Beat cream cheese until fluffy. Put the coconut chunks and stevia inside a blender and puree. Combine using the Cream cheese and set in serving plates. Top with berries. Serve.

NUTRITIONS

- *Calories: 200*
- *Fat: 4 g*
- *Carbohydrates: 17 g*
- *Protein: 22 g*

244. COCONUT PANNA COTTA

PREPARATION	COOKING	SERVES
5 MIN	20 MIN	2

INGREDIENTS

- 2 cups skimmed milk
- 1/2 cup water
- 1 tsp. sugar-free coconut extract
- 1 envelope powdered grass-fed – organic gelatin – sugar-free
- 2 scoops whey protein isolate
- 4 tbsp. stevia/xylitol/yacon syrup
- 1/3 cup fresh raspberries
- 2 tbsp. fresh mint

DIRECTIONS

1. In a non-stick pan, pour the milk, stevia, water, and coconut extract. Bring to a boil. Slowly add the gelatin and stir well until the mixtures start to thicken.
2. When ready, divide the mix among the small silicon cups. Refrigerate overnight to relax and hang up.
3. Remove through the fridge and thoroughly turn each cup over ahead of a serving plate. Garnish with raspberries and fresh mint, serve and revel in.

NUTRITIONS

- Calories: 130
- Fat: 3 g
- Carbohydrates: 14 g
- Protein: 29 g

245. BLUEBERRY LEMON CAKE

PREPARATION	COOKING	SERVES
10 MIN	40 MIN	4

INGREDIENTS

For the cake:
- 2/3 cup almond flour
- 5 eggs
- 1/3 cup almond milk, unsweetened
- ¼ cup erythritol
- 2 tsp. vanilla extract
- Juice of 2 lemons
- 1 tsp. lemon zest
- ½ tsp. baking soda
- Pinch of salt
- ½ cup fresh blueberries

- 2 tbsp. butter, melted

For the frosting:
- ½ cup heavy cream
- Juice of 1 lemon
- 1/8 cup erythritol

DIRECTIONS

1. Warm oven to 350F. In a bowl, add the almond flour, eggs, and almond milk and mix well until smooth.
2. Add the erythritol, a pinch of salt, baking soda, lemon zest, lemon juice, and vanilla extract. Mix and combine well. Fold in the blueberries.
3. Use the butter to grease the pans. Pour the batter into the greased pans, then put on a baking sheet for even baking.
4. Put in the oven to bake until cooked through and slightly brown on the top, about 35 to 40 minutes.
5. Let cool before removing from the pan. Mix the erythritol, lemon juice, and heavy cream. Mix well. Pour frosting on top. Serve.

NUTRITIONS

- Calories:274
- Fat: 23 g
- Carbohydrates: 8 g
- Protein: 9 g

246. RICH CHOCOLATE MOUSSE

PREPARATION	COOKING	SERVES
10 MIN	0 MIN	3

INGREDIENTS

- ¼ cup low-fat coconut cream
- 2 cups fat-free Greek-style yogurt, strained
- 4 tsp. powered cocoa, no added sugar
- 2 tbsp. stevia/xylitol/bacon syrup
- 1 tsp. natural vanilla extract

DIRECTIONS

1. Mix all the fixings in a medium mixing bowl. Put individual serving bowls or glasses and refrigerate. Serve cold.

NUTRITIONS

- Calories: 269
- Fat: 3 g
- Carbohydrates: 20 g
- Protein: 43 g

247. RASPBERRY CHEESECAKE

PREPARATION	COOKING	SERVES
10 MIN	25 MIN	6

INGREDIENTS

- 2/3 cup coconut oil, melted
- ½ cup cream cheese
- 6 eggs
- 3 tbsp. granulated sweetener
- 1 tsp. vanilla extract
- ½ tsp. baking powder
- ¾ cup raspberries

DIRECTIONS

1. In a bowl, beat together the coconut oil and cream cheese until smooth. Beat in eggs, then beat in the sweetener, vanilla, and baking powder until smooth.
2. Spoon the batter into the baking dish and smooth out the top. Scatter the raspberries on top. Bake for 25 to 30 minutes or until the center is firm. Cool, slice, and serve.

NUTRITIONS

- *Calories: 176*
- *Fat: 18 g*
- *Carbohydrates: 3 g*
- *Protein: 6 g*

248. VANILLA BEAN FRAPPUCCINO

PREPARATION	COOKING	SERVES
3 MIN	6 MIN	4

INGREDIENTS

- 3 cups unsweetened vanilla almond milk, chilled
- 2 tsp. swerve
- 1 1/2 cups heavy cream, cold
- 1 vanilla bean
- 1/4 tsp. xanthan gum
- Unsweetened chocolate shavings to garnish

DIRECTIONS

1. Combine the almond milk, swerve, heavy cream, vanilla bean, and xanthan gum in the blender and process on high speed for 1 minute until smooth.
2. Pour into tall shake glasses, sprinkle with chocolate shavings, and serve immediately.

NUTRITIONS

- Calories: 193
- Fats: 14 g
- Carbohydrates: 6 g
- Protein: 15 g

249. VANILLA AVOCADO POPSICLES

PREPARATION	COOKING	SERVES
20 MIN	0 MIN	6

INGREDIENTS

- 2 avocados
- 1 tsp. vanilla
- 1 cup almond milk
- 1 tsp. liquid stevia
- 1/2 cup unsweetened cocoa powder

DIRECTIONS

1. In the blender, add all the listed ingredients and blend smoothly. Pour blended mixture into the Popsicle molds and place in the freezer until set. Serve and enjoy.

NUTRITIONS

- Calories: 130
- Fat: 12 g
- Carbs: 7 g
- Protein: 3 g

250. RASPBERRY ICE CREAM

PREPARATION	COOKING	SERVES
10 MIN	0 MIN	2

INGREDIENTS

- 1 cup frozen raspberries
- 1/2 cup heavy cream
- 1/8 tsp. stevia powder

DIRECTIONS

1. Blend all the listed fixings in a blender until smooth. Serve immediately and enjoy.

NUTRITIONS

- Calories: 144
- Fat: 11 g
- Carbs: 10 g
- Protein: 2 g

251. BLUEBERRIES STEW

PREPARATION	COOKING	SERVES
10 MIN	10 MIN	4

INGREDIENTS

- 2 cups blueberries
- 3 tablespoons stevia
- 1 and ½ cups pure apple juice
- 1 teaspoon vanilla extract

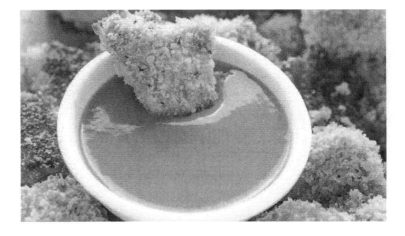

DIRECTIONS

1. In a pan, combine the blueberries with stevia and the other ingredients, bring to a simmer and cook over medium-low heat for 10 minutes. Divide into cups and serve cold.

NUTRITIONS

- *Calories: 192*
- *Fat: 5.4g*
- *Carbs 9.4g*
- *Protein 4.5g*

252. MANDARIN CREAM

PREPARATION	COOKING	SERVES
20 MIN	0 MIN	8

INGREDIENTS

- 2 mandarins, peeled and cut into segments
- Juice of 2 mandarins
- 2 tablespoons stevia
- 4 eggs, whisked
- ¾ cup stevia
- ¾ cup almonds, ground

DIRECTIONS

1. In a blender, combine the mandarins with the mandarin's juice and the other ingredients, whisk well, divide into cups and keep in the fridge for 20 minutes before serving.

NUTRITIONS

- Calories: 106
- Fat: 3.4g
- Carbs 2.4g
- Protein 4g

253. CREAMY MINT STRAWBERRY MIX

PREPARATION	COOKING	SERVES
10 MIN	30 MIN	6

INGREDIENTS

- Cooking spray
- ¼ cup stevia
- 1 and ½ cup of almond flour
- 1 teaspoon baking powder
- 1 cup almond milk
- 1 egg, whisked
- 2 cups strawberries, sliced
- 1 tablespoon mint, chopped
- 1 teaspoon lime zest, grated
- ½ cup whipping cream

DIRECTIONS

1. In a bowl, combine the almond with the strawberries, mint, and the other ingredients except for the cooking spray and whisk well.
2. Grease 6 ramekins with the cooking spray, pour the strawberry mix inside, introduce in the oven and bake at 350 degrees F for 30 minutes. Cooldown and serve.

NUTRITIONS

- *Calories: 200*
- *Fat: 6.3g*
- *Carbs 6.5g*
- *Protein 8g*

254. VANILLA CAKE

PREPARATION	COOKING	SERVES
10 MIN	25 MIN	10

INGREDIENTS

- 3 cups almond flour
- 3 teaspoons baking powder
- 1 cup olive oil
- 1 and ½ cup of almond milk
- 1 and 2/3 cup stevia
- 2 cups of water
- 1 tablespoon lime juice
- 2 teaspoons vanilla extract
- Cooking spray

DIRECTIONS

1. Mix the almond flour with the baking powder, the oil, the rest of the ingredients except the cooking spray in a bowl, and whisk well.
2. Pour the mix into a cake pan greased with the cooking spray, introduce in the oven and bake at 370 degrees F for 25 minutes. Leave the cake to cool down, cut, and serve!

NUTRITIONS

- *Calories: 200*
- *Fat: 7.6g*
- *Carbs 5.5g*
- *Protein 4.5g*

255. PUMPKIN CREAM

PREPARATION	COOKING	SERVES
5 MIN	5 MIN	2

INGREDIENTS

- 2 cups canned pumpkin flesh
- 2 tablespoons stevia
- 1 teaspoon vanilla extract
- 2 tablespoons water
- A pinch of pumpkin spice

DIRECTIONS

1. In a pan, combine the pumpkin flesh with the other ingredients, simmer for 5 minutes, divide into cups and serve cold.

NUTRITIONS

- *Calories: 192*
- *Fat: 3.4g*
- *Carbs 7.6g*
- *Protein 3.5g*

256. CHIA AND BERRIES SMOOTHIE BOWL

PREPARATION	COOKING	SERVES
5 MIN	0 MIN	2

INGREDIENTS

- 1 and ½ cup of almond milk
- 1 cup blackberries
- ¼ cup strawberries, chopped
- 1 and ½ tablespoons chia seeds
- 1 teaspoon cinnamon powder

DIRECTIONS

1. In a blender, combine the blackberries with the strawberries and the rest of the ingredients, pulse well, divide into small bowls and serve cold.

NUTRITIONS

- *Calories: 182*
- *Fat: 3.4g*
- *Carbs 8.4g*
- *Protein 3g*

257. MINTY COCONUT CREAM

PREPARATION	COOKING	SERVES
4 MIN	0 MIN	2

INGREDIENTS

- 1 banana, peeled
- 2 cups coconut flesh, shredded
- 3 tablespoons mint, chopped
- 1 and ½ cups of coconut water
- 2 tablespoons stevia
- ½ avocado pitted and peeled

DIRECTIONS

1. In a blender, combine the coconut with the banana and the rest of the ingredients, pulse well, divide into cups and serve cold.

NUTRITIONS

- *Calories: 193*
- *Fat: 5.4g*
- *Carbs 7.6g*
- *Protein 3g*

258. GRAPES STEW

PREPARATION	COOKING	SERVES
10 MIN	10 MIN	4

INGREDIENTS

- 2/3 cup stevia
- 1 tablespoon olive oil
- 1/3 cup coconut water
- 1 teaspoon vanilla extract
- 1 teaspoon lemon zest, grated
- 2 cup red grapes, halved

DIRECTIONS

1. Heat-up a pan with the water over medium heat, add the oil, stevia, and the rest of the ingredients, toss, simmer for 10 minutes, divide into cups and serve.

NUTRITIONS

- Calories: 122
- Fat: 3.7g
- Carbs 2.3g
- Protein 0.4g

259. COCOA SWEET CHERRY CREAM

PREPARATION	COOKING	SERVES
2 HOURS	0 MIN	4

INGREDIENTS

- ½ cup of cocoa powder
- ¾ cup red cherry jam
- ¼ cup stevia
- 2 cups of water
- 1-pound cherries pitted and halved

DIRECTIONS

1. In a blender, mix the cherries with the water and the rest of the ingredients, pulse well, divide into cups and keep in the fridge for 2 hours before serving.

NUTRITIONS

- *Calories: 162*
- *Fat: 3.4g*
- *Carbs 5g*
- *Protein 1g*

260. APPLE COUSCOUS PUDDING

PREPARATION	COOKING	SERVES
10 MIN	25 MIN	4

INGREDIENTS

- ½ cup couscous
- 1 and ½ cups of milk
- ¼ cup apple, cored and chopped
- 3 tablespoons stevia
- ½ teaspoon rose water
- 1 tablespoon orange zest, grated

DIRECTIONS

1. Heat a pan with the milk over medium heat, add the couscous and the rest of the ingredients, whisk, simmer for 25 minutes, divide into bowls and serve.

NUTRITIONS

- *Calories: 150*
- *Fat: 4.5g*
- *Carbs 7.5g*
- *Protein 4g*

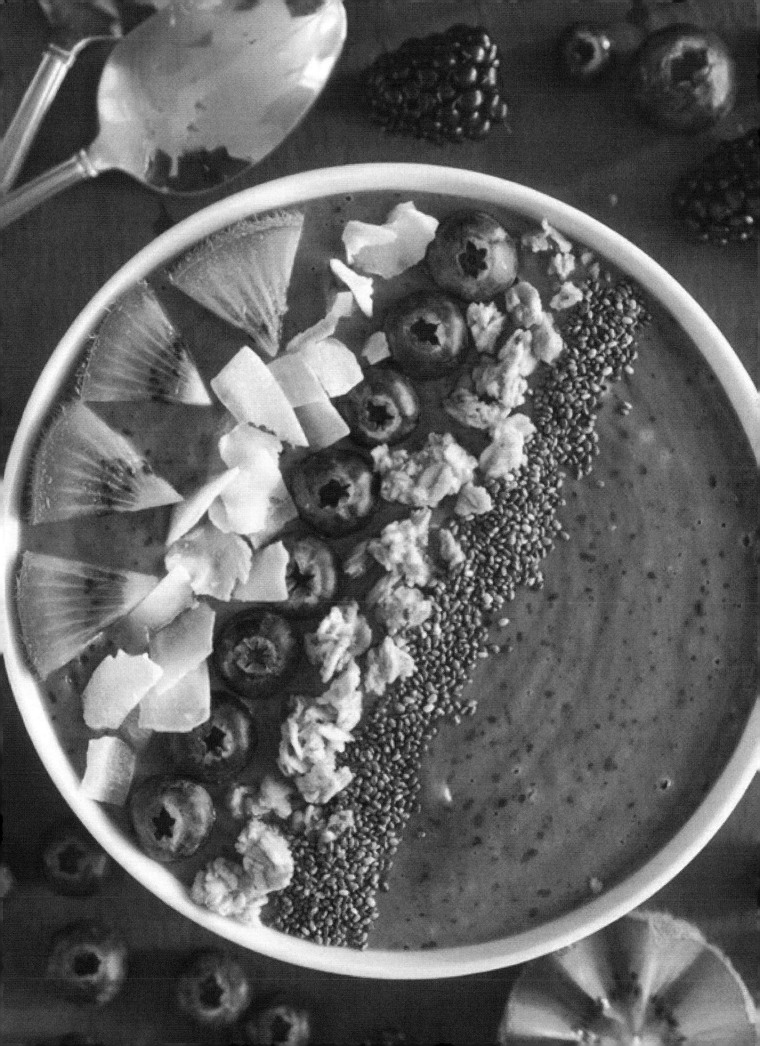

CONCLUSION

Thank you for reaching the end of this book.

Remember that Mediterranean Diet Pyramid is divided into 5 main sections, each with its own distinctive style. Sections between the pyramid peak and the peak are related to other scientific works on the Mediterranean diet.

Here are some more tips for you to remember:

First, the pyramid has a central peak. This is because the Mediterranean Diet Pyramid starts with our brain, the most important organ in our body.

Second, the Mediterranean Diet Pyramid is divided into 5 main sections: protein, carbohydrates, vitamin and mineral food groups, non-meat or fish and fruits and vegetables. The pyramid looks like as below when you are reading it:

Third, each section of the Mediterranean Diet Pyramid has its own distinctive style. For example:

1. Fruits and Vegetables: Each fruit and vegetable has it's own shade of color that represents its body function benefits. For example: dark green indicates that it is rich in carotenoids; deep red indicates that it is rich in flavonoids; yellow/orange indicates that it contains flavonolactones; blue/purple indicates that it contains anthocyanins; purple/dark purple indicates that it contains quercetin; magenta red indicates that it has high naringenin content.

2. Protein: Each protein has its own shade of color that represents its body function benefits. For example: dark green indicates that it is rich in Omega 3 fatty acids; orange indicates that it is rich in Omega 6 fatty acids; red/purple indicates that it is rich in lipoic acid; yellow/gold indicate that it contains CoQ10, which helps produce energy; pinks indicate that it has high cysteine content; maroon indicates that it has high arginine content.

3. Carbs: The shades of each carbohydrate represent their body function benefits. For example: dark green indicates that they are rich in beta-carotene and vitamin A; blue/purple indicates that they are rich in anthocyanins or quercetin; yellow represents complex carbohydrates.

4. Minerals and vitamins: Each mineral and vitamin has its own shade of color based on scientific studies made for determining whether a certain food group should be eaten with another food group to enhance their absorption.

5. Non-fish meats: Each non-fish meat (such as turkey or chicken breast, etc.) has its own unique style.

6. Other: For each food category, the pyramid shows the best choice or title (i.e. Best Protein), and then second best choice is shown as another title (i.e. Protein 2).

Fourth, the pyramid is divided into two parts: the 1) pyramid peak and 2) the section of the pyramid to the end. This is because Mediterranean diet has two different types of meals: breakfast and dinner. The general foods that you eat for breakfast are different from those you will eat for dinner.

So, when eating your meals, first make sure to start with food that is found at the top of this pyramid (i.e. protein). Then, if there's more time after finishing your protein foods, eat at least one food from each section (i.e. carbohydrates, vitamins and minerals or fruits and vegetables) in line with your energy level and health condition as long as you want to satisfy your hunger until you reach their max level. And then finally finish up with non-fish meats (or other kinds of meats that are not eaten for most people in U.S.

It is recommended that you use this book as a list for reading (personalised learning). Select those pearls of wisdom and read them each day. Make notes on the pages about your thoughts, struggles, progress and successes through a personal journal. Each time you read it, you'll gain greater insight into how to make practical changes that will help you live in harmony with nature.

INDEX RECIPES

1. BASIC CREPES — 10

2. BREAKFAST EGG MUFFINS — 11

3. BROCCOLI & CHEESE OMELET — 12

4. CHIA BERRY OVERNIGHT OATS — 13

5. CRUSTLESS SPINACH QUICHE — 14

6. DEEP DISH SPINACH QUICHE — 15

7. DELICIOUS SCRAMBLED EGGS — 16

8. EGG WHITE SCRAMBLE WITH CHERRY TOMATOES & SPINACH — 17

9. EGGS BAKED IN TOMATOES — 18

10. FETA FRITTATA — 19

11. TASTY BREAKFAST DONUTS — 20

12. CHEESY SPICY BACON BOWLS — 21

13. GOAT, CHEESE, ZUCCHINI, AND KALE QUICHE — 22

14. CREAM CHEESE EGG BREAKFAST — 23

15. AVOCADO RED PEPPERS ROASTED SCRAMBLED EGGS — 24

16. MUSHROOM QUICKIE SCRAMBLE — 25

17. COCONUT COFFEE AND GHEE — 26

18. YUMMY VEGGIE WAFFLES — 27

19. OMEGA 3 BREAKFAST SHAKE — 28

20. LIME BACON THYME MUFFINS — 29

21. AMARANTH PORRIDGE — 30

22. GLUTEN-FREE PANCAKES — 31

23. MUSHROOM & SPINACH OMELET — 32

24. WHOLE-WHEAT BLUEBERRY MUFFINS — 33

25. HEMP SEED PORRIDGE — 34

26. WALNUT CRUNCH BANANA BREAD — 35

27. STRAWBERRY & ASPARAGUS SALAD — 38

28. BERRIES & SPINACH SALAD — 39

29. EGGS & VEGGIE SALAD — 40

30. CHICKEN STUFFED AVOCADO — 41

31. CHICKEN LETTUCE WRAPS — 42

32. CHICKEN BURGERS — 43

33. BEEF BURGERS — 44

34. MEATBALLS WITH SALAD — 45

35. STUFFED BELL PEPPERS — 46

36. SHRIMP WITH ZOODLES — 47

37. SHRIMP WITH ASPARAGUS — 48

38. SHRIMP WITH BELL PEPPERS — 49

39. SHRIMP WITH SPINACH — 50

40. SCALLOPS WITH BROCCOLI — 51

41. CAULIFLOWER WITH PEAS — 52

42. BROCCOLI WITH BELL PEPPERS — 53

43. 3-VEGGIES COMBO — 54

44. TOFU WITH BROCCOLI — 55

45. TOFU WITH KALE — 56

46. TOFU WITH PEAS — 57

47. ZUCCHINI SALMON SALAD — 60

48. PAN-FRIED SALMON — 61

49. GRILLED SALMON WITH PINEAPPLE SALSA — 62

50. MEDITERRANEAN CHICKPEA SALAD — 63

51. WARM CHORIZO CHICKPEA SALAD — 64

52. GREEK ROASTED FISH — 65

53. TOMATO FISH BAKE	66
54. GARLICKY TOMATO CHICKEN CASSEROLE	67
55. CHICKEN CACCIATORE	68
56. FENNEL WILD RICE RISOTTO	69
57. WILD RICE PRAWN SALAD	70
58. CHICKEN BROCCOLI SALAD WITH AVOCADO DRESSING	71
59. SEAFOOD PAELLA	72
60. HERBED ROASTED CHICKEN BREASTS	73
61. MARINATED CHICKEN BREASTS	74
62. BALSAMIC BEEF AND MUSHROOMS MIX	75
63. OREGANO PORK MIX	76
64. SIMPLE BEEF ROAST	77
65. CHICKEN BREAST SOUP	78
66. CAULIFLOWER CURRY	79
67. PISTACHIO-CRUSTED WHITEFISH	82
68. GRILLED FISH ON LEMONS	83
69. WEEKNIGHT SHEET PAN FISH DINNER	84
70. CRISPY POLENTA FISH STICKS	85
71. CRISPY HOMEMADE FISH STICKS RECIPE	86
72. SAUCED SHELLFISH IN WHITE WINE	87
73. PISTACHIO SOLE FISH	88
74. SPEEDY TILAPIA WITH RED ONION AND AVOCADO	89
75. SALMON SKILLET SUPPER	90
76. TUSCAN TUNA AND ZUCCHINI BURGERS	91
77. SICILIAN KALE AND TUNA BOWL	92
78. MEDITERRANEAN COD STEW	93
79. STEAMED MUSSELS IN WHITE WINE SAUCE	94
80. ORANGE AND GARLIC SHRIMP	95
81. ROASTED SHRIMP-GNOCCHI BAKE	96
82. SPICY SHRIMP PUTTANESCA	97
83. BAKED COD WITH VEGETABLES	98
84. SLOW COOKER SALMON IN FOIL	99
85. DILL CHUTNEY SALMON	100
86. GARLIC-BUTTER PARMESAN SALMON AND ASPARAGUS	101
87. LEMON ROSEMARY ROASTED BRANZINO	102
88. GRILLED LEMON PESTO SALMON	103
89. STEAMED TROUT WITH LEMON HERB CRUST	104
90. WASABI TUNA ASIAN SALAD	106
91. LEMON GREEK SALAD	107
92. BROCCOLI SALAD	108
93. POTATO CARROT SALAD	109
94. MARINATED VEGGIE SALAD	110
95. MEDITERRANEAN SALAD	111
96. POTATO TUNA SALAD	112
97. HIGH PROTEIN SALAD	113
98. RICE AND VEGGIE BOWL	114
99. SQUASH BLACK BEAN BOWL	115
100. PEA SALAD	116
101. SNAP PEA SALAD	117
102. CUCUMBER TOMATO CHOPPED SALAD	118
103. ZUCCHINI PASTA SALAD	119
104. EGG AVOCADO SALAD	120
105. LEAN TURKEY PAPRIKASH	122
106. POLLO FAJITAS	123
107. CHUNKY CHICKEN QUESADILLA	124
108. CHICKEN FETTUCCINE WITH SHIITAKE MUSHROOMS	125

294

109. CHICKEN YAKITORI	126	138. CHICKEN CAPER	158
110. MUSCLE MEATBALLS	127	139. TURKEY SAUSAGE SPAGHETTI	159
111. ORANGE AND HONEY-GLAZED CHICKEN	128	140. SPICY TURKEY AND CAULIFLOWER	160
112. THAI BASIL CHICKEN	129	141. SPINACH-CHICKEN NOODLES	161
113. CHICKEN CURRY	130	142. DIJON CHICKEN VEGGIES	162
114. ITALIAN PARMESAN CHICKEN	131	143. SESAME GINGER CHICKEN	163
115. CHICKEN AND BROCCOLI STIR-FRY	132	144. CREAMY GARLIC SAUCE TURKEY	164
116. GREEK PITA PIZZA	133	145. TOMATO ROTISSERIE	165
117. BOW-TIE PASTA SALAD WITH CHICKEN AND CHICKPEAS	134	146. BALSAMIC STRAWBERR CHICKEN	166
118. GREEK STYLE QUESADILLAS	135	147. CAULIFLOWER TOMATO SHAKSHUKA	167
119. LIGHT PAPRIKA MOUSSAKA	136	148. TURKEY SHRIMP	168
120. CUCUMBER BOWL WITH SPICES AND GREEK YOGURT	137	149. BROCCOLI CHICKEN THIGHS	169
121. SWEET POTATO BACON MASH	138	150. BELL PEPPER CASHEW CHICKEN	170
122. PROSCIUTTO WRAPPED MOZZARELLA BALLS	139	151. TOMATO PUTTANESCA	171
123. MEDITERRANEAN BURRITO	140	152. HERBED LEMON CHICKEN	172
124. TENDER LAMB CHOPS	142	153. PHOENIX CHICKEN SOUP	173
125. SMOKY PORK & CABBAGE	143	154. BELL PEPPER TURKEY SONOMA	174
126. SEASONED PORK CHOPS	144	155. GRILLED CHICKEN	175
127. BEEF STROGANOFF	145	156. CREAMY CHICKEN ASPARAGUS	176
128. LEMON BEEF	146	157. TACO TOMATO SEASONED TURKEY	177
129. HERB PORK ROAST	147	158. SHRIMP WITH GARLIC	180
130. GREEK BEEF ROAST	148	159. SABICH SANDWICH	181
131. TOMATO PORK CHOPS	149	160. SALMON WITH VEGETABLES	182
132. GREEK PORK CHOPS	150	161. CRISPY FISH	183
133. PORK CACCIATORE	151	162. MOULES MARINIERES	184
134. PORK WITH TOMATO & OLIVES	152	163. STEAMED MUSSELS WITH COCONUT-CURRY	185
135. PORK ROAST	153	164. TUNA NOODLE CASSEROLE	186
136. EASY BEEF KOFTA	154	165. SEARED SCALLOPS	187
137. LEMON PEPPER PORK TENDERLOIN	155	166. BLACK COD	188
		167. MISO-GLAZED SALMON	189

168. ARUGULA AND SWEET POTATO SALAD 190

169. NICOISE SALAD 191

170. SHRIMP CURRY 192

171. SALMON PASTA 193

172. CRAB LEGS 194

173. CRUSTY PESTO SALMON 195

174. BUTTERY COD 196

175. SESAME TUNA STEAK 197

176. LEMON GARLIC SHRIMP 198

177. FOIL PACKET SALMON 199

178. BABY CORN IN CHILI-TURMERIC SPICE 202

179. BAKED CHEESY EGGPLANT WITH MARINARA 203

180. BAKED POLENTA WITH CHILI-CHEESE 204

181. BAKED PORTOBELLO PASTA 'N CHEESE 205

182. BAKED POTATO TOPPED WITH CREAM CHEESE' N OLIVES 206

183. MEXICAN BAKED ZUCCHINI 207

184. BANANA PEPPER STUFFED WITH TOFU' N SPICES 208

185. BELL PEPPER-CORN WRAPPED IN TORTILLA 209

186. BLACK BEAN BURGER WITH GARLIC-CHIPOTLE 210

187. BROWN RICE, SPINACH 'N TOFU FRITTATA 211

188. BRUSSELS SPROUTS WITH BALSAMIC OIL 212

189. BUTTERED CARROT-ZUCCHINI WITH MAYO 213

190. ROASTED TOMATO SOUP 216

191. CHEESEBURGER SOUP 217

192. QUICK LENTIL CHILI 218

193. CREAMY CAULIFLOWER SOUP 219

194. CRACKPOT CHICKEN TACO SOUP 220

195. THYME TOMATO SOUP 221

196. MUSHROOM & JALAPEÑO STEW 222

197. LIME-MINT SOUP 223

198. SAVORY SPLIT PEA SOUP 224

199. AVOCADO BLUEBERRY SMOOTHIE 226

200. VEGAN BLUEBERRY SMOOTHIE 227

201. BERRY PEACH SMOOTHIE 228

202. CANTALOUPE BLACKBERRY SMOOTHIE 229

203. CANTALOUPE KALE SMOOTHIE 230

204. MIX BERRY CANTALOUPE SMOOTHIE 231

205. AVOCADO KALE SMOOTHIE 232

206. APPLE KALE CUCUMBER SMOOTHIE 233

207. CUCUMBER SMOOTHIE 234

208. CAULIFLOWER VEGGIE SMOOTHIE 235

209. SOURSOP SMOOTHIE 236

210. CUCUMBER-GINGER WATER 237

211. STRAWBERRY MILKSHAKE 238

212. CACTUS SMOOTHIE 239

213. PRICKLY PEAR JUICE 240

214. EASY SALMON BURGER 242

215. SALMON SANDWICH WITH AVOCADO AND EGG 243

216. SALMON SPINACH AND COTTAGE CHEESE SANDWICH 244

217. SALMON FETA AND PESTO WRAP 245

218. SALMON CREAM CHEESE AND ONION ON BAGEL 246

219. GREEK BAKLAVA 247

220. GLAZED BANANAS IN PHYLLO NUT CUPS 248

221. SALMON APPLE SALAD SANDWICH 249

222. SMOKED SALMON AND CHEESE ON RYE BREAD 250

223. BULGUR LAMB MEATBALLS 251

224. CUCUMBER BITES 252

225. STUFFED AVOCADO 253

226. HUMMUS WITH GROUND LAMB 254

227. WRAPPED PLUMS 255

228. VEGGIE FRITTERS 256

229. WHITE BEAN DIP 257

230. EGGPLANT DIP 258

231. CUCUMBER ROLLS 259

232. OLIVES AND CHEESE STUFFED TOMATOES 260

233. TOMATO SALSA 261

234. CHILI MANGO AND WATERMELON SALSA 262

235. CREAMY SPINACH AND SHALLOTS DIP 263

236. FETA ARTICHOKE DIP 264

237. AVOCADO DIP 265

238. GOAT CHEESE AND CHIVES SPREAD 266

239. BOUNTY BARS 268

240. SHAKE CAKE 269

241. AVOCADO KALE BOWL 270

242. HOMEMADE COCONUT ICE CREAM 271

243. BERRIES WITH COCONUT CREAM 272

244. COCONUT PANNA COTTA 273

245. BLUEBERRY LEMON CAKE 274

246. RICH CHOCOLATE MOUSSE 275

247. RASPBERRY CHEESECAKE 276

248. VANILLA BEAN FRAPPUCCINO 277

249. VANILLA AVOCADO POPSICLES 278

250. RASPBERRY ICE CREAM 279

251. BLUEBERRIES STEW 280

252. MANDARIN CREAM 281

253. CREAMY MINT STRAWBERRY MIX 282

254. VANILLA CAKE 283

255. PUMPKIN CREAM 284

256. CHIA AND BERRIES SMOOTHIE BOWL 285

257. MINTY COCONUT CREAM 286

258. GRAPES STEW 287

259. COCOA SWEET CHERRY CREAM 288

260. APPLE COUSCOUS PUDDING 289

THE 2021 COMPLETE MEDITERRANEAN COOKBOOK

LOSE WEIGHT AND START TO EAT HEALTHY WITH THE MEDITERRANEAN DIET | 250+ QUICK AND EASY RECIPES FOR EVERYDAY COOKING| FOR BEGINNERS AND NOT | FEEL BETTER

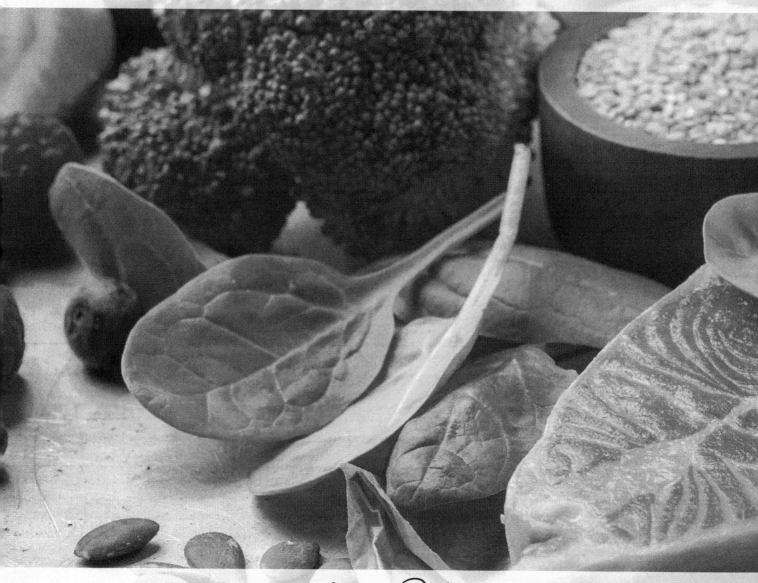

Jennifer Paul

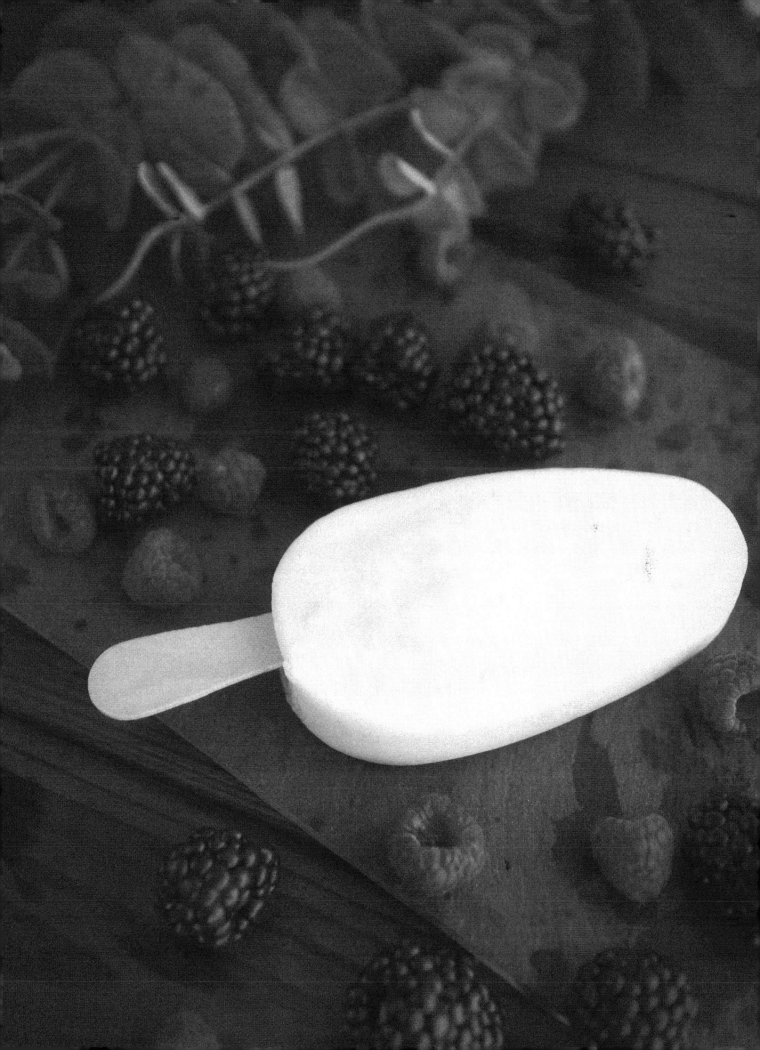

INTRODUCTION

Thank you for getting this book.

Let us begin with some basics of Mediterranean Diet.

This diet, Mediterranean diet, is a dietary pattern typical of the Mediterranean region, which includes Southern Europe, Western Asia and Northern Africa.

It is rich in olive oil, vegetables, fruits, nuts and legumes. There is a considerable amount of seafood in the diet as well. Dairy products are used infrequently but not completely excluded. Meat and poultry are consumed in small amounts or used as condiments or side dishes.

The main characteristic of this diet is its high consumption of plant food: cereal grains (52%), legumes (25%), fruits (16%), vegetables (12%) and nuts (2%). Fish was consumed in low quantities as seafood in coastal regions. Meat was reserved for special occasions; it took the form of a variety of fowl such as chicken, turkey and duck; pork was consumed on rare occasions because pigs were kept mainly by peasants who had no other choice than raising them for financial reasons such as taxes or tithe payments.

There is a wide range of desserts and sweetened drinks. There were also some dishes with a high fat content such as meat stews, roasts and sausages.

It should be noted that people from Mediterranean regions were not wealthy even in the recent past, so they had to make do with what was available to them at all times.

It originates from the French word "diet" which means "food", and the first reference to it is from the Greek word "medimnoia".

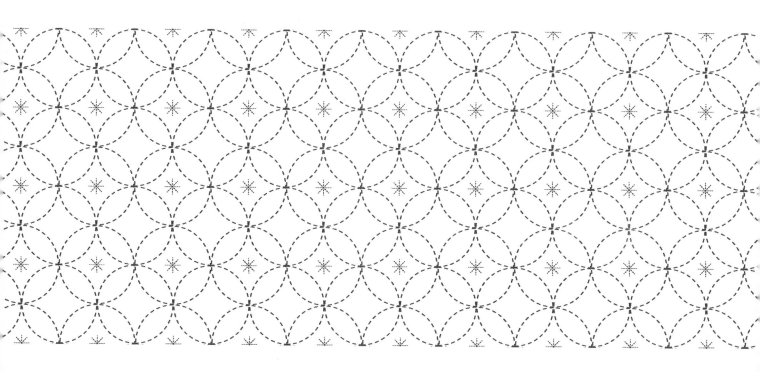

Who started Mediterranean Diet?

Now for the million-dollar question: who started Mediterranean Diet? The Mediterranean region has always been known as the cradle of civilization, and many ancient civilizations such as Egyptian, Greek and Roman have been credited with developing a diet rich in vegetables, grains, fruits and seafood.

Mediterranean Diet – the Proven Benefits

In addition to this diet being high in nutrients, it contains less saturated fats and cholesterol than other diets. In fact, regular intake of certain components of this diet is believed to lower blood pressure (antioxidants), boost immunity (omega 3 fatty acids) and fight inflammation (olive oil). It also seems to be a great way to prevent or reduce risk factors for heart disease and stroke (monounsaturated fat from olive oil), diabetes (whole grains), Alzheimer's disease (olive oil polyphenols) and even breast cancer.

Studies show that while consuming a typical American diet, there is a 20% increase in the risk of developing heart disease. On the other hand, participants at a Mediterranean-style diet lowered their risk by 15%.

Although these studies are over 15 years old, its conclusions still hold true today.

Why does this diet work? [In my opinion] The power of this diet lies in its high concentration of antioxidants and micronutrients which fight free radicals. Antioxidants neutralize toxic molecules that can cause inflammation and cell damage, so eating Mediterranean can help your body's cells stay healthy and youthful (and therefore less likely to be damaged by chronic disease, or cancer).

In addition to this, eating lots of omega 3s from fish and nuts keeps your artery walls healthy for longer – so you'll be less likely to find yourself afflicted with arterial blockages. Fish oil supplements are even better because they contain the most bioavailable form of omega 3s – EPA (eicosapentaenoic acid) and DHA (docosahexaenoic acid).

Let us now see the meals you can have on this diet.

CHAPTER 1:
BREAKFAST RECIPES

1. BEEF WITH BROCCOLI PLUS CAULIFLOWER RICE

PREPARATION	COOKING	SERVES
5 MIN	15 MIN	2

INGREDIENTS

- 1-pound raw beef round steak, cut into strips.
- 1 tablespoon + 2 teaspoons low sodium soy sauce
- 1 Splenda packet
- ½ cup of water
- 1 ½ cup broccoli florets
- 1 teaspoon sesame or olive oil
- 2 cups cooked, grated cauliflower or frozen riced cauliflower

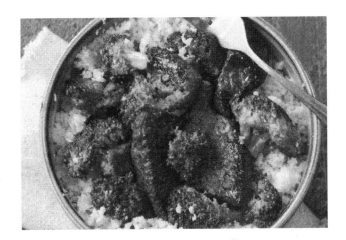

DIRECTIONS

1. Stir steak with soy sauce and let sit for about 15 minutes.
2. Heat oil over medium-high heat and stir-fry beef for 3-5 minutes or until browned.
3. Remove from pan.
4. Place broccoli, Splenda and water. Cook for 5 minutes or until broccoli starts to turn tender, stirring sometimes.
5. Add beef back in and heat up thoroughly.
6. Serve the dish with cauliflower rice.

NUTRITIONS

- *Calories 201;*
- *Protein 23g;*
- *Fat 4;*
- *Carbs 2*

2. GRILLED CHICKEN POWER BOWL WITH GREEN GODDESS DRESSING

PREPARATION	COOKING	SERVES
5 MIN	15 MIN	4

INGREDIENTS

- 1 ½ boneless, skinless chicken breasts
- ¼ teaspoon each salt & pepper
- 1 cup diced or cubed kabocha squash
- 1 cup diced zucchini
- 1 cup diced yellow summer squash
- 1 cup diced broccoli
- 8 cherry tomatoes, halved
- 4 radishes, sliced thin
- 1 cup shredded red cabbage
- ¼ cup hemp or pumpkin seeds

Green Goddess Dressing:
- ½ cup low-fat plain Greek yogurt
- 1 cup fresh basil
- 1 clove garlic
- 4 tbsp. lemon juice
- ¼ tsp each salt & pepper

DIRECTIONS

1. Preheat oven to 350°F.
2. Season chicken with salt and pepper.
3. Roast chicken for 12 minutes until it reaches a temperature of 165°F. When done, dismiss from the oven and set aside to rest for about 5 minutes. Cut into bite-sized pieces and keep warm.
4. While the chicken is resting, steam riced kabocha squash, yellow summer squash, zucchini, and broccoli in a covered microwave-proof bowl for about 5 minutes until tender.
5. For the dressing, arrange the ingredients in a blender and puree until smooth.
6. To serve, place an equal amount of Veggie Mix into four individual bowls. Add an equal amount of cherry tomatoes, radishes, and chopped cabbage to each bowl, along with a quarter of the chicken and a tablespoon of seeds. Dress up. Enjoy!

NUTRITIONS

- *Calories: 300;*
- *Protein: 43 g;*
- *Carbohydrate: 12 g;*
- *Fat: 10 g*

305

3. BACON CHEESEBURGER

PREPARATION	COOKING	SERVES
5 MIN	15 MIN	4

INGREDIENTS

- 1-pound lean ground beef
- ¼ cup chopped yellow onion
- 1 clove garlic, minced
- 1 tablespoon yellow mustard
- 1 tablespoon Worcestershire sauce
- ½ teaspoon salt
- Cooking spray
- 4 ultra-thin slices of cheddar cheese, cut into 6 equal-sized rectangular pieces
- 3 pieces of turkey bacon, each cut into 8 evenly-sized rectangular pieces
- 24 dill pickle chips
- 4-6 green leaf
- lettuce leaves, torn into 24 small square-shaped pieces
- 12 cherry tomatoes, sliced in half

DIRECTIONS

1. Preheat oven to 400°F.
2. Combine the garlic, salt, onion, Worcestershire sauce, and beef in a medium-sized bowl, and mix well.
3. Form mixture into 24 small meatballs. Put meatballs onto a foil-lined baking sheet and cook for 12-15 minutes. Leave oven on.
4. Top every meatball with a piece of cheese, then go back to the oven until cheese melts for about 2 to 3 minutes. Let meatballs cool.
5. To assemble bites: on a toothpick, layer a cheese-covered meatball, piece of bacon, piece of lettuce, pickle chip, and a tomato half.

NUTRITIONS

- Calories 234;
- Protein 20g;
- Fat 3g;
- Carbs 12g

4. CHEESEBURGER PIE

PREPARATION	COOKING	SERVES
25 MIN	90 MIN	4

INGREDIENTS

- 1 large spaghetti squash
- 1-pound lean ground beef
- ¼ cup diced onion
- 2 eggs
- 1/3 cup low-fat, plain Greek yogurt
- 2 tablespoon Tomato sauce
- ½ teaspoon Worcestershire sauce
- 2/3 cup reduced-fat, shredded cheddar cheese
- 2 ounces dill pickle slices
- Cooking spray

DIRECTIONS

1. Preheat oven to 400°F.
2. Slice spaghetti squash in half lengthwise; dismiss pulp and seeds. Spray cooking spray.
3. Place the cut pumpkin halves on a foil-lined baking sheet and bake for 30 minutes. Once cooked, let it cool before scraping the pulp from the squash with a fork to remove the spaghetti-like strings. Set aside.
4. Push squash strands in the bottom and up sides of the greased pie pan, creating an even layer.
5. Meanwhile, set up pie filling. In a lightly greased, medium-sized skillet, cook beef and onion over medium heat for 8 to 10 minutes, sometimes stirring, until meat is brown. Drain and remove from heat.
6. Whisk together the eggs, tomato paste, Greek yogurt and Worcestershire sauce and add the ground beef mixture. Pour the pie filling over the pumpkin rind.
7. Sprinkle the meat filling with cheese, and then fill with pickled cucumber slices.
8. Bake for 40 minutes.

NUTRITIONS

- Calories: 270;
- Protein: 23 g;
- Carbohydrate: 10 g;
- Fat: 23 g

5. CRISPY APPLES

PREPARATION	COOKING	SERVES
10 MIN	10 MIN	4

INGREDIENTS

- 2 tbsp. cinnamon powder
- 5 apples
- ½ tablespoon nutmeg powder
- 1 tablespoon maple syrup
- ½ cup water
- 4 tablespoon butter
- ¼ cup flour
- ¾ cup oats
- ¼ cup brown sugar

DIRECTIONS

1. Get the apples in a pan, put in nutmeg, maple syrup, cinnamon and water.
2. Mix in butter with flour, sugar, salt and oat, turn, put a spoonful of the blend over apples, get into the air fryer and cook at 350°F for 10 minutes.
3. Serve while warm.

NUTRITIONS

- Calories: 387;
- Total Fat: 5.6g;
- Total carbs: 12.4g

6. TURKEY CAPRESE MEATLOAF CUPS

PREPARATION	COOKING	SERVES
20 MIN	45 MIN	6

INGREDIENTS

- 1 large egg
- 2 pounds ground turkey breast
- 3 pieces of sun-dried tomatoes, drained and chopped
- ¼ cup fresh basil leaves, chopped
- 5 ounces low-fat fresh mozzarella, shredded
- ½ teaspoon garlic powder
- ¼ teaspoon salt and ½ teaspoon pepper, to taste

DIRECTIONS

1. Preheat oven to 400°F.
2. Beat the egg in a big mixing bowl.
3. Add the remaining ingredients and mix everything with your hands until evenly combined.
4. Spray a 12-cup muffin tin and divide the turkey mixture among the muffin cups, pressing the mix in. Cook in the preheated oven till the turkey is well-cooked for about 25-30 minutes.
5. Chill the meatloaves entirely and store them in a container in the fridge for up to 5 days.

NUTRITIONS

- *Calories 181;*
- *Protein 43g;*
- *Fat 11;*
- *Carbs 9*

7. ZUCCHINI NOODLES WITH CREAMY AVOCADO PESTO

PREPARATION	COOKING	SERVES
10 MIN	20 MIN	4

INGREDIENTS

- 6 cups of spiralized zucchini
- 1 tablespoon olive oil
- 6 ounces of avocado
- 1 basil leaves
- 3 garlic cloves
- 1/3-ounce pine nuts
- 2 tablespoon lemon juice
- ½ teaspoon salt
- ¼ teaspoon black pepper

DIRECTIONS

1. Spiralize the courgettes and set them aside on paper towels so that the excess water is absorbed.
2. In a food processor, put avocados, lemon juice, basil leaves, garlic, pine nuts, and sea salt and pulse until chopped. Then put olive oil in a slow stream till emulsified and creamy.
3. Drizzle olive oil in a skillet over medium-high heat and put zucchini noodles, cooking for about 2 minutes till tender.
4. Put zucchini noodles into a big bowl and toss with avocado pesto. Season with cracked pepper and a little Parmesan and serve.

NUTRITIONS

- Calories 115;
- Protein 30g;
- Fat 0g;
- Carbs 3g

8. AVOCADO CHICKEN SALAD

PREPARATION	COOKING	SERVES
5 MIN	10 MIN	2

INGREDIENTS

- 10 ounces diced cooked chicken
- ½ cup 2% Plain Greek yogurt
- 3 ounces chopped avocado
- 12 teaspoon garlic powder
- ¼ teaspoon salt
- 1/8 teaspoon pepper
- 1 tablespoon + 1 teaspoon lime juice
- ¼ cup fresh cilantro, chopped

DIRECTIONS

1. Combine all ingredients in a medium-sized bowl. Refrigerate until ready to serve.
2. Cut the chicken salad in half and serve with your favorite greens.

NUTRITIONS

- *Calories 265;*
- *Protein 35g;*
- *Fat 13;*
- *Carbs 5*

9. RICOTTA RAMEKINS

PREPARATION	COOKING	SERVES
10 MIN	60 MIN	4

INGREDIENTS

- 6 eggs, whisked
- 1 and ½ pounds ricotta cheese, soft
- ½ pound stevia
- 1 teaspoon vanilla extract
- ½ teaspoon baking powder
- Cooking spray

DIRECTIONS

1. In a bowl, mix the eggs with the ricotta and the other ingredients except for the cooking spray and whisk well.
2. Grease 4 ramekins with the cooking spray, pour the ricotta cream in each and bake at 360 degrees F for 1 hour.
3. Serve cold.

NUTRITIONS

- Calories 180;
- Fat 5.3;
- Fiber 5.4;
- Carbs 11.5;
- Protein 4

10. CHICKEN LO MEIN

PREPARATION	COOKING	SERVES
15 MIN	30 MIN	4

INGREDIENTS

- 2 tablespoon+ 2 teaspoon sesame oil, divided
- 790grams boneless. skinless chicken breasts, sliced
- ¼ teaspoon ground black pepper
- 2 tablespoons soy sauce
- 2 tablespoons oyster sauce
- 1 garlic clove, minced
- 2 teaspoons peeled and minced fresh ginger-root
- 2 spring onions, trimmed and sliced with white and green parts separated
- 110 grams fresh mushrooms, divided
- 1 medium red bell pepper, membranes and seeds removed
- 2 medium zucchinis (400g), cut, sliced

DIRECTIONS

1. In a skillet, heat one teaspoon sesame oil over medium-high heat. Put the sliced chicken, season with black pepper, and cook until the chicken is done (internal temperature about 165°F). Dismiss from wok or skillet and set aside.
2. While the chicken cooks, prepare the sauce by combining the oyster sauce, soy sauce, and 2 tablespoons of sesame oil in a bowl and whisking together. Set aside.
3. With the same skillet used to cook the chicken, heat 1 teaspoon sesame oil and put the garlic, ginger, and white spring onion pieces; cook until fragrant, about 1 minute. Put the mushrooms and bell peppers and continue to cook until just tender, about 3 minutes. Add zucchini noodles and toss to combine.
4. Pour in the sauce and put the chicken; cook until zucchini is tender and the mixture is heated for 5 minutes.
5. Garnish with green parts of spring onions.

NUTRITIONS

- *Calories: 312;*
- *Protein: 9g;*
- *Fat: 10;*
- *Carbs: 22*

313

11. PANCAKES WITH BERRIES

PREPARATION	COOKING	SERVES
5 MIN	20 MIN	2

INGREDIENTS

Pancake:
- 1 egg
- 50 grams spelled flour
- 50 grams of almond flour
- 15 grams of coconut flour
- 150 milliliters of water
- salt

Filling:
- 40 grams of mixed berries
- 10 grams of chocolate
- 5 grams of powdered sugar
- 4 tablespoons yogurt

DIRECTIONS

1. Put the flour, egg, and some salt in a blender jar.
2. Add 150 ml of water.
3. Mix everything with a whisk.
4. Mix everything into a batter.
5. Heat a coated pan and put in half of the batter.
6. Once the pancake is firm, turn it over. Take out the pancake, add the second half of the batter to the pan and repeat.
7. Melt chocolate over a water bath.
8. Let the pancakes cool.
9. Brush the pancakes with the yogurt.
10. Wash the berry and let it drain.
11. Put berries on the yogurt.
12. Roll up the pancakes.
13. Sprinkle them with powdered sugar.
14. Decorate the whole thing with the melted chocolate.

NUTRITIONS

- kcal: 298;
- Carbohydrates: 26 g;
- Protein: 21 g;
- Fat: 9 g

12. OMELETTE À LA MARGHERITA

PREPARATION	COOKING	SERVES
10 MIN	20 MIN	2

INGREDIENTS

- 3 eggs
- 50 grams parmesan cheese
- 2 tablespoons heavy cream
- 1 tablespoon olive oil
- 1 teaspoon oregano
- nutmeg
- salt
- pepper

For covering:
- 3 - 4 stalks of basil
- 1 tomato
- 100 grams grated mozzarella

DIRECTIONS

1. Mix the cream and eggs in a medium bowl.
2. Add the grated parmesan, nutmeg, oregano, pepper and salt and stir everything.
3. Heat the oil in a pan.
4. Add 1/2 of the egg and cream to the pan.
5. Let the omelet set over medium heat, turn it, and then remove it. Repeat with the second half of the egg mixture.
6. Cut the tomatoes into slices and place them on top of the omelets.
7. Scatter the mozzarella over the tomatoes.
8. Place the omelets on a baking sheet.
9. Cook at 180 degrees for 5 to 10 minutes. Then take the omelets out and decorate them with the basil leaves.

NUTRITIONS

- *kcal: 402;*
- *Carbohydrates: 7 g;*
- *Protein: 21 g;*
- *Fat: 34 g*

13. OMELET WITH TOMATOES AND SPRING ONIONS

PREPARATION	COOKING	SERVES
5 MIN	25 MIN	6

INGREDIENTS

- 6 eggs
- 2 tomatoes
- 2 spring onions
- 1 shallot
- 2 tablespoons butter
- 1 tablespoon olive oil
- 1 pinch of nutmeg
- salt
- pepper

DIRECTIONS

1. Whisk the eggs in a bowl. Mix them and season them with salt and pepper.
2. Peel the shallot and chop it up.
3. Clean the onions and cut them into rings.
4. Wash the tomatoes and cut them into pieces.
5. Heat butter and oil in a pan. Braise half of the shallots in it.
6. Add half the egg mixture.
7. Let everything set over medium heat.
8. Scatter a few tomatoes and onion rings on top.
9. Repeat with the second half of the egg mixture. In the end, spread the grated nutmeg over the whole thing.

NUTRITIONS

- kcal: 263;
- Carbohydrates: 8 g;
- Protein: 20.3 g;
- Fat: 24 g

14. COCONUT CHIA PUDDING WITH BERRIES

PREPARATION	COOKING	SERVES
20 MIN	45 MIN	2

INGREDIENTS

- 150 grams raspberries and blueberries
- 60 grams chia seeds
- 500 milliliters coconut milk
- 1 teaspoon agave syrup
- ½ teaspoon ground bourbon vanilla

DIRECTIONS

1. Put the chia seeds, agave syrup, and vanilla in a bowl. Pour in the coconut milk.
2. Mix thoroughly and let it soak for 30 minutes.
3. Meanwhile, wash the berries and let them drain well.
4. Divide the coconut chia pudding between two glasses.
5. Put the berries on top.

NUTRITIONS

- *kcal: 662;*
- *Carbohydrates: 18 g;*
- *Protein: 8 g*
- *Fat: 55 g*

15. EEL ON SCRAMBLED EGGS AND BREAD

PREPARATION	COOKING	SERVES
15 MIN	10 MIN	2

INGREDIENTS

- 4 eggs
- 1 shallot
- 4 slices of low carb bread
- 2 sticks of dill
- 200 grams smoked eel
- 1 tablespoon oil
- salt
- White pepper

DIRECTIONS

1. Mix the eggs in a bowl and season with salt and pepper.
2. Peel the shallot and cut it into fine cubes. Chop the dill.
3. Remove the skin from the eel and cut it into pieces.
4. Heat the oil in a pan and steam the shallot in it.
5. Add the eggs in and let them set.
6. Use the spatula to turn the eggs several times.
7. Reduce the heat and add the dill. Stir everything.
8. Spread the scrambled eggs over four slices of bread.
9. Put the eel pieces on top. Add some fresh dill and serve everything.

NUTRITIONS

- kcal: 830;
- Carbohydrates: 8 g;
- Protein: 45 g;
- Fat: 64 g

16. CHIA SEED GEL WITH POMEGRANATE AND NUTS

PREPARATION	COOKING	SERVES
5 MIN	10 MIN	3

INGREDIENTS

- 20 grams hazelnuts
- 20 grams walnuts
- 120 milliliters almond milk
- 4 tablespoons chia seeds
- 4 tablespoons pomegranate seeds
- 1 teaspoon agave syrup
- Some lime juices

DIRECTIONS

1. Finely chop the nuts.
2. Mix the almond milk with the chia seeds. Let everything soak for 10 to 20 minutes.
3. Occasionally stir the mixture with the chia seeds. Stir in the agave syrup.
4. Pour 2 tablespoons of each mixture into a dessert glass.
5. Layer the chopped nuts on top. Cover the nuts with 1 tablespoon each of the chia mass.
6. Sprinkle the pomegranate seeds on top and serve everything.

NUTRITIONS

- kcal: 248;
- Carbohydrates: 7 g;
- Protein: 1 g;
- Fat: 19 g

17. LAVENDER BLUEBERRY CHIA SEED PUDDING

PREPARATION	COOKING	SERVES
1H 10 MIN	0 MIN	4

INGREDIENTS

- 100 grams blueberries
- 70 grams of organic quark
- 50 grams of soy yogurt
- 30 grams hazelnuts
- 200 milliliters almond milk
- 2 tablespoons chia seeds
- 2 teaspoons agave syrup
- 2 teaspoons of lavender

DIRECTIONS

1. Bring the almond milk to a boil along with the lavender.
2. Let the mixture simmer for 10 minutes at a reduced temperature. Let them cool down afterward.
3. If the milk is cold, add the blueberries and puree everything.
4. Mix the whole thing with the chia seeds and agave syrup.
5. Let everything soak in the refrigerator for an hour.
6. Mix the yogurt and curd cheese. Add both to the crowd.
7. Divide the pudding into glasses.
8. Finely chop the hazelnuts and sprinkle them on top.

NUTRITIONS

- kcal: 252;
- Carbohydrates: 12 g;
- Protein: 1 g;
- Fat: 11 g

18. YOGURT WITH GRANOLA AND PERSIMMON

PREPARATION	COOKING	SERVES
5 MIN	5 MIN	1

INGREDIENTS

- 150grams Greek-style yogurt
- 20grams oatmeal
- 60grams fresh persimmons
- 30 milliliters of tap water

DIRECTIONS

1. Put the oatmeal in the pan without any fat.
2. Toast them, constantly stirring, until golden brown.
3. Then put them on a plate and let them cool down briefly.
4. Peel the persimmon and put it in a bowl with the water. Mix the whole thing into a fine puree.
5. Put the yogurt, the toasted oatmeal, and then puree in layers in a glass and serve.

NUTRITIONS

- kcal: 286;
- Carbohydrates: 29 g;
- Protein: 1 g;
- Fat: 11 g

19. SMOOTHIE BOWL WITH SPINACH, MANGO AND MUESLI

PREPARATION	COOKING	SERVES
10 MIN	0 MIN	1

INGREDIENTS

- 150grams yogurt
- 30grams apple
- 30grams mango
- 30grams low carb muesli
- 10grams spinach
- 10grams chia seeds

DIRECTIONS

1. Soak the spinach leaves and let them drain.
2. Peel the mango and cut it into strips.
3. Remove apple core and cut it into pieces.
4. Put everything except the mango together with the yogurt in a blender and make a fine puree out of it.
5. Put the spinach smoothie in a bowl.
6. Add the muesli, chia seeds, and mango. Serve the whole thing

NUTRITIONS

- *kcal: 362;*
- *Carbohydrates: 21 g;*
- *Protein: 12 g;*
- *Fat: 21 g*

20. ALKALINE BLUEBERRY SPELT PANCAKES

PREPARATION	COOKING	SERVES
6 MIN	20 MIN	3

INGREDIENTS

- 2 cups Spelt Flour
- 1 cup Coconut Milk
- 1/2 cup Alkaline Water
- 2 tablespoons Grapeseed Oil
- 1/2 cup Agave
- 1/2 cup Blueberries
- 1/4 teaspoon Sea Moss

DIRECTIONS

1. Mix the spelt flour, agave, grapeseed oil, hemp seeds, and sea moss in a bowl.
2. Add in 1 cup of hemp milk and alkaline water to the mixture until you get the consistency mixture you like.
3. Crimp the blueberries into the batter.
4. Heat the skillet to moderate heat, then lightly coat it with the grapeseed oil.
5. Pour the batter into the skillet, then let them cook for approximately 5 minutes on every side.
6. Serve and Enjoy.

NUTRITIONS

- *Calories: 203 kcal;*
- *Fat: 1.4g;*
- *Carbs: 41.6g;*
- *Proteins: 4.8g*

21. ALKALINE BLUEBERRY MUFFINS

PREPARATION	COOKING	SERVES
10 MIN	20 MIN	3

INGREDIENTS

- 1 cup Coconut Milk
- 3/4 cup Spelt Flour
- 3/4 Teff Flour
- 1/2 cup Blueberries
- 1/3 cup Agave
- 1/4 cup Sea Moss Gel
- 1/2 tsp. Sea Salt
- Grapeseed Oil

DIRECTIONS

1. Adjust the temperature of the oven to 365 degrees.
2. Grease 6 regular-size muffin cups with muffin liners.
3. In a bowl, mix sea salt, sea moss, agave, coconut milk, and flour gel until they are properly blended.
4. You then crimp in blueberries.
5. Coat the muffin pan lightly with the grapeseed oil.
6. Pour in the muffin batter. Bake for at least 30 minutes until it turns golden brown.
7. Serve.

NUTRITIONS

- *Calories: 160 kcal;*
- *Fat: 5g;*
- *Carbs: 25g;*
- *Proteins: 2g*

22. CRUNCHY QUINOA MEAL

PREPARATION	COOKING	SERVES
5 MIN	25 MIN	2

INGREDIENTS

- 3 cups of coconut milk
- 1 cup rinsed quinoa
- 1/8 tsp. ground cinnamon
- 1 cup raspberry
- 1/2 cup chopped coconuts

DIRECTIONS

1. In a saucepan, pour milk and bring to a boil over moderate heat.
2. Add the quinoa to the milk, and then bring it to a boil once more.
3. You then let it simmer for at least 15 minutes on medium heat until the milk is reduced.
4. Stir in the cinnamon, then mix properly.
5. Cover it, then cook for 8 minutes until the milk is completely absorbed.
6. Add the raspberry and cook the meal for 30 seconds.
7. Serve and enjoy.

NUTRITIONS

- Calories: 271 kcal;
- Fat: 3.7g;
- Carbs: 54g;
- Proteins: 6.5g

23. COCONUT PANCAKES

PREPARATION	COOKING	SERVES
5 MIN	15 MIN	4

INGREDIENTS

- 1 cup coconut flour
- 2 tablespoons arrowroot powder
- 1 teaspoon baking powder
- 1 cup of coconut milk
- 3 tablespoons coconut oil

DIRECTIONS

1. In a medium container, mix in all the dry ingredients.
2. Add the coconut milk and 2 tbsps. of the coconut oil, then mix properly.
3. In a skillet, melt 1 tsp of coconut oil.
4. Pour a ladle of the batter into the skillet, then swirl the pan to spread the batter evenly into a smooth pancake.
5. Cook it for like 3 minutes on medium heat until it becomes firm.
6. Turn the pancake to the other side, then cook it for another 2 minutes until it turns golden brown.
7. Cook the remaining pancakes in the same process. Serve.

NUTRITIONS

- *Calories: 377 kcal;*
- *Fat: 14.9g;*
- *Carbs: 60.7g;*
- *Protein: 6.4g*

24. QUINOA PORRIDGE

PREPARATION	COOKING	SERVES
5 MIN	25 MIN	2

INGREDIENTS

- 2 cups of coconut milk
- 1 cup rinsed quinoa
- 1/8 teaspoon ground cinnamon
- 1 cup fresh blueberries

DIRECTIONS

1. In a saucepan, boil the coconut milk over high heat.
2. Add the quinoa to the milk, then bring the mixture to a boil. Let it simmer for 15 minutes on medium heat until the milk is reducing.
3. Add the cinnamon, then mix it properly in the saucepan.
4. Cover the saucepan and cook for at least 8 minutes until the milk is completely absorbed.
5. Add in the blueberries, then cook for 30 more seconds.
6. Serve.

NUTRITIONS

- Calories: 271 kcal;
- Fat: 3.7g;
- Carbs: 54g;
- Protein: 6.5g

25. AMARANTH PORRIDGE

PREPARATION	COOKING	SERVES
5 MIN	30 MIN	2

INGREDIENTS

- 2 cups of coconut milk
- 2 cups alkaline water
- 1 cup amaranth
- 2 tablespoons coconut oil
- 1 tablespoon ground cinnamon

DIRECTIONS

1. In a saucepan, mix the milk with water, then boil the mixture.
2. You stir in the amaranth, then reduce the heat to medium.
3. Cook on medium heat, then let it simmer for at least 30 minutes as you stir it occasionally. Turn off the heat.
4. Add in cinnamon and coconut oil, then stir.
5. Serve.

NUTRITIONS

- Calories: 434 kcal;
- Fat: 35g;
- Carbs: 27g;
- Protein: 6.7g

26. BANANA BARLEY PORRIDGE

PREPARATION	COOKING	SERVES
15 MIN	5 MIN	2

INGREDIENTS

- 1 cup divided unsweetened coconut milk
- 1 small peeled and sliced banana
- 1/2 cup barley
- 3 drops liquid Stevia
- 1/4 cup chopped coconuts

DIRECTIONS

1. In a bowl, properly mix barley with half of the coconut milk and Stevia. Cover the mixing bowl, then refrigerate for about 6 hours.
2. In a saucepan, mix the barley mixture with coconut milk. Cook for about 5 minutes on moderate heat.
3. Then top it with the chopped coconuts and the banana slices. Serve.

NUTRITIONS

- Calories: 159kcal;
- Fat: 8.4g;
- Carbs: 19.8g;
- Proteins: 4.6g

27. ZUCCHINI MUFFINS

PREPARATION	COOKING	SERVES
10 MIN	25 MIN	16

INGREDIENTS

- 1 tablespoon ground flaxseed
- 3 tablespoons. alkaline water
- 1/4 cup walnut butter
- 3 medium over-ripe bananas
- 2 small grated zucchinis
- 1/2 cup coconut milk
- 1 teaspoon vanilla extract
- 2 cups coconut flour
- 1 tablespoon baking powder
- 1 teaspoon cinnamon
- 1/4 teaspoon sea salt

DIRECTIONS

1. Tune the temperature of your oven to 375°F.
2. Grease the muffin tray with the cooking spray.
3. In a bowl, mix the flaxseed with water.
4. In a glass bowl, mash the bananas, then stir in the remaining ingredients.
5. Properly mix and then divide the mixture into the muffin tray.
6. Bake it for 25 minutes. Serve.

NUTRITIONS

- *Calories: 127 kcal;*
- *Fat: 6.6g;*
- *Carbs: 13g;*
- *Protein: 0.7g*

28. MILLET PORRIDGE

PREPARATION	COOKING	SERVES
10 MIN	20 MIN	2

INGREDIENTS

- Sea salt
- 1 tbsp. finely chopped coconuts
- 1/2 cup unsweetened coconut milk
- 1/2 cup rinsed and drained millet
- 1-1/2 cups alkaline water
- 3 drops liquid Stevia

DIRECTIONS

1. Sauté the millet in a non-stick skillet for about 3 minutes. Add salt and water, then stir.
2. Let the meal boil, then reduce the amount of heat.
3. Cook for 15 minutes, then add the remaining ingredients. Stir.
4. Cook the meal for 4 extra minutes.
5. Serve the meal with a topping of the chopped nuts.

NUTRITIONS

- Calories: 219 kcal;
- Fat: 4.5g;
- Carbs: 38.2g;
- Protein: 6.4g

29. JACKFRUIT VEGETABLE FRY

PREPARATION	COOKING	SERVES
5 MIN	5 MIN	6

INGREDIENTS

- 2 finely chopped small onions
- 2 cups finely chopped cherry tomatoes
- 1/8 teaspoon ground turmeric
- 1 tablespoon olive oil
- 2 seeded and chopped red bell peppers
- 3 cups seeded and chopped firm jackfruit
- 1/8 teaspoon cayenne pepper
- 2 tablespoons chopped fresh basil leaves
- Salt

DIRECTIONS

1. In a greased skillet, sauté the onions and bell peppers for about 5 minutes.
2. Add the tomatoes, then stir. Cook for 2 minutes.
3. Then add the jackfruit, cayenne pepper, salt, and turmeric. Cook for about 8 minutes.
4. Garnish the meal with basil leaves.
5. Serve warm.

NUTRITIONS

- *Calories: 236 kcal;*
- *Fat: 1.8g;*
- *Carbs: 48.3g;*
- *Protein: 7g*

30. ZUCCHINI PANCAKES

PREPARATION	COOKING	SERVES
15 MIN	8 MIN	8

INGREDIENTS

- 12 tbsps. alkaline water
- 6 large grated zucchinis
- Sea salt
- 4 tbsps. ground Flax Seeds
- 2 tsp. olive oil
- 2 finely chopped jalapeño peppers
- 1/2 cup finely chopped scallions

DIRECTIONS

1. In a bowl, mix water and the flax seeds, then set it aside.
2. Pour oil into a large non-stick skillet, then heat it on medium heat.
3. Then add the black pepper, salt, and zucchini.
4. Cook for 3 minutes, then transfer the zucchini into a large bowl.
5. Add the flaxseed and the scallion mixture, then properly mix it.
6. Preheat a griddle, then grease it lightly with the cooking spray.
7. Pour 1/4 of the zucchini mixture into the griddle, then cook for 3 minutes.
8. Flip the side carefully, then cook for 2 more minutes.
9. Repeat the procedure with the remaining mixture in batches.
10. Serve.

NUTRITIONS

- Calories: 71 kcal;
- Fat: 2.8g;
- Carbs: 9.8g;
- Protein: 3.7g

31. SQUASH HASH

PREPARATION	COOKING	SERVES
2 MIN	10 MIN	2

INGREDIENTS

- 1 tsp. onion powder
- 1/2 cup finely chopped onion
- 2 cups spaghetti squash
- 1/2 tsp. sea salt

DIRECTIONS

1. Using paper towels, squeeze extra moisture from spaghetti squash.
2. Place the squash into a bowl, then add the salt, onion, and the onion powder. Stir properly to mix them.
3. Spray a non-stick cooking skillet with cooking spray, then place it over moderate heat.
4. Add the spaghetti squash to the pan. Cook the squash for about 5 minutes.
5. Flip the hash browns using a spatula.
6. Cook for 5 minutes until the desired crispness is reached.
7. Serve.

NUTRITIONS

- *Calories: 44 kcal;*
- *Fat: 0.6g;*
- *Carbs: 9.7g;*
- *Protein: 0.9g*

32. HEMP SEED PORRIDGE

PREPARATION	COOKING	SERVES
5 MIN	6 MIN	6

INGREDIENTS

- 3 cups cooked hemp seed
- 1 packet Stevia
- 1 cup of coconut milk

DIRECTIONS

1. In a saucepan, mix the rice and the coconut milk over moderate heat for about 5 minutes as you stir it constantly.
2. Remove the pan from the burner, then add the Stevia. Stir.
3. Serve in 6 bowls. Enjoy.

NUTRITIONS

- Calories: 236 kcal;
- Fat: 1.8g;
- Carbs: 48.3g
- Protein: 7g

33. PUMPKIN SPICE QUINOA

PREPARATION	COOKING	SERVES
10 MIN	0 MIN	2

INGREDIENTS

- 1 cup cooked quinoa
- 1 cup unsweetened coconut milk
- 1 large mashed banana
- 1/4 cup pumpkin puree
- 1 tsp. pumpkin spice
- 2 tsp. chia seeds

DIRECTIONS

1. In a container, mix all the ingredients.
2. Seal the lid, then shake the container properly to mix.
3. Refrigerate overnight.
4. Serve.

NUTRITIONS

- Calories: 212 kcal;
- Fat: 11.9g;
- Carbs: 31.7g;
- Protein: 7.3g

34. SCRAMBLED EGGS WITH SOY SAUCE AND BROCCOLI SLAW

PREPARATION	COOKING	SERVES
5 MIN	10 MIN	2

INGREDIENTS

- 1 tablespoon peanut oil, divided
- 4 large eggs
- ½ to 1 tablespoon soy sauce, tamari, or Bragg's liquid aminos
- 1 tablespoon water
- 1 cup shredded broccoli slaw or other shredded vegetables
- Kosher salt
- Chopped fresh cilantro for serving
- Hot sauce, for serving

DIRECTIONS

1. In a medium non-stick skillet or cast-iron skillet over medium heat, heat 2 teaspoons of peanut oil, swirling to coat the skillet.
2. In a small bowl, whip the eggs, soy sauce, and water until smooth. Pour the eggs into the pan and let the bottom set. Using a wooden spoon, spread the eggs from one side to the other a couple of times so the uncooked portions on top pool into the bottom. Cook until the eggs are set.
3. In a medium container, stir together the broccoli slaw, the remaining 1 teaspoon of peanut oil, and a salt touch. Divide the slaw between 2 plates.
4. Top with the eggs and scatter cilantro on each serving. Serve with hot sauce.

NUTRITIONS

- Calories: 22g;
- Total fat: 4g;
- Cholesterol: 374mg;
- Fiber: 2g;
- Protein: 12g;
- Sodium: 737mg

35. MANGO COCONUT OATMEAL

PREPARATION	COOKING	SERVES
5 MIN	5 MIN	2

INGREDIENTS

- 1½ cups water
- ½ cup 5-minute steel cut oats
- ¼ cup unsweetened canned coconut milk, plus more for serving (optional)
- 1 tablespoon pure maple syrup
- 1 teaspoon sesame seeds
- Dash ground cinnamon
- 1 mango, stripped, pitted, and divide into slices
- 1 tablespoon unsweetened coconut flakes

DIRECTIONS

1. In a frying pan over high heat, boil water. Put the oats and lower the heat. Cook, occasionally stirring, for 5 minutes.
2. Put in the coconut milk, maple syrup, and salt to combine.
3. Get two bowls and sprinkle with the sesame seeds and cinnamon. Top with sliced mango and coconut flakes.

NUTRITIONS

- Calories: 373;
- Total fat: 11g;
- Cholesterol: 0mg;
- Fiber: 2g;
- Protein: 12g;
- Sodium: 167mg

36. WHOLE-WHEAT BLUEBERRY MUFFINS

PREPARATION	COOKING	SERVES
5 MIN	25 MIN	8

INGREDIENTS

- 1/2 cup plant-based milk
- 1/2 cup unsweetened applesauce
- 1/2 cup maple syrup
- 1 teaspoon vanilla extract
- 2 cups whole-wheat flour
- 1/2 teaspoon baking soda
- 1 cup blueberries

DIRECTIONS

1. Preheat the oven to 375°F.
2. In a large bowl, mix the milk, applesauce, maple syrup, and vanilla.
3. Stir in the flour and baking soda until no dry flour is left, and the batter is smooth.
4. Gently fold in the blueberries until they are evenly distributed throughout the batter.
5. In a muffin tin, fill 8 muffin cups three-quarters full of batter.
6. Bake for 25 minutes, or until you can stick a knife into the center of a muffin and it comes out clean. Allow cooling before serving.

Tip: Both frozen and fresh blueberries will work great in this recipe. The only difference will be that muffins using fresh blueberries will cook slightly quicker than those using frozen.

NUTRITIONS

- Fat: 1 g;
- Carbohydrates: 45 g;
- Fiber: 2 g;
- Protein: 4 g

37. WALNUT CRUNCH BANANA BREAD

PREPARATION	COOKING	SERVES
5 MIN	1H 30 MIN	1

INGREDIENTS

- 4 ripe bananas
- 1/4 cup maple syrup
- 1 tablespoon apple cider vinegar
- 1 teaspoon vanilla extract
- 11/2 cups whole-wheat flour
- 1/2 teaspoon ground cinnamon
- 1/2 teaspoon baking soda
- 1/4 cup walnut pieces (optional)

DIRECTIONS

1. Preheat the oven to 350°F.
2. In a large bowl, use a fork or mixing spoon to mash the bananas until they reach a puréed consistency (small bits of banana are acceptable). Stir in the maple syrup, apple cider vinegar, and vanilla.
3. Stir in the flour, cinnamon, and baking soda. Fold in the walnut pieces (if using).
4. Gently pour the batter into a loaf pan, filling it no more than three-quarters of the way full. Bake for 1 hour, or until you can stick a knife into the middle and it comes out clean.
5. Transfer from the oven then let cooling on the countertop for a minimum of 30 minutes before serving.

NUTRITIONS

- Fat: 1g;
- Carbohydrates: 40 g;
- Fiber: 5 g;
- Protein: 4 g

38. PLANT-POWERED PANCAKES

PREPARATION	COOKING	SERVES
5 MIN	15 MIN	8

INGREDIENTS

- 1 cup whole-wheat flour
- 1 teaspoon baking powder
- 1/2 teaspoon ground cinnamon
- 1 cup plant-based milk
- 1/2 cup unsweetened applesauce
- 1/4 cup maple syrup
- 1 teaspoon vanilla extract

DIRECTIONS

1. In a large bowl, combine the flour, baking powder, and cinnamon.
2. Stir in the milk, applesauce, maple syrup, and vanilla until no dry flour is left and the batter is smooth.
3. Heat a large, non-stick skillet or griddle over medium heat. For each pancake, pour 1/4 cup of batter onto the hot skillet. Once bubbles form over the top of the pancake and the sides begin to brown, flip and cook for 1 to 2 minutes more.
4. Repeat until all of the batters are used, and serve.

NUTRITIONS

- *Fat: 2 g;*
- *Carbohydrates: 44 g;*
- *Fiber: 5 g;*
- *Protein: 5 g*

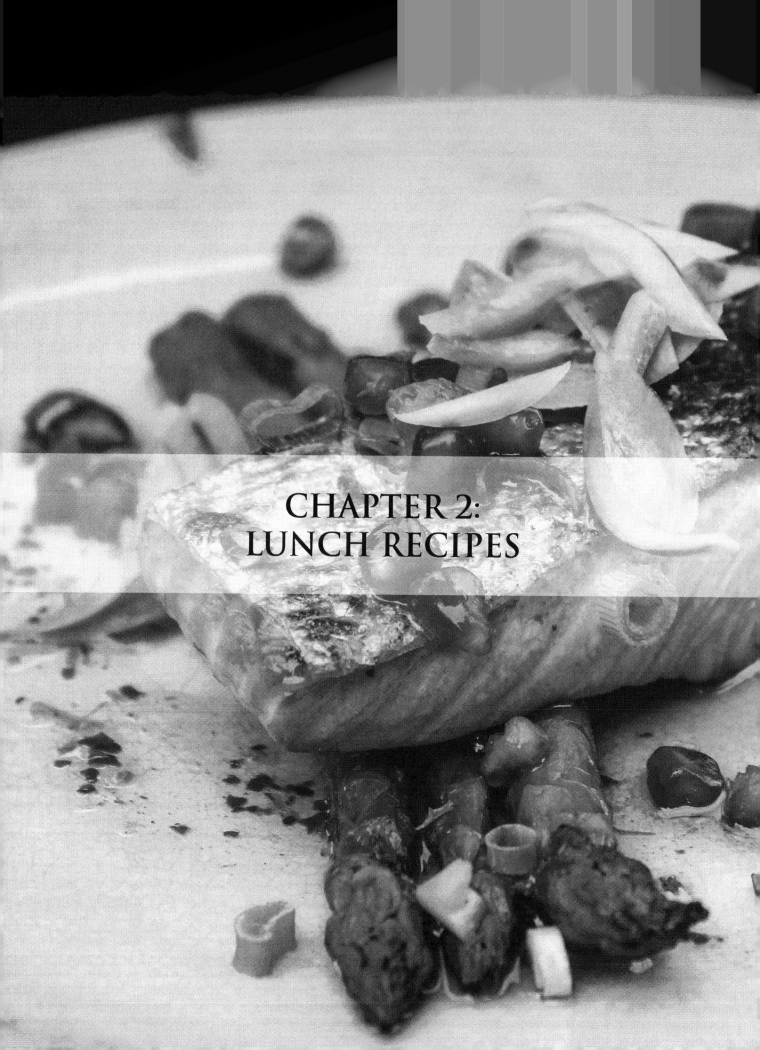

CHAPTER 2:
LUNCH RECIPES

39. BOK CHOY WITH TOFU STIR FRY

PREPARATION	COOKING	SERVES
15 MIN	15 MIN	4

INGREDIENTS

- Super-firm tofu: 1 lb. (drained and pressed)
- Coconut oil; one tablespoon
- Clove of garlic; 1 (minced)
- Baby bok choy; 3 heads (chopped)
- Low-sodium vegetable broth.
- Maple syrup; 2 teaspoons
- Bragg's liquid aminos
- Sambal oelek; 1 to 2 teaspoons (similar chili sauce)
- Scallion or green onion; 1 (chopped)
- Freshly grated ginger; 1 teaspoon
- Quinoa/rice, for serving

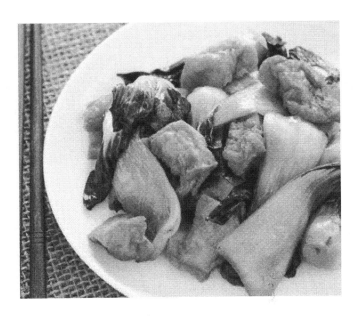

DIRECTIONS

1. With paper towels, Pat pressed the tofu dry and cut it into tiny pieces of bite-size around 1/2 inch wide.
2. Heat coconut oil in a wide skillet onto a warm.
3. Remove tofu and stir-fry until painted softly.
4. Stir-fry for 1-2 minutes before the choy of the Bok starts to wilt.
5. When this occurs, you'll want to apply the vegetable broth and all the remaining ingredients to the skillet.
6. Hold the mixture stir-frying until all components are well coated and the bulk of the liquid evaporates, around 5-6 minutes.
7. Serve over brown rice or quinoa.

NUTRITIONS

- Calories: 263.7 Cal;
- Fat 4.2 g;
- Cholesterol: 0.3 mg;
- Sodium: 683.6 mg;
- Potassium: 313.7 mg;
- Carbohydrate: 35.7 g

40. SALMON WITH VEGETABLES

PREPARATION	COOKING	SERVES
10 MIN	15 MIN	4

INGREDIENTS

- 2 tablespoons olive oil
- 2 carrots
- 1 head fennel
- 2 squash
- ¼ onion
- 1-inch ginger
- 1 cup white wine
- 2 cups of water
- 2 parsley sprigs
- 2 tarragon sprigs
- 6 oz. salmon fillets
- 1 cup cherry tomatoes
- 1 scallion

DIRECTIONS

1. In a skillet, heat olive oil, add fennel, squash, onion, ginger, carrot and cook until vegetables are soft
2. Add wine, water, parsley and cook for another 4-5 minutes
3. Season salmon fillets and place in the pan
4. Cook for 4-5 minutes per side or until it is ready
5. Transfer salmon to a bowl, spoon tomatoes and scallion around salmon and serve

NUTRITIONS

- Calories: 301;
- Total Carbohydrate: 2 g;
- Cholesterol: 13 mg;
- Total Fat: 17 g;
- Fiber: 4 g;
- Protein: 8 g;
- Sodium: 201 mg

41. EASIEST TUNA COBBLER EVER

PREPARATION	COOKING	SERVES
15 MIN	25 MIN	4

INGREDIENTS

- Water, cold (1/3 cup)
- Tuna, canned, drained (10 ounces)
- Sweet pickle relish (2 tablespoons)
- Mixed vegetables, frozen (1 ½ cups)
- Soup, cream of chicken, condensed (10 ¾ ounces)
- Pimientos, sliced, drained (2 ounces)
- Lemon juice (1 teaspoon)
- Paprika

DIRECTIONS

1. Preheat the air fryer at 375 degrees Fahrenheit.
2. Mist cooking spray into a round casserole (1 ½ quart).
3. Mix the frozen vegetables with milk, soup, lemon juice, relish, pimientos, and tuna in a saucepan. Cook for six to eight minutes over medium heat.
4. Fill the casserole with the tuna mixture.
5. Mix the biscuit mix with cold water to form a soft dough. Beat for half a minute before dropping by four spoonsful into the casserole.
6. Dust the dish with paprika before air-frying for twenty to twenty-five minutes.

NUTRITIONS

- *Calories 320;*
- *Fat 10 g;*
- *Protein 20 g;*
- *Carbohydrates 30 g*

42. DELICIOUSLY HOMEMADE PORK BUNS

PREPARATION	COOKING	SERVES
20 MIN	25 MIN	8

INGREDIENTS

- Green onions, sliced thinly (3 pieces)
- Egg, beaten (1 piece)
- Pulled pork, diced, w/ barbecue sauce (1 cup)
- Buttermilk biscuits, refrigerated (16 1/3 ounces)
- Soy sauce (1 teaspoon)

DIRECTIONS

1. Preheat the air fryer at 325 degrees Fahrenheit.
2. Use parchment paper to line your baking sheet.
3. Combine pork with green onions.
4. Separate and press the dough to form 8 four-inch rounds.
5. Fill each biscuit round's center with two tablespoons of pork mixture. Cover with the dough edges and seal by pinching. Arrange the buns on the sheet and brush with a mixture of soy sauce and egg.
6. Cook in the air fryer for twenty to twenty-five minutes.

NUTRITIONS

- Calories 240;
- Fat 0 g;
- Protein 0 g;
- Carbohydrates 20 g

43. PEPPER PESTO LAMB

PREPARATION	COOKING	SERVES
15 MIN	1H 15 MIN	12

INGREDIENTS

Pesto:
- Rosemary leaves, fresh (1/4 cup)
- Garlic cloves (3 pieces)
- Parsley, fresh, packed firmly (3/4 cup)
- Mint leaves, fresh (1/4 cup)
- Olive oil (2 tablespoons)

Lamb:
- Red bell peppers, roasted, drained (7 ½ ounces)
- Leg of lamb, boneless, rolled (5 pounds)
- Seasoning, lemon pepper (2 teaspoons)

DIRECTIONS

1. Preheat the oven to 325 degrees Fahrenheit.
2. Mix the pesto ingredients in the food processor.
3. Unroll the lamb and cover the cut side with pesto. Top with roasted peppers before rolling up the lamb and tying with kitchen twine.
4. Coat lamb with seasoning (lemon pepper) and air-fry for one hour.

NUTRITIONS

- *Calories 310;*
- *Fat 10 g;*
- *Protein 40.0 g;*
- *Carbohydrates 0 g*

44. CHICKEN GOULASH

PREPARATION	COOKING	SERVES
10 MIN	17 MIN	6

INGREDIENTS

- 4 oz. chive stems
- 2 green peppers, chopped
- 1 teaspoon olive oil
- 14 oz. ground chicken
- 2 tomatoes
- ½ cup chicken stock
- 2 garlic cloves, sliced
- 1 teaspoon salt
- 1 teaspoon ground black pepper
- 1 teaspoon mustard

DIRECTIONS

1. Chop chives roughly.
2. Spray the air fryer basket tray with the olive oil.
3. Preheat the air fryer to 365 F.
4. Put the chopped chives in the air fryer basket tray.
5. Add the chopped green pepper and cook the vegetables for 5 minutes.
6. Add the ground chicken.
7. Chop the tomatoes into small cubes and add them to the air fryer mixture too.
8. Cook the mixture for 6 minutes more.
9. Add the chicken stock, sliced garlic cloves, salt, ground black pepper, and mustard.
10. Mix well to combine.
11. Cook the goulash for 6 minutes more.

NUTRITIONS

- *Calories: 161;*
- *Fat: 6.1g;*
- *Carbs: 6g;*
- *Protein: 20.3g*

45. GRILLED MAHI MAHI WITH JICAMA SLAW

PREPARATION	COOKING	SERVES
20 MIN	10 MIN	4

INGREDIENTS

- 1 teaspoon each for pepper and salt, divided
- 1 tablespoon of lime juice, divided
- 2 tablespoon + 2 teaspoons of extra virgin olive oil
- 4 raw mahi-mahi fillets, which should be about 8 oz. each
- ½ cucumber, which should be thinly cut into long strips like matchsticks (it should yield about 1 cup)
- 1 jicama, which should be thinly cut into long strips like matchsticks (it should yield about 3 cups)
- 1 cup of alfalfa sprouts
- 2 cups of coarsely chopped watercress

DIRECTIONS

1. Combine ½ teaspoon of both pepper and salt, 1 teaspoon of lime juice, and 2 teaspoons of oil in a small bowl. Then brush the mahi-mahi fillets all through with the olive oil mixture.
2. Grill the mahi-mahi on medium-high heat until it becomes done in about 5 minutes, turn it to the other side, and let it be done for about 5 minutes. (You will have an internal temperature of about 1450F).
3. For the slaw, combine the watercress, cucumber, jicama, and alfalfa sprouts in a bowl. Now combine ½ teaspoon of both pepper and salt, 2 teaspoons of lime juice, and 2 tablespoons of extra virgin oil in a small bowl. Drizzle it over slaw and toss together to combine.

NUTRITIONS

- Calories: 320;
- Protein: 44g;
- Carbohydrate: 10g;
- Fat: 11 g

46. PORK CACCIATORE

PREPARATION	COOKING	SERVES
10 MIN	6 HOURS	6

INGREDIENTS

- 1 ½ lb. pork chops
- 1 teaspoon dried oregano
- 1 cup beef broth
- 3 tablespoon tomato paste
- 14 oz. can tomato, diced
- 2 cups mushrooms, sliced
- 1 small onion, diced
- 1 garlic clove, minced
- 2 tablespoon olive oil
- ¼ teaspoon pepper
- ½ teaspoon salt

DIRECTIONS

1. Heat oil in a pan over medium heat.
2. Add pork chops to the pan and cook until brown on both sides.
3. Transfer pork chops into the crockpot.
4. Pour remaining ingredients over the pork chops.
5. Cover and cook on low heat for 6 hours.
6. Serve and enjoy.

NUTRITIONS

- Calories: 440;
- Fat: 33 g;
- Carbohydrates: 6 g;
- Sugar: 3 g;
- Protein: 28 g;
- Cholesterol: 97 mg

47. PORK WITH TOMATO & OLIVES

PREPARATION	COOKING	SERVES
10 MIN	30 MIN	6

INGREDIENTS

- 6 pork chops, boneless and cut into thick slices
- 1/8 teaspoon ground cinnamon
- 1/2 cup olives, pitted and sliced
- 8 oz. can tomato, crushed
- 1/4 cup beef broth
- 2 garlic cloves, chopped
- 1 large onion, sliced
- 1 tablespoon olive oil

DIRECTIONS

1. Heat olive oil in a pan over medium heat.
2. Place pork chops in a pan and cook until lightly brown and set aside.
3. Cook onion and garlic in the same pan over medium heat, until onion is softened.
4. Add broth and bring to boil over high heat.
5. Return pork to pan and stir in crushed tomatoes and remaining ingredients.
6. Cover and simmer for 20 minutes.
7. Serve and enjoy.

NUTRITIONS

- *Calories: 321;*
- *Fat: 23 g;*
- *Carbohydrates: 7 g;*
- *Sugar: 1 g;*
- *Protein: 19 g;*
- *Cholesterol: 70 mg*

48. PORK ROAST

PREPARATION	COOKING	SERVES
10 MIN	1H 35 MIN	6

INGREDIENTS

- 3 lbs. pork roast, boneless
- 1 cup of water
- 1 onion, chopped
- 3 garlic cloves, chopped
- 1 tablespoon black pepper
- 1 rosemary sprig
- 2 fresh oregano sprigs
- 2 fresh thyme sprigs
- 1 tablespoon olive oil
- 1 tablespoon kosher salt

DIRECTIONS

1. Preheat the oven to 350 F.
2. Season pork roast with pepper and salt.
3. Heat olive oil in a stockpot and sear pork roast on each side, about 4 minutes.
4. Add onion and garlic. Pour in the water, oregano, and thyme and bring to boil for a minute.
5. Cover pot and roast in the preheated oven for 1 1/2 hours. Serve and enjoy.

NUTRITIONS

- *Calories: 502;*
- *Fat: 23.8 g;*
- *Carbohydrates: 3 g;*
- *Sugar: 0.8 g;*
- *Protein: 65 g;*
- *Cholesterol: 195 mg*

49. SALMON BURGERS

PREPARATION	COOKING	SERVES
10 MIN	15 MIN	4

INGREDIENTS

- 1 lb. salmon fillets
- 1 onion
- ¼ dill fronds
- 1 tablespoon honey
- 1 tablespoon horseradish
- 1 tablespoon mustard
- 1 tablespoon olive oil
- 2 toasted split rolls
- 1 avocado

DIRECTIONS

1. Place salmon fillets in a blender and blend until smooth, transfer to a bowl, add onion, dill, honey, horseradish and mix well
2. Season with salt and pepper then make 4 patties
3. In a bowl, combine mustard, honey, mayonnaise and dill
4. In a skillet, heat oil, add salmon patties and cook for 2-3 minutes per side
5. When ready, remove from heat
6. Divided lettuce and onion between the buns
7. Place salmon patty on top and spoon mustard mixture and avocado slices
8. Serve when ready

NUTRITIONS

- Calories: 189;
- Total Carbohydrate: 6 g;
- Cholesterol: 3 mg;
- Total Fat: 7g;
- Fiber: 4 g;
- Protein: 12 g;
- Sodium: 293 mg

50. SEARED SCALLOPS

PREPARATION	COOKING	SERVES
15 MIN	20 MIN	4

INGREDIENTS

- 1 lb. sea scallops
- 1 tablespoon canola oil

DIRECTIONS

1. Season scallops and refrigerate for a couple of minutes
2. In a skillet, heat oil, add scallops and cook for 1-2 minutes per side
3. When ready, remove from heat and serve

NUTRITIONS

- *Calories: 283;*
- *Total Carbohydrate: 10 g;*
- *Cholesterol: 3 mg;*
- *Total Fat: 8 g;*
- *Fiber: 2 g;*
- *Protein: 9 g;*
- *Sodium: 271 mg*

51. BLACK COD

PREPARATION	COOKING	SERVES
15 MIN	20 MIN	4

INGREDIENTS

- ¼ cup miso paste
- ¼ cup sake
- 1 tablespoon mirin
- 1 teaspoon soy sauce
- 1 tablespoon olive oil
- 4 black cod fillets

DIRECTIONS

1. In a bowl, combine miso, soy sauce, oil and sake
2. Rub mixture over cod fillets and let it marinate for 20-30 minutes
3. Adjust broiler and broil cod filets for 10-12 minutes
4. When fish is cook remove and serve

NUTRITIONS

- Calories: 231;
- Total Carbohydrate: 2 g;
- Cholesterol: 13 mg;
- Total Fat: 15 g;
- Fiber: 2 g;
- Protein: 8 g;
- Sodium: 298 mg

52. MISO-GLAZED SALMON

PREPARATION	COOKING	SERVES
10 MIN	40 MIN	4

INGREDIENTS

- ¼ cup red miso
- ¼ cup sake
- 1 tablespoon soy sauce
- 1 tablespoon vegetable oil
- 4 salmon fillets

DIRECTIONS

1. In a bowl, combine sake, oil, soy sauce and miso
2. Rub mixture over salmon fillets and marinate for 20-30 minutes
3. Preheat a broiler
4. Broil salmon for 5-10 minutes
5. When ready, remove and serve

NUTRITIONS

- *Calories: 198;*
- *Total Carbohydrate: 5 g;*
- *Cholesterol: 12 mg;*
- *Total Fat: 10 g;*
- *Fiber: 2 g;*
- *Protein: 6 g;*
- *Sodium: 257 mg*

53. CUCUMBER-BASIL SALSA ON HALIBUT POUCHES

PREPARATION	COOKING	SERVES
10 MIN	17 MIN	4

INGREDIENTS

- 1 lime, thinly sliced into 8 pieces
- 2 cups mustard greens, stems removed
- 2 teaspoon olive oil
- 4 – 5 radishes trimmed and quartered
- 4 4-oz skinless halibut filets
- 4 large fresh basil leaves
- Cayenne pepper to taste – optional
- Pepper and salt to taste

Salsa Ingredients:
- 1 ½ cups diced cucumber
- 1 ½ finely chopped fresh basil leaves
- 2 teaspoons fresh lime juice
- Pepper and salt to taste

DIRECTIONS

1. Preheat oven to 400oF
2. Prepare parchment papers by making 4 pieces of 15 x 12-inch rectangles. Lengthwise, fold in half and unfold pieces on the table.
3. Season halibut fillets with pepper, salt and cayenne—if using cayenne.
4. Just to the right of the fold, place ½ cup of mustard greens. Add a basil leaf on the center of mustard greens and topped with 1 lime slice. Around the greens, layer ¼ of the radishes. Drizzle with ½ teaspoon of oil, season with pepper and salt. Top it with a slice of halibut fillet.
5. Just as you would make a calzone, fold the parchment paper over your filling and crimp the edges of the parchment paper beginning from one end to the other end. To seal the end of the crimped parchment paper, pinch it.
6. Repeat the remaining ingredients until you have 4 pieces of parchment papers filled with halibut and greens.
7. Place pouches in a pan and bake in the oven until halibut is flaky around 15 to 17 minutes.
8. While waiting for halibut pouches to cook, make your salsa by mixing all salsa ingredients in a medium bowl.
9. Once halibut is cooked, please remove it from the oven and make a tear on top. Be careful of the steam as it is very hot. Equally, divide salsa and spoon ¼ of salsa on top of halibut through the slit you have created.

NUTRITIONS

- Calories: 335.4
- Protein: 20.2g
- Fat: 16.3g
- Carbs: 22.1g

54. CURRY SALMON WITH MUSTARD

PREPARATION	COOKING	SERVES
10 MIN	8 MIN	4

INGREDIENTS

- ¼ teaspoon ground red pepper or chili powder
- ¼ teaspoon ground turmeric
- ¼ teaspoon salt
- 1 teaspoon honey
- 1/8 teaspoon garlic powder or a minced clove garlic
- 2 teaspoons. whole grain mustard
- 4 pcs 6-oz salmon fillets

DIRECTIONS

1. In a small bowl, mix salt, garlic powder, red pepper, turmeric, honey and mustard.
2. Preheat oven to broil and grease a baking dish with cooking spray.
3. Place salmon on a baking dish with skin side down and spread evenly mustard mixture on top of salmon.
4. Pop in the oven and broil until flaky, around 8 minutes.

NUTRITIONS

- Calories: 324;
- Fat: 18.9 g;
- Protein: 34 g;
- Carbs: 2.9 g

55. DIJON MUSTARD AND LIME MARINATED SHRIMP

PREPARATION	COOKING	SERVES
10 MIN	10 MIN	8

INGREDIENTS

- ½ cup fresh lime juice and lime zest as garnish
- ½ cup of rice vinegar
- ½ teaspoon hot sauce
- 1 bay leaf
- 1 cup of water
- 1 lb. uncooked shrimp, peeled and deveined
- 1 medium red onion, chopped
- 2 tablespoon capers
- 2 tablespoon Dijon mustard
- 3 whole cloves

DIRECTIONS

1. Mix hot sauce, mustard, capers, lime juice and onion in a shallow baking dish and set aside.
2. Bring to a boil in a large saucepan bay leaf, cloves, vinegar and water.
3. Once boiling, add shrimps and cook for a minute while stirring continuously.
4. Drain shrimps and pour shrimps into onion mixture.
5. For an hour, refrigerate while covered the shrimps.
6. Then serve shrimps cold and garnished with lime zest.

NUTRITIONS

- *Calories: 232.2;*
- *Protein: 17.8g;*
- *Fat: 3g;*
- *Carbs: 15g*

56. WW SALAD IN A JAR

PREPARATION	COOKING	SERVES
10 MIN	5 MIN	1

INGREDIENTS

- 1-ounce favorite greens
- 1-ounce red bell pepper; chopped.
- 4 ounces' rotisserie chicken; roughly chopped.
- 4 tablespoons extra virgin olive oil
- 1/2 scallion; chopped.
- 1-ounce cucumber; chopped.
- 1-ounce cherry tomatoes; halved
- Salt and black pepper to the taste.

DIRECTIONS

1. In a bowl, mix greens with bell pepper, tomatoes, scallion, cucumber, salt, pepper and olive oil and toss to coat well.
2. Transfer this to a jar, top with chicken pieces and serve for breakfast.

NUTRITIONS

- Calories: 180
- Fat: 12
- Fiber: 4
- Carbs: 5
- Protein: 17

57. YUMMY SMOKED SALMON

PREPARATION	COOKING	SERVES
10 MIN	10 MIN	3

INGREDIENTS

- 4 eggs; whisked
- 1/2 teaspoon avocado oil
- 4 ounces smoked salmon; chopped

For the sauce:
- 1/2 cup cashews; soaked; drained
- 1/4 cup green onions; chopped.
- 1 teaspoon garlic powder
- 1 cup of coconut milk
- 1 tablespoon lemon juice
- Salt and black pepper to the taste

DIRECTIONS

1. In your blender, mix cashews with coconut milk, garlic powder and lemon juice and blend well.
2. Add salt, pepper and green onions, blend again well, transfer to a bowl and keep in the fridge for now.
3. Heat a pan with the oil over medium-low heat; add eggs, whisk a bit and cook until they are almost done
4. Introduce in your preheated broiler and cook until eggs set.
5. Divide eggs on plates, top with smoked salmon and serve with the green onion sauce on top.

NUTRITIONS

- *Calories: 200*
- *Fat: 10*
- *Fiber: 2*
- *Carbs: 11*
- *Protein: 15*

58. ASPARAGUS FRITTATA RECIPE

PREPARATION	COOKING	SERVES
20 MIN	20 MIN	4

INGREDIENTS

- Bacon slices, chopped: 4
- Salt and black pepper
- Eggs (whisked): 8
- Asparagus (trimmed and chopped): 1 bunch
-

DIRECTIONS

1. Heat a pan, add bacon, stir and cook for 5 minutes.
2. Add asparagus, salt, and pepper, stir and cook for another 5 minutes.
3. Add the chilled eggs, spread them in the pan, let them stand in the oven and bake for 20 minutes at 350° F.
4. Share and divide between plates and serve for breakfast.

NUTRITIONS

- Calories 251
- Carbs 16
- Fat 6
- Fiber 8
- Protein 7

59. AVOCADOS STUFFED WITH SALMON

PREPARATION	COOKING	SERVES
5 MIN	5 MIN	2

INGREDIENTS

- Avocado (pitted and halved): 1
- Olive oil: 2 tablespoons
- Lemon juice: 1
- Smoked salmon (flaked): 2 ounces
- Goat cheese (crumbled): 1 ounce
- Salt and black pepper

DIRECTIONS

1. Combine the salmon with lemon juice, oil, cheese, salt, and pepper in your food processor and pulsate well.
2. Divide this mixture into avocado halves and serve.
3. Dish and Enjoy!

NUTRITIONS

- Calories: 300
- Fat: 15
- Fiber: 5
- Carbs: 8
- Protein: 16

60. ONION AND ZUCCHINI PLATTER

PREPARATION	COOKING	SERVES
15 MIN	45 MIN	4

INGREDIENTS

- 3 large zucchinis, julienned
- 1 cup cherry tomatoes, halved
- 1/2 cup basil
- 2 red onions, thinly sliced
- 1/4 teaspoon salt
- 1 teaspoon cayenne pepper
- 2 tablespoons lemon juice

DIRECTIONS

1. Create zucchini Zoodles by using a vegetable peeler and shaving the zucchini with a peeler lengthwise until you get to the core and seeds
2. Turn zucchini and repeat until you have long strips. Discard seeds
3. Lay strips on a cutting board and slice lengthwise to your desired thickness
4. Mix Zoodles in a bowl alongside onion, basil, tomatoes, and toss
5. Sprinkle salt and cayenne pepper on top. Drizzle lemon juice
6. Serve and enjoy!

NUTRITIONS

- Calories: 156
- Fat: 8g
- Carbohydrates: 6g
- Protein: 7g

61. LEMON FLAVORED SPROUTS

PREPARATION	COOKING	SERVES
10 MIN	0 MIN	4

INGREDIENTS

- 1-pound Brussel sprouts, trimmed and shredded
- 8 tablespoons olive oil
- 1 lemon, juiced and zested
- Salt and pepper to taste
- 3/4 cup spicy almond and seed mix

DIRECTIONS

1. Take a bowl and mix in lemon juice, salt, pepper and olive oil
2. Mix well
3. Stir in shredded Brussel sprouts and toss
4. Let it sit for 10 minutes
5. Add nuts and toss

NUTRITIONS

- Calories: 382
- Fat: 36g
- Carbohydrates: 9g
- Protein: 7g

62. AVOCADO AND CAPRESE SALAD

PREPARATION	COOKING	SERVES
15 MIN	19 MIN	6

INGREDIENTS

- 2 avocados, cubed
- 1 cup cherry tomatoes, halved
- 8 ounces cashew cheese
- 2 tablespoons finely chopped fresh basil
- 2 tablespoons olive oil
- 2 tablespoons balsamic vinegar
- 1 tablespoon salt
- Fresh ground black pepper

DIRECTIONS

1. Take a bowl and add the listed ingredient.
2. Toss them well until thoroughly mixed
3. Season with pepper according to your taste
4. Serve and enjoy!

NUTRITIONS

- Calories: 358
- Fat: 30g
- Carbohydrates: 9g
- Protein: 14g

63. CILANTRO AND KIDNEY BEANS

PREPARATION	COOKING	SERVES
6 MIN	0 MIN	4

INGREDIENTS

- 1 can (15 ounces) kidney beans, drained and rinsed
- 1/2 English cucumber, chopped
- 1 medium heirloom tomato, chopped
- 1 bunch fresh cilantro, stems removed and chopped
- 1 red onion, chopped
- Juice of 1 large lime
- 3 tablespoons Dijon mustard
- 1/2 teaspoon fresh garlic paste
- 1 teaspoon Sumac
- Salt and pepper as needed

DIRECTIONS

1. Take a medium-sized bowl and add kidney beans, chopped up veggies and cilantro
2. Take a small bowl and make the vinaigrette by adding lime juice, oil, fresh garlic, pepper, mustard, and sumac
3. Pour the vinaigrette over the salad and give it a gentle stir
4. Add some salt and pepper
5. Cover and allow it to chill for half an hour

NUTRITIONS

- *Calories: 74*
- *Fat: 0.7g*
- *Carbohydrates: 16g*
- *Protein: 21g*

64. GINGER SOUP

PREPARATION	COOKING	SERVES
10 MIN	10 MIN	4

INGREDIENTS

- 1 Can Diced Tomatoes
- 1 Can Peppers
- 6 cups Vegetable Broth
- 3 Cups Green Onions, Diced
- 2 Cups Mushrooms, Sliced
- 3 Teaspoons Garlic, minced
- 3 Teaspoons Ginger, Fresh & Grated
- 4 Tablespoons Tamari
- 2 Cups Bok Choy, Chopped
- 1 Tablespoon Cilantro, Chopped
- 3 Tablespoons Carrot Grated

DIRECTIONS

1. Add all ingredients except for your carrot and green onion into a saucepan, and then bring it to a boil using medium-high heat.
2. Lower to medium-low, cooking for six minutes.
3. Stir in your carrots and green onions, cooking for another two minutes.
4. Serve with cilantro.

NUTRITIONS

- *Calories: 65*
- *Protein: 7 Grams*
- *Fat: 2 Grams*
- *Net Carbs: 5 Grams*

65. SCALLOPS IN BACON SAUCE

PREPARATION	COOKING	SERVES
15 MIN	10 MIN	4

INGREDIENTS

- 2 Cups Heavy Whipping Cream
- 2 Tablespoons Butter
- 8 Bacon Slices
- ½ Cup Parmesan Cheese, Grated
- 2 Tablespoons Ghee
- 16 Scallops, Large & Patted Dry
- Sea Salt & Black Pepper to Taste

DIRECTIONS

1. Place a skillet over medium-high heat, and then cook your bacon. It should take eight minutes.
2. Lower the heat to medium, then add in parmesan cheese, butter and cream. Season with salt and pepper, and then reduce to low. Cook, stirring constantly. It should thicken and reduce by half in ten minutes.
3. Put another skillet over medium-high heat, heating until your ghee begins to sizzle.
4. Season your scallops with salt and pepper, adding them to the skillet. Cook for a minute per side. Make sure you don't crowd your scallops.
5. Serve with your cream sauce with crumbled bacon on top.

NUTRITIONS

- Calories: 728
- Protein: 24 Grams
- Fat: 73 Grams
- Net Carbs: 10 Grams

66. FISH TACO BOWLS

PREPARATION	COOKING	SERVES
10 MIN	15 MIN	4

INGREDIENTS

- 4 Tilapia Fillets, 5 Ounces Each
- 8 Teaspoons Tajin Seasoning Salt, Divided
- 2 Tablespoons Olive Oil
- 4 Cups Coleslaw Cabbage Mix
- 2 Tablespoons Red Pepper Miso Mayonnaise + Some for Serving
- 2 Avocados, Mashed
- Sea Salt & Black Pepper to Taste

DIRECTIONS

1. Start by heating your oven to 425, lining a baking sheet with foil.
2. Rub your tilapia down with olive oil and season it.
3. Bake for fifteen minutes, and then allow it to cool.
4. In a bowl, combine your mayonnaise and coleslaw, and top with fish to serve. Add in your mashed avocado.

NUTRITIONS

- Calories: 315
- Protein: 16 Grams
- Fat: 24 Grams
- Net Carbs: 5 Grams

67. BUTTERY GARLIC SHRIMP

PREPARATION	COOKING	SERVES
10 MIN	15 MIN	4

INGREDIENTS

- 6 Tablespoons Butter
- 1 lb. Shrimp, Cooked
- 2 Lemons, Halved
- ½ Teaspoon Red Pepper Flakes
- 4 Cloves Garlic, Crushed
- Sea Salt & Black Pepper to Taste

DIRECTIONS

1. Begin by warming your oven to 425, and then place your butter in an eight-inch baking dish. The butter should melt.
2. Sprinkle your shrimp with salt and pepper, and then slice your lemon halves into thin slices.
3. Add your shrimp, garlic and butter into your baking dish. Sprinkle with red pepper flakes, cooking for fifteen minutes. Stir halfway through, and then squeeze the lemon wedges across the dish before serving.

NUTRITIONS

- Calories: 329
- Protein: 32 Grams
- Fat: 20 Grams
- Net Carbs: 4 Grams

68. SALMON STEW

PREPARATION	COOKING	SERVES
8 MIN	12 MIN	2

INGREDIENTS

- 1-pound salmon fillet, sliced
- 1 onion, chopped
- Salt, to taste
- 1 tablespoon butter, melted
- 1 cup fish broth
- ½ teaspoon red chili powder

DIRECTIONS

1. Season the salmon fillets with salt and red chili powder.
2. Put butter and onions in a skillet and sauté for about 3 minutes.
3. Add seasoned salmon and cook for about 2 minutes on each side.
4. Add fish broth and secure the lid.
5. Cook for about 7 minutes on medium heat and open the lid.
6. Dish out and serve immediately.
7. Transfer the stew to a bowl and set aside to cool for meal prepping. Divide the mixture into 2 containers. Cover the containers and refrigerate for about 2 days. Reheat in the microwave before serving.

NUTRITIONS

- Calories: 272
- Carbs: 4.4g
- Protein: 32.1g
- Fat: 14.2g
- Sugar: 1.9g

373

69. ASPARAGUS SALMON FILLETS

PREPARATION	COOKING	SERVES
10 MIN	20 MIN	2

INGREDIENTS

- 1 teaspoon olive oil
- 4 asparagus stalks
- 2 salmon fillets
- ¼ cup butter
- ¼ cup champagne
- Salt and freshly ground black pepper, to taste

DIRECTIONS

1. Preheat the oven to 355 degrees and grease a baking dish.
2. Put all the ingredients in a bowl and mix well.
3. Put this mixture in the baking dish and transfer it to the oven.
4. Bake for about 20 minutes and dish out.
5. Place the salmon fillets in a dish and set aside to cool for meal prepping. Divide it into 2 containers and close the lid. Refrigerate for 1 day and reheat in microwave before serving.

NUTRITIONS

- Calories: 475
- Carbs: 1.1g
- Protein: 35.2g
- Fat: 36.8g
- Sugar: 0.5g
- Sodium: 242mg

70. CRISPY BAKED CHICKEN

PREPARATION	COOKING	SERVES
30 MIN	10 MIN	2

INGREDIENTS

- 2 chicken breasts, skinless and boneless
- 2 tablespoons butter
- ¼ teaspoon turmeric powder
- Salt and black pepper, to taste
- ¼ cup sour cream

DIRECTIONS

1. Preheat the oven to 360 degrees and grease a baking dish with butter.
2. Season the chicken with turmeric powder, salt and black pepper in a bowl.
3. Put the chicken on the baking dish and transfer it to the oven.
4. Bake for about 10 minutes and dish out to serve topped with sour cream.
5. Transfer the chicken to a bowl and set aside to cool for meal prepping. Divide it into 2 containers and cover the containers. Refrigerate for up to 2 days and reheat in microwave before serving.

NUTRITIONS

- Calories: 304
- Carbs: 1.4g
- Protein: 26.1g
- Fat: 21.6g
- Sugar: 0.1g
- Sodium: 137mg

71. SOUR AND SWEET FISH

PREPARATION	COOKING	SERVES
15 MIN	0 MIN	2

INGREDIENTS

- 1 tablespoon vinegar
- 2 drops stevia
- 1-pound fish chunks
- ¼ cup butter, melted
- Salt and black pepper, to taste

DIRECTIONS

1. Put butter and fish chunks in a skillet and cook for about 3 minutes.
2. Add stevia, salt and black pepper and cook for about 10 minutes, stirring continuously.
3. Dish out in a bowl and serve immediately.
4. Place fish in a dish and set aside to cool for meal prepping. Divide it into 2 containers and refrigerate for up to 2 days. Reheat in the microwave before serving.

NUTRITIONS

- Calories: 258
- Carbs: 2.8g
- Protein: 24.5g
- Fat: 16.7g
- Sugar: 2.7g
- Sodium: 649mg

72. CREAMY CHICKEN

PREPARATION	COOKING	SERVES
12 MIN	13 MIN	2

INGREDIENTS

- ½ small onion, chopped
- ¼ cup sour cream
- 1 tablespoon butter
- ¼ cup mushrooms
- ½ pound chicken breasts

DIRECTIONS

1. Heat butter in a skillet and add onions and mushrooms.
2. Sauté for about 5 minutes and add chicken breasts and salt.
3. Secure the lid and cook for about 5 more minutes.
4. Add sour cream and cook for about 3 minutes.
5. Open the lid and dish it out in a bowl to serve immediately.
6. Transfer the creamy chicken breasts to a dish and set aside to cool for meal prepping.
7. Divide them into 2 containers and cover their lid. Refrigerate for 2-3 days and reheat in microwave before serving.

NUTRITIONS

- Calories: 335
- Carbs: 2.9g
- Protein: 34g
- Fat: 20.2g
- Sugar: 0.8g
- Sodium: 154mg

73. PAPRIKA BUTTER SHRIMP

PREPARATION	COOKING	SERVES
15 MIN	15 MIN	2

INGREDIENTS

- ¼ tablespoon smoked paprika
- 1/8 cup sour cream
- ½ pound shrimp
- 1/8 cup butter
- Salt and black pepper, to taste

DIRECTIONS

1. Preheat the oven to 390 degrees and grease a baking dish.
2. Mix all the ingredients in a large bowl and transfer them into the baking dish.
3. Place in the oven then bake for approximately 15 minutes.
4. Place paprika shrimp in a dish and set aside to cool for meal prepping. Divide it into 2 containers and cover the lid. Refrigerate for 1-2 days and reheat in microwave before serving.

NUTRITIONS

- Calories: 330
- Carbs: 1.5g
- Protein: 32.6g
- Fat: 21.5g
- Sugar: 0.2g
- Sodium: 458mg

74. ALMOND FLOUR BURGER WITH GOAT CHEESE

PREPARATION	COOKING	SERVES
10 MIN	20 MIN	2

INGREDIENTS

- 2 almond flour bagels
- 2 tablespoon of fresh goat cheese
- 4 slices of smoked salmon
- 2 pinch Salt and pepper
- 4 Radishes
- Dill

DIRECTIONS

1. Cut the gluten-free bagel in half. Put the two halves in the toaster to make them crisp.
2. Spread both slices of fresh goat cheese and add salmon.
3. Garnish the bagel with the radish and dill.
4. A pinch of salt and pepper and it's ready
5. Put each burger in a container and store in the refrigerator

NUTRITIONS

- Calories: 325
- Fat: 29 g
- Carbs: 4 g
- Protein 12 g
- Sugar: 0.9 g

75. SAUSAGE SKILLET WITH CABBAGE

PREPARATION	COOKING	SERVES
5 MIN	13 MIN	2

INGREDIENTS

- 1 tablespoon. olive oil
- 3/4 cup shredded green cabbage
- 3/4 cup grated red cabbage
- 1/4 cup diced onion
- 1/4 cup spicy sausages
- 1/4 cup grated mozzarella
- 1 tablespoon. fresh and chopped parsley
- Salt and pepper to taste

DIRECTIONS

1. Place a large skillet on a stove over medium-high heat and heat olive oil. Immerse the cabbage and onion in the heated oil. Let stand for about 8-10 minutes or until vegetables are tender.
2. Chop the sausage into bite-size pieces. Mix with cabbage and onion and let stand another 8 minutes.
3. Spread the cheese over the top
4. Cover the skillet with a lid and set aside for 5 minutes to melt.
5. Remove the lid and mix your Ingredients. Garnish with salt, pepper, and parsley before serving.
6. To assemble the dish, divide the mixture between 2 containers; then store it in the refrigerator

NUTRITIONS

- *Calories: 316*
- *Fat: 27.2 g*
- *Carbs: 4.9 g*
- *Protein 12.8 g*
- *Sugar: 1.3 g*

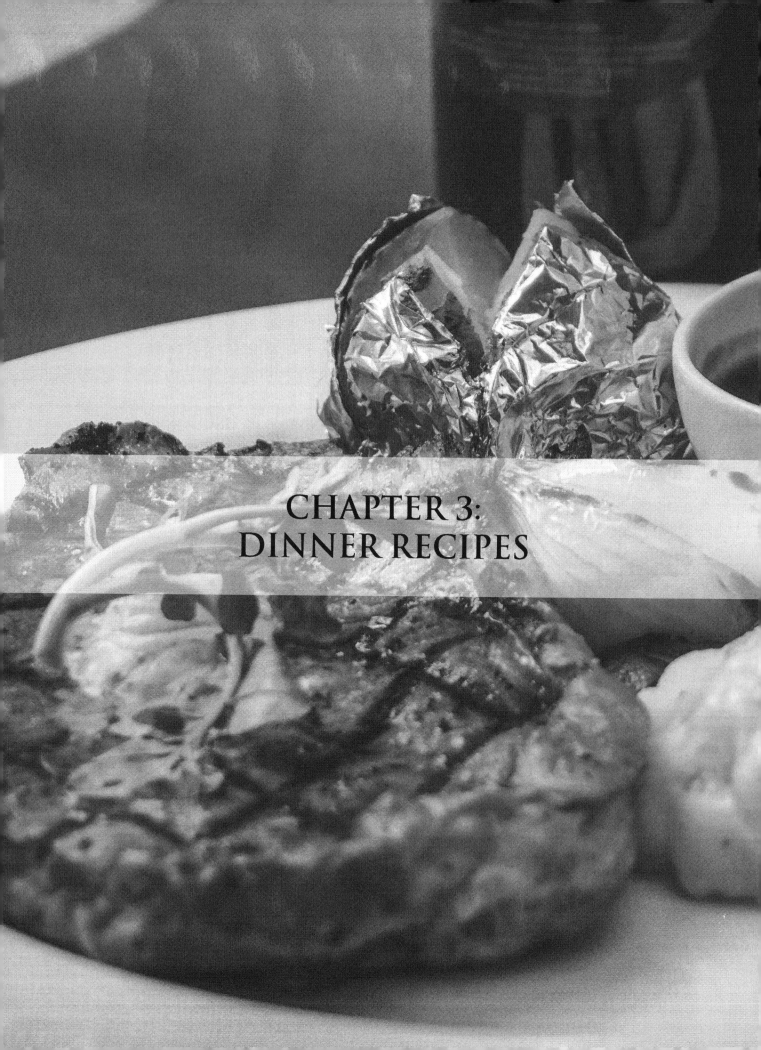

CHAPTER 3:
DINNER RECIPES

76. AIR FRYER ASPARAGUS

PREPARATION	COOKING	SERVES
5 MIN	8 MIN	1

INGREDIENTS

- Nutritional yeast
- Olive oil non-stick spray
- One bunch of asparagus

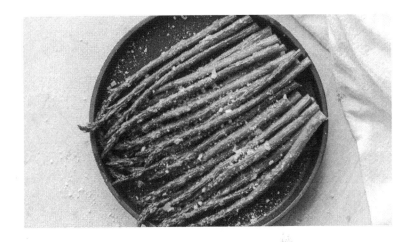

DIRECTIONS

1. Preparing the Ingredients. Wash asparagus. Do not forget to trim off thick, woody ends.
2. Spray asparagus with olive oil spray and sprinkle with yeast.
3. Air Frying. In your Instant Crisp Air Fryer, lay asparagus in a singular layer. Set the temperature to 360°F. While the time limit to 8 minutes.

NUTRITIONS

- Calories: 17;
- Fat: 4g;
- Protein: 9g

77. AVOCADO FRIES

PREPARATION	COOKING	SERVES
10 MIN	7 MIN	1

INGREDIENTS

- One avocado
- 1/8 teaspoon salt
- 1/4 cup panko breadcrumbs
- Bean liquid (aquafaba) from a 15-ounces can consist of white or garbanzo beans

DIRECTIONS

1. Preparing the Ingredients. Peel, pit, and slice up avocado.
2. Toss salt and breadcrumbs together in a bowl. Place aquafaba into another bowl.
3. Dredge slices of avocado first in aquafaba and then in panko, making sure you can even coating.
4. Air Frying. Place coated avocado slices into a single layer in the Instant Crisp Air Fryer. Set temperature to 390°F and set time to 5 minutes.
5. Serve with your favorite keto dipping sauce!

NUTRITIONS

- Calories: 102;
- Fat: 22g;
- Protein: 9g;
- Sugar: 1g

78. BELL-PEPPER CORN WRAPPED IN TORTILLA

PREPARATION	COOKING	SERVES
5 MIN	15 MIN	1

INGREDIENTS

- 1/4 small red bell pepper, chopped
- 1/4 small yellow onion, diced
- 1/4 tablespoon water
- 1/2 cobs grilled corn kernels
- One large tortilla
- One-piece commercial vegan nuggets, chopped
- Mixed greens for garnish

DIRECTIONS

1. Preparing the Ingredients. Preheat the Instant Crisp Air Fryer to 400°F.
2. In a skillet heated over medium heat, water sautés the vegan nuggets and the onions, bell peppers, and corn kernels. Set aside.
3. Place filling inside the corn tortillas.
4. Air Frying. Lock the air fryer lid. Fold the tortillas and place inside the Instant Crisp Air Fryer and cook for 15 minutes until the tortilla wraps are crispy.
5. Serve with mixed greens on top.

NUTRITIONS

- *Calories: 548;*
- *Fat: 20.7g;*
- *Protein: 46g*

79. CAULIFLOWER RICE

PREPARATION	COOKING	SERVES
5 MIN	20 MIN	1

INGREDIENTS

Round 1:
- 1/2 teaspoon turmeric
- 1/2 cup diced carrot
- 1/8 cup diced onion
- 1/2 tablespoon low-sodium soy sauce
- 1/8 block of extra firm tofu

Round 2:
- ½ cup frozen peas
- 1/4 minced garlic cloves
- ½ cup chopped broccoli
- 1/2 tablespoon minced ginger
- 1/4 tablespoon rice vinegar
- 1/4 teaspoon toasted sesame oil
- 1/2 tablespoon reduced-sodium soy sauce
- 1/2 cup rice cauliflower

DIRECTIONS

1. Preparing the Ingredients. Crush tofu in a large bowl and toss with all the Round one ingredient.
2. Air Frying. Lock the air fryer lid—preheat the Instant Crisp Air Fryer to 370 degrees. Also, set the temperature to 370°F, set the time to 10 minutes, and cook 10 minutes, making sure to shake once.
3. In another bowl, toss ingredients from Round 2 together.
4. Add Round 2 mixture to Instant Crisp Air Fryer and cook another 10 minutes to shake 5 minutes.
5. Enjoy!

NUTRITIONS

- Calories: 67;
- Fat: 8g;
- Protein: 3g;
- Sugar: 0g

80. STUFFED MUSHROOMS

PREPARATION	COOKING	SERVES
7 MIN	8 MIN	1

INGREDIENTS

- 1/2 Rashers Bacon, Diced
- ½ Onion, Diced
- ½ Bell Pepper, Diced
- 1/2 Small Carrot, Diced
- 2 Medium Size Mushrooms (Separate the caps & stalks)
- 1/4 cup Shredded Cheddar Plus Extra for the top
- 1/4 cup Sour Cream

DIRECTIONS

1. Preparing the Ingredients. Chop the mushrooms stalks finely and fry them up with the bacon, onion, pepper, and carrot at 350 ° for 8 minutes.
2. Also, check when the veggies are tender, stir in the sour cream & the cheese. Keep on the heat until the cheese has melted and everything is mixed nicely.
3. Now grab the mushroom caps and heap a plop of filling on each one.
4. Place in the fryer basket and top with a little extra cheese.

NUTRITIONS

- Calories: 285;
- Fat: 20.5g;
- Protein: 8.6g

81. ZUCCHINI OMELET

PREPARATION	COOKING	SERVES
10 MIN	10 MIN	1

INGREDIENTS

- 1/2 teaspoon butter
- 1/2 zucchini, julienned
- One egg
- 1/8 teaspoon fresh basil, chopped
- 1/8 teaspoon red pepper flakes, crushed
- Salted and newly ground black pepper, to taste

DIRECTIONS

1. Preparing the Ingredients. Preheat the Instant Crisp Air Fryer to 355 degrees F.
2. Melt butter on a medium heat using a skillet.
3. Add zucchini and cook for about 3-4 minutes.
4. In a bowl, add the eggs, basil, red pepper flakes, salt, and black pepper and beat well.
5. Add cooked zucchini and gently stir to combine.
6. Air Frying. Transfer the mixture into the Instant Crisp Air Fryer pan. Lock the air fryer lid.
7. Cook for about 10 minutes. Also, you may opt to wait until it is done thoroughly.

NUTRITIONS

- Calories: 285;
- Fat: 20.5g;
- Protein: 8.6g

82. CHEESY CAULIFLOWER FRITTERS

PREPARATION	COOKING	SERVES
10 MIN	7 MIN	1

INGREDIENTS

- ½ cup chopped parsley
- 1 cup Italian breadcrumbs
- 1/3 cup shredded mozzarella cheese
- 1/3 cup shredded sharp cheddar cheese
- 1 egg
- 2 minced garlic cloves
- 3 chopped scallions
- 1 head of cauliflower

DIRECTIONS

1. Preparing the Ingredients. Cut the cauliflower up into florets. Wash well and pat dry.
2. Place into a food processor and pulse 20-30 seconds till it looks like rice.
3. Place the cauliflower rice in a bowl and mix with pepper, salt, egg, cheeses, breadcrumbs, garlic, and scallions.
4. With hands, form 15 patties of the mixture, then add more breadcrumbs if needed.
5. Air Frying. With olive oil, spritz patties, and put the fitters into your Instant Crisp Air Fryer.
6. Pile it in a single layer. Lock the air fryer lid. Set temperature to 390°F, and set time to 7 minutes, flipping after 7 minutes.

NUTRITIONS

- *Calories: 209;*
- *Fat: 17g;*
- *Protein: 6g;*
- *Sugar: 0.5*

83. ZUCCHINI PARMESAN CHIPS

PREPARATION	COOKING	SERVES
10 MIN	8 MIN	1

INGREDIENTS

- ½ teaspoon paprika
- ½ cup grated parmesan cheese
- ½ cup Italian breadcrumbs
- 1 lightly beaten egg
- 2 thinly sliced zucchinis

DIRECTIONS

1. Preparing the Ingredients. Use a very sharp knife or mandolin slicer to slice zucchini as thinly as you can. Pat off extra moisture.
2. Beat egg with a pinch of pepper and salt and a bit of water.
3. Combine paprika, cheese, and breadcrumbs in a bowl.
4. Dip slices of zucchini into the egg mixture and then into the breadcrumb mixture. Press gently to coat.
5. Air Frying. With olive oil cooking spray, mist encrusted zucchini slices. Put into your Instant Crisp Air Fryer in a single layer. Latch the air fryer lid. Set temperature to 350°F and set time to 8 minutes.
6. Sprinkle with salt and serve with salsa.

NUTRITIONS

- Calories: 211;
- Fat: 16g;
- Protein: 8g;
- Sugar: 0g

84. JALAPENO CHEESE BALLS

PREPARATION	COOKING	SERVES
10 MIN	8 MIN	1

INGREDIENTS

- 1-ounce cream cheese
- 1/6 cup shredded mozzarella cheese
- 1/6 cup shredded Cheddar cheese
- 1/2 jalapeños, finely chopped
- ½ cup breadcrumbs
- 2 eggs
- ½ cup all-purpose flour
- Salt
- Pepper
- Cooking oil

DIRECTIONS

1. Preparing the Ingredients. Combine the cream cheese, mozzarella, Cheddar, and jalapeños in a medium bowl. Mix well.
2. Form the cheese mixture into balls about an inch thick. You may also use a small ice cream scoop. It works well.
3. Arrange the cheese balls on a sheet pan and place in the freezer for 15 minutes. It will help the cheese balls maintain their shape while frying.
4. Spray the Instant Crisp Air Fryer basket with cooking oil. Place the breadcrumbs in a small bowl. In another small bowl, beat the eggs. In the third small bowl, combine the flour with salt and pepper to taste, and mix well. Remove the cheese balls from the freezer. Plunge the cheese balls in the flour, then the eggs, and then the breadcrumbs.
5. Air Frying. Place the cheese balls in the Instant Crisp Air Fryer. Spray with cooking oil. Lock the air fryer lid—Cook for 8 minutes.
6. Open the Instant Crisp Air Fryer and flip the cheese balls. Cook for additional 4 minutes. Cool before serving.

NUTRITIONS

- Calories: 96;
- Fat: 6g;
- Protein: 4g;
- Sugar: 0g

85. COCONUT BATTERED CAULIFLOWER BITES

PREPARATION	COOKING	SERVES
5 MIN	20 MIN	1

INGREDIENTS

- Salt and pepper to taste
- 1 flax egg or 1 tablespoon flaxseed meal + 3 tablespoon water
- 1 small cauliflower, cut into florets
- 1 teaspoon mixed spice
- ½ teaspoon mustard powder
- 2 tablespoons maple syrup
- 1 clove of garlic, minced
- 2 tablespoons soy sauce
- 1/3 cup oats flour
- 1/3 cup plain flour
- 1/3 cup desiccated coconut

DIRECTIONS

1. Preparing the Ingredients.
2. In a mixing bowl, mix oats, flour, and desiccated coconut. Season with salt and pepper to taste. Set aside.
3. In another bowl, place the flax egg and add a pinch of salt to taste. Set aside.
4. Season the cauliflower with mixed spice and mustard powder.
5. Dredge the florets in the flax egg first, then in the flour mixture.
6. Air Frying. Place inside the Instant Crisp Air Fryer, lock the air fryer lid and cook at 400°F or 15 minutes.
7. Meanwhile, place the maple syrup, garlic, and soy sauce in a saucepan and heat over medium flame. Wait for it to boil and adjust the heat to low until the sauce thickens.
8. After 15 minutes, take out the Instant Crisp Air Fryer's florets and place them in the saucepan.
9. Toss to coat the florets and place inside the Instant Crisp Air Fryer and cook for another 5 minutes.

NUTRITIONS

- Calories: 154;
- Fat: 2.3g;
- Protein: 4.69g

86. CRISPY JALAPENO COINS

PREPARATION	COOKING	SERVES
10 MIN	5 MIN	1

INGREDIENTS

- 1 egg
- 2-3 tbsp. coconut flour
- 1 sliced and seeded jalapeno
- Pinch of garlic powder
- Pinch of onion powder
- Bit of Cajun seasoning (optional)
- Pinch of pepper and salt

DIRECTIONS

1. Preparing the Ingredients. Ensure your Instant Crisp Air Fryer is preheated to 400 degrees.
2. Mix all dry ingredients.
3. Pat jalapeno slices dry. Dip coins into the egg wash and then into the dry mixture. Toss to coat thoroughly.
4. Add coated jalapeno slices to Instant Crisp Air Fryer in a singular layer. Spray with olive oil.
5. Air Frying. Lock the air fryer lid. Set temperature to 350°F and set time to 5 minutes. Cook just till crispy.

NUTRITIONS

- *Calories: 128;*
- *Fat: 8g;*
- *Protein: 7g;*
- *Sugar: 0g*

87. CRISPY ROASTED BROCCOLI

PREPARATION	COOKING	SERVES
10 MIN	8 MIN	1

INGREDIENTS

- ¼ teaspoon Masala
- ½ teaspoon red chili powder
- ½ teaspoon salt
- ¼ teaspoon turmeric powder
- 1 tablespoon chickpea flour
- 1 tablespoon yogurt
- 1/2-pound broccoli

DIRECTIONS

1. Preparing the Ingredients. Cut broccoli up into florets. Immerse in a bowl of water with two teaspoons of salt for at least half an hour to remove impurities.
2. Take out broccoli florets from water and let drain. Wipe down thoroughly.
3. Mix all other ingredients to create a marinade.
4. Toss broccoli florets in the marinade. Cover and chill for 15-30 minutes.
5. Air Frying. Preheat the Instant Crisp Air Fryer to 390 degrees.
6. Place marinated broccoli florets into the fryer, lock the air fryer lid, set the temperature to 350°F, and set the time to 10 minutes. Florets will be crispy when done.

NUTRITIONS

- *Calories: 96;*
- *Fat: 1.3g;*
- *Protein: 7g;*
- *Sugar: 4.5g*

88. TURKEY STUFFED BELL PEPPERS

PREPARATION	COOKING	SERVES
10 MIN	25 MIN	1

INGREDIENTS

- 1 Whole Bell Peppers (We used Red & Green)
- One 4-ounce Trifecta Turkey Burger
- 1/8 Red Onion (diced)
- 1/2 Medium Tomato (chopped)
- 1/4 Cup of Panko Breadcrumbs
- 1/4 Cup of Low-Fat Shredded Cheddar Cheese
- 1/2 Tsp Italian Seasoning
- 1/2 tsp of Ground Cumin
- 1/2 Clove of Garlic
- Salt & Pepper

DIRECTIONS

1. Preheat oven to 325 degrees. Then, cut the bell peppers in half, remove seeds, and clean.
2. In a large bowl, crumble the Trifecta turkey burgers and mix with the onions, breadcrumbs, tomato, garlic, and seasoning.
3. Next, you need to add half of the cheese to the bowl (save another half for the top). Add a dash of salt and pepper. Mix well together.
4. Spray a baking sheet with non-stick cooking spray.
5. Then add the bell pepper halves. Fill each bell peppers with the stuffing. Heat for 15-20 minutes.
6. Remove the bell peppers from heat and add the rest of the cheese to the peppers' top. Place back in the oven for 3-5 minutes or until cheese is melted.

NUTRITIONS

- *Calories: 350;*
- *Protein: 51 g;*
- *Carbohydrates: 10 g;*
- *Fats: 10 g*

89. LEAN CROCKPOT PULLED PORK

PREPARATION	COOKING	SERVES
15 MIN	480 MIN	1

INGREDIENTS

- 1 Boneless Pork Chops
- 1/2 15ounces Cans Tomato Sauce, No Sugar Added
- 1/3 tablespoon Onion Powder
- 1/2 tablespoon garlic powder
- 1/4 tablespoon Cumin
- 1/2 teaspoon Cinnamon
- 1/4 teaspoon Chili Powder
- 1/8 teaspoon Cayenne Pepper

DIRECTIONS

1. Trim extra fat from pork and add to crockpot.
2. Make sure to add the tomato sauce and seasonings to a bowl and mix.
3. Pour the sauce over the pork chops
4. Cook for 8 to 12 hours on low heat or until meat is thoroughly tender and starts to fall apart.
5. Lastly, pull the pork apart with a fork and enjoy!

NUTRITIONS

- Calories: 250;
- Carbohydrates: 14.5 g;
- Fats: 15.9 g;
- Protein: 25 g

90. EASY CREAMY CAJUN SHRIMP PASTA

PREPARATION	COOKING	SERVES
5 MIN	15 MIN	1

INGREDIENTS

- 2 ounces linguine pasta
- 1/4 teaspoon olive oil
- 1/4-pound raw shrimp
- 1/4 tablespoon Cajun
- 1-ounce sausage
- 1/8 red peppers
- 1/8 green peppers
- 1/8 onions
- 1/2 tomatoes
- 1/2 tablespoon butter
- 1/2 Whip cream

- 1/2 Almond milk
- 1-ounce cream cheese
- 1/2 shredded Parmesan Reggiano

DIRECTIONS

1. Cook the pasta as per package instructions.
2. Place the shrimp in a bowl along with 1/2 tablespoon of Cajun or creole seasoning.
3. Mix to ensure the shrimp is fully coated.
4. Heat a skillet or pan on medium-high heat. I use a cast-iron skillet. Next, add 1 teaspoonful of olive oil to the pan.
5. While it is hot, add the shrimp to the pan. Then cook each side for 2-3 minutes until it turns bright pink. Remove the shrimp and set aside.
6. The next step will be adding a teaspoon of olive oil to the pan along with the chopped sausage, onions, green peppers, and red peppers.
7. Sauté for 3-4 minutes until the vegetables are soft and the onions are translucent and fragrant. Make sure to remove the vegetables from the pan and set them aside.
8. You also need to reduce the heat on the pan to medium. Do not forget to add the butter to the pan and allow it to melt.
9. The next step will be adding the heavy cream, almond milk, cream cheese, the remaining 1/2 tablespoon of Cajun or creole seasoning, and parmesan Reggiano cheese.
10. Just continue stirring the sauce until all the cheese has fully melted.
11. The cream cheeses may take some time to melt. Add in the fire-roasted tomatoes and stir. Allow the mixture to cook for 2 minutes.
12. Next, you need to add the shrimp, sausage, vegetables, and pasta to the pan and stir. Allow the pasta to cook for 4-5 minutes until combined. Serve.

NUTRITIONS

- Calories: 384;
- Protein: 7 g;
- Carbohydrates: 22 g;
- Fats: 28 g

91. FALL CHICKEN NOODLE STIR FRY

PREPARATION	COOKING	SERVES
5 MIN	10 MIN	1

INGREDIENTS

- 2 ounces Trifecta Chicken Breast
- 1/4 cup of Butternut Squash Cubes
- One egg, whole,
- 1 ounce of brown rice Pad Thai Noodles
- 1/2 tablespoon of Fish Sauce
- 1/4 teaspoon sesame oil, untoasted
- 1/4 tablespoon of Teriyaki Sauce
- 1/4 tablespoon of Sriracha
- 1/2 teaspoon of garlic
- One serving of fresh bean sprouts

Ingredients Needed for One Person:
- One lean
- Two green
- One condiment

DIRECTIONS

1. First, cook the noodles as indicated by the package.
2. In the microwave, eat up the pre-cooked butternut squash.
3. The next step is cooking for 3-5 minutes, or you may opt to wait when the squash softens.
4. Meanwhile, in a non-stick skillet, heat the oil over medium heat. Then add the garlic, Trifecta chicken, and butternut squash. You may cut up the chicken in the skillet and heat until golden.
5. Scramble the eggs to the skillet. Wait for the noodles to become 75%-80% cooked through.
6. You may now add the noodles to the skillet. It may be followed by adding the fish sauce, teriyaki sauce, and Sriracha. Stir often.
7. Proceed by adding the bean sprouts. Cook for an additional minute to two until bean sprouts are heated through. Serve on a bowl.
8. If desired, top with red pepper flakes and cilantro.

NUTRITIONS

- Protein: 51 g;
- Calories: 350;
- Carbohydrates: 10 g;
- Fats: 10 g

92. HEALTHY SALMON CHOWDER

PREPARATION	COOKING	SERVES
10 MIN	10 MIN	1

INGREDIENTS

- 1/4 tablespoon olive oil
- 1/4 small onion, diced
- 1/4 cup chopped cilantro leaves or stems
- ½ chipotle peppers in adobo, diced
- 1/2 medium head of cauliflower, chopped
- 1/2 cups chicken broth (low sodium)
- 1 cup baby spinach
- 1/4 cup frozen corn
- 4 ounces Trifecta salmon
- 1-oz low-fat Greek yogurt
- Finishing salt
- Chili flakes

DIRECTIONS

1. Heat oil, chopped onion, cilantro stems, and sauté until brown, 3 to 4 minutes.
2. Add chipotle peppers and cauliflower. Cook for 1 to 2 minutes.
3. You may now add the chicken broth and wait for it to simmer.
4. Wait for it to cook for 5 minutes, or until cauliflower is tender.
5. Over medium-high heat, adds spinach and corn. Let cook for 1 to 2 minutes.
6. Crumble salmon into bite-size chunks, then add to the pot.
7. Reduce heat to a gentle simmer.
8. Do not forget to remove from heat and stir in Greek yogurt.
9. Finally, serve warm with finishing salt and chili flakes if desired

NUTRITIONS

- *Calories: 350;*
- *Protein: 51 g;*
- *Carbohydrates: 10 g;*
- *Fats: 10 g*

93. FLAT IRON STEAK FAJITA BOWLS

PREPARATION	COOKING	SERVES
5 MIN	5 MIN	1

INGREDIENTS

- 4 ounces of Trifecta Flat Iron Steak
- Fresh Cilantro
- 1/4 cup of White Corn
- 1/2 Yellow Onion
- 1/2 cup of Trifecta Bell Peppers
- 1/2 cup of Trifecta Brown Rice
- Green Leaf Lettuce
- Jalapenos (optional)
- Red Pepper Flakes
- Avocado (optional)

DIRECTIONS

1. Cut the onion and combine Trifecta bell peppers.
2. Next, cut the Trifecta flat iron steak into strips.
3. Heat a skillet and then spray with non-stick spray.
4. Grill the steak and vegetables until cooked.
5. Heat two cups of Trifecta brown rice in a microwave.
6. (For best results, place a wet paper towel on top of the bowl of rice before heating)
7. Drain the can of corn and rinse.
8. On a plate, portion out the base layer of rice, steak, and fajita veggies.
9. If desired, top with lettuce, corn, jalapenos, and red pepper flakes.

NUTRITIONS

- *Calories: 352;*
- *Protein: 20 g;*
- *Carbohydrates: 4.1 g;*
- *Fats: 12 g*

94. REAL SIMPLE AND CLEAN MEATBALLS

PREPARATION	COOKING	SERVES
5 MIN	25 MIN	1

INGREDIENTS

- 1/2 pounds of lean grass-fed ground beef
- 1/2 medium onion
- One clove garlic
- One egg
- 1/4 cup quinoa flour
- Salt and pepper to taste

DIRECTIONS

1. Preheat your oven to 350 degrees.
2. Then, cut the onion into small pieces, add the minced garlic.
3. Next will be adding the meat, onion, garlic, egg, quinoa flour, salt, and pepper in a large mixing bowl and mix until well combined.
4. Next, using your hands, grab a small amount of the meat mixture and work it into a ball, about 1 inch in diameter.
5. Put the meatball on a baking sheet that has been sprayed with non-stick spray. Then repeat this process with the remaining meat mixture. It should yield about 25 meatballs.
6. Lastly, put the meatballs in the oven for 25 minutes. Serve with your favorite sauce and veggies!

NUTRITIONS

- Calories: 350;
- Protein: 51 g;
- Carbohydrates: 10 g;
- Fats: 10 g

95. HIGH PROTEIN LOW CARB SHRIMP CEVICHE

PREPARATION	COOKING	SERVES
5 MIN	1 MIN	1

INGREDIENTS

- One 5-ounce package Trifecta Shrimp
- 1/2 Red Bell Pepper
- 1/2 Small Cucumber
- 1 to 2 Radishes
- 1/2 large tomato
- 1/4 Jalapeno
- 1/8 cup Fresh Cilantro, Diced (Stems and Leaves)
- 1/4 tablespoon Olive Oil
- ½ lime, juice, and zest
- 1/4 teaspoon salt

DIRECTIONS

1. Start to dice all veggies into bite-size. Finely chop cilantro stems and leaves, leaving some leaves for garnish.
2. Mix the oil with lime juice, lime zest, salt, and cilantro in a bowl. Make sure to add a dash of honey or sugar if needed for taste.
3. Make sure to drain Trifecta shrimp and mix it in a bowl with veggies.
4. Last, toss shrimp and veggies in the cilantro dressing and serve.

NUTRITIONS

- *Calories: 529;*
- *Protein: 34 g;*
- *Carbohydrates: 68 g;*
- *Fats: 13 g*

96. BAKED RICOTTA WITH PEARS

PREPARATION	COOKING	SERVES
5 MIN	25 MIN	4

INGREDIENTS

- Non-stick cooking spray
- 1 (16-ounce) container whole-milk ricotta cheese
- 2 large eggs
- 1/4 cup white whole-wheat flour or whole-wheat pastry flour
- 1 tablespoon sugar
- 1 teaspoon vanilla extract
- 1/4 teaspoon ground nutmeg
- 1 pear, cored and diced
- 2 tablespoons water
- 1 tablespoon honey

DIRECTIONS

1. Preheat the oven to 400°F. Spray four 6-ounce ramekins with non-stick cooking spray.
2. In a large bowl, beat together the ricotta, eggs, flour, sugar, vanilla, and nutmeg.
3. Spoon into the ramekins.
4. Bake for 22 to 25 minutes, or until the ricotta is just about set.
5. Remove from the oven and cool slightly on racks.
6. While the ricotta is baking, in a small saucepan over medium heat, simmer the pear in the water for 10 minutes, until slightly softened.
7. Remove from the heat, and stir in the honey.
8. Serve the ricotta ramekins topped with the warmed pear.

NUTRITIONS

- *Calories: 312 Cal*
- *Fat: 17g*
- *Cholesterol: 163mg*
- *Sodium: 130mg*
- *Carbohydrates: 23g*
- *Fiber: 2g*
- *Protein: 17g*

97. PESTO ZUCCHINI NOODLES

PREPARATION	COOKING	SERVES
10 MIN	30 MIN	4

INGREDIENTS

- 4 zucchinis, spiralized
- 1 tablespoon avocado oil
- 2 garlic cloves, chopped
- 2/3 cup olive oil
- 1/3 cup parmesan cheese, grated
- 2 cups fresh basil
- 1/3 cup almonds
- 1/8 tsp. black pepper
- 3/4 tsp. sea salt

DIRECTIONS

1. Add zucchini noodles into a colander and sprinkle with 1/4 teaspoon of salt.
2. Cover and let sit for 30 minutes.
3. Drain zucchini noodles well and pat dry.
4. Preheat the oven to 400 F.
5. Place almonds on a parchment-lined baking sheet and bake for 6-8 minutes.
6. Transfer toasted almonds into the food processor and process until coarse.
7. Add olive oil, cheese, basil, garlic, pepper, and remaining salt in a food processor with almonds and process until pesto texture.
8. Heat avocado oil in a large pan over medium-high heat, add zucchini noodles and cook for 4-5 minutes.
9. Pour pesto over zucchini noodles, mix well and cook for 1 minute.
10. Serve immediately with baked salmon.

NUTRITIONS

- Calories: 525 Cal
- Fat: 47.4 g
- Carbohydrates: 9.3 g
- Sugar: 3.8 g
- Protein: 16.6 g
- Cholesterol: 30 mg

98. STEWED HERBED FRUIT

PREPARATION	COOKING	SERVES
15 MIN	6-8 HOURS	1

INGREDIENTS

- 2 cups dried apricots
- 2 cups prunes
- 2 cups dried unsulfured pears
- 2 cups dried apples
- 1 cup dried cranberries
- 1/4 cup honey
- 6 cups of water
- 1 teaspoon dried thyme leaves
- 1 teaspoon dried basil leaves

DIRECTIONS

1. In a 6-quart slow cooker, mix all of the ingredients.
2. Cover and cook on low for 6 to 8 hours, or until the fruits have absorbed the liquid and are tender.
3. Store in the refrigerator for up to 1 week.
4. You can freeze the fruit in 1-cup portions for more extended storage.

NUTRITIONS

- *Calories: 242 Cal*
- *Carbohydrates: 61 g*
- *Sugar: 43 g*
- *Fiber: 9 g*
- *Fat: 0 g*
- *Saturated Fat: 0 g*
- *Protein: 2 g*
- *Sodium: 11 mg*

99. HERBED WILD RICE

PREPARATION	COOKING	SERVES
10 MIN	4-6 HOURS	8

INGREDIENTS

- 3 cups wild rice, rinsed and drained
- 6 cups Roasted Vegetable Broth
- 1 onion, chopped
- 1/2 teaspoon salt
- 1/2 teaspoon dried thyme leaves
- 1/2 teaspoon dried basil leaves
- 1 bay leaf
- 1/3 cup chopped fresh flat-leaf parsley

DIRECTIONS

1. In a 6-quart slow cooker, mix the wild rice, vegetable broth, onion, salt, thyme, basil, and bay leaf.
2. Cover and cook on low for 4 to 6 hours, or until the wild rice is tender but still firm.
3. You can cook this dish longer until the wild rice pops, taking about 7 to 8 hours.
4. Remove and discard the bay leaf.
5. Stir in the parsley and serve.

NUTRITIONS

- Calories: 258 Cal
- Carbohydrates: 54 g
- Sugar: 3 g
- Fiber: 5 g
- Fat: 2 g
- Saturated Fat: 0 g
- Protein: 6 g
- Sodium: 257 mg

100. BUFFALO CHICKEN SLIDERS

PREPARATION	COOKING	SERVES
10 MIN	15 MIN	2

INGREDIENTS

- Chicken breasts (2 lb., cooked, shredded)
- Wing sauce (1 cup)
- Ranch dressing mix (1 pack)
- Blue cheese dressing (1/4 cup, low fat)
- Lettuce (for topping)
- Buns (12, slider)

DIRECTIONS

1. Add the chicken breasts (shredded, cooked) in a large bowl along with the ranch dressing and wing sauce.
2. Stir well to incorporate, then place a piece of lettuce onto each slider roll.
3. Top off using a chicken mixture.
4. Drizzle blue cheese dressing over chicken, then top off using top buns of slider rolls
5. Serve.

NUTRITIONS

- Calories: 300 Cal
- Fat: 14 g
- Cholesterol: 25 mg

101. HIGH PROTEIN CHICKEN MEATBALLS

PREPARATION	COOKING	SERVES
5 MIN	25 MIN	2

INGREDIENTS

- Chicken (1 lb., lean, ground)
- Oats (3/4 cup, rolled)
- Onions (2, grated)
- All-spice (2 tsp. ground)
- Salt and black pepper (dash)

DIRECTIONS

1. Heat a skillet (large) over medium heat, then grease using cooking spray.
2. Add in the onions (grated), chicken (lean, ground), oats (rolled), allspice (earth) and a dash of salt and black pepper in a large-sized bowl. Stir well to incorporate.
3. Shape mixture into meatballs (small).
4. Place into the skillet (greased). Cook for roughly 5 minutes until golden brown on all sides.
5. Remove meatballs from heat, then serve immediately.

NUTRITIONS

- Calories: 519 Cal
- Protein: 57g
- Carbohydrates: 32 g
- Fat: 15 g

102. BARLEY RISOTTO

PREPARATION	COOKING	SERVES
15 MIN	7-8 HOURS	8

INGREDIENTS

- 2 1/4 cups hulled barley, rinsed
- 1 onion, finely chopped
- 4 garlic cloves, minced
- 1 (8-ounce) package button mushrooms, chopped
- 6 cups low-sodium vegetable broth
- 1/2 teaspoon dried marjoram leaves
- 1/8 teaspoon freshly ground black pepper
- 2/3 cup grated Parmesan cheese
-

DIRECTIONS

1. In a 6-quart slow cooker, mix the barley, onion, garlic, mushrooms, broth, marjoram, and pepper.
2. Cover and cook on low for 7 to 8 hours, or until the barley has absorbed most of the liquid and is tender, and the vegetables are tender.
3. Stir in the Parmesan cheese and serve.

NUTRITIONS

- Calories: 288 Cal
- Carbohydrates: 45 g
- Sugar: 2 g
- Fiber: 9 g
- Fat: 6 g
- Saturated Fat: 3 g
- Protein: 13 g
- Sodium: 495 mg

103. RISOTTO WITH GREEN BEANS, SWEET POTATOES, AND PEAS

PREPARATION	COOKING	SERVES
20 MIN	4-5 HOURS	8

INGREDIENTS

- 1 large sweet potato, peeled and chopped
- 1 onion, chopped
- 5 garlic cloves, minced
- 2 cups short-grain brown rice
- 1 teaspoon dried thyme leaves
- 7 cups low-sodium vegetable broth
- 2 cups green beans, cut in half crosswise
- 2 cups frozen baby peas
- 3 tablespoons unsalted butter
- 1/2 cup grated Parmesan cheese

DIRECTIONS

1. In a 6-quart slow cooker, mix the sweet potato, onion, garlic, rice, thyme, and broth.
2. Cover and cook on low for 3 to 4 hours, or until the rice is tender.
3. Stir in the green beans and frozen peas.
4. Cover and cook on low for 30 to 40 minutes or until the vegetables are tender.
5. Stir in the butter and cheese. Cover and cook on low for 20 minutes, then stir and serve.

NUTRITIONS

- *Calories: 385 Cal*
- *Carbohydrates: 52 g*
- *Sugar: 4 g*
- *Fiber: 6 g*
- *Fat: 10 g*
- *Saturated Fat: 5 g*
- *Protein: 10 g*
- *Sodium: 426 mg*

104. MAPLE LEMON TEMPEH CUBES

PREPARATION	COOKING	SERVES
10 MIN	30-40 MIN	4

INGREDIENTS

- Tempeh; 1 packet
- Coconut oil; 2 to 3 teaspoons
- Lemon juice; 3 tablespoons
- Maple syrup; 2 teaspoons
- Bragg's Liquid Aminos or low-sodium tamari or (optional); 1 to 2 teaspoons
- Water; 2 teaspoons
- Dried basil; 1/4 teaspoon
- Powdered garlic; 1/4 teaspoon
- Black pepper (freshly grounded); to taste

DIRECTIONS

1. Heat your oven to 400 ° C. Cut your tempeh block into squares in bite form.
2. Heat coconut oil over medium to high heat in a non-stick skillet.
3. When melted and heated, add the tempeh and cook on one side for 2-4 minutes, or until the tempeh turns down into a golden-brown color.
4. Flip the tempeh bits, and cook for 2-4 minutes.
5. Mix the lemon juice, tamari, maple syrup, basil, water, garlic, and black pepper while tempeh is browning.
6. Drop the mixture over tempeh, then swirl to cover the tempeh.
7. Sauté for 2-3 minutes, then turn the tempeh and sauté 1-2 minutes more.
8. The tempeh, on both sides, should be soft and orange.

NUTRITIONS

- Carbohydrates: 22 Cal
- Fats: 17 g
- Sugar: 5 g
- Protein: 21 g
- Fiber: 9 g

105. BOK CHOY WITH TOFU STIR-FRY

PREPARATION	COOKING	SERVES
15 MIN	15 MIN	4

INGREDIENTS

- Super-firm tofu; 1 lb. (drained and pressed)
- Coconut oil; one tablespoon
- Clove of garlic; 1 (minced)
- Baby bok choy; 3 heads (chopped)
- Low-sodium vegetable broth;
- Maple syrup; 2 teaspoons
- Bragg's liquid aminos
- Sambal oiled; 1 to 2 teaspoons (similar chili sauce)
- Scallion or green onion; 1 (chopped)
- Freshly grated ginger; 1 teaspoon
- Quinoa/rice, for serving

DIRECTIONS

1. With paper towels, Pat pressed the tofu dry and cut it into tiny pieces of bite-size around 1/2 inch wide.
2. Heat coconut oil in a wide skillet onto a warm.
3. Remove tofu and stir-fry until painted softly.
4. Stir-fry for 1-2 minutes before the choy of the Bok starts to wilt.
5. When this occurs, you'll want to apply the vegetable broth and all the remaining ingredients to the skillet.
6. Hold the mixture stir-frying until all components are well coated, and the bulk of the liquid evaporates, around 5-6 min.
7. Serve over brown rice or quinoa.

NUTRITIONS

- Calories: 263.7 Cal
- Fat 4.2 g
- Cholesterol: 0.3 mg
- Sodium: 683.6 mg
- Potassium: 313.7 mg
- Carbohydrate: 35.7 g

106. THREE-BEAN MEDLEY

PREPARATION	COOKING	SERVES
15 MIN	6-8 HOURS	8

INGREDIENTS

- 1 1/4 cups dried kidney beans, rinsed and drained
- 1 1/4 cups dried black beans, rinsed and drained
- 1 1/4 cups dried black-eyed peas, rinsed and drained
- 1 onion, chopped
- 1 leek, chopped
- 2 garlic cloves, minced
- 2 carrots, peeled and chopped
- 6 cups low-sodium vegetable broth
- 1 1/2 cups water
- 1/2 teaspoon dried thyme leaves

DIRECTIONS

1. In a 6-quart slow cooker, mix all of the ingredients.
2. Cover and cook on low for 6 to 8 hours, or until the beans are tender and the liquid is absorbed.

NUTRITIONS

- Calories: 284 Cal
- Carbohydrates: 56 g
- Sugar: 6 g
- Fiber: 19 g
- Fat: 0 g
- Saturated Fat: 0 g
- Protein: 1 9g
- Sodium: 131 mg

107. HERBED GARLIC BLACK BEANS

PREPARATION	COOKING	SERVES
10 MIN	7-9 HOURS	8

INGREDIENTS

- 3 cups dried black beans, rinsed and drained
- 2 onions, chopped
- 8 garlic cloves, minced
- 6 cups low-sodium vegetable broth
- 1/2 teaspoon salt
- 1 teaspoon dried basil leaves
- 1/2 teaspoon dried thyme leaves
- 1/2 teaspoon dried oregano leaves

DIRECTIONS

1. In a 6-quart slow cooker, mix all the ingredients.
2. Cover and cook on low for 7 to 9 hours, or until the beans have absorbed the liquid and are tender.
3. Remove and discard the bay leaf

NUTRITIONS

- Calories: 250 Cal
- Carbohydrates: 47 g
- Sugar: 3 g
- Fiber: 17 g
- Fat: 0 g
- Saturated Fat: 0 g
- Protein: 15 g
- Sodium: 253 mg

108. QUINOA WITH VEGETABLES

PREPARATION	COOKING	SERVES
10 MIN	5-6 HOURS	8

INGREDIENTS

- 2 cups quinoa, rinsed and drained
- 2 onions, chopped
- 2 carrots, peeled and sliced
- 1 cup sliced cremini mushrooms
- 3 garlic cloves, minced
- 4 cups low-sodium vegetable broth
- 1/2 teaspoon salt
- 1 teaspoon dried marjoram leaves
- 1/8 teaspoon freshly ground black pepper

DIRECTIONS

1. In a 6-quart slow cooker, mix all of the ingredients.
2. Cover and cook on low for 5 to 6 hours, or until the quinoa and vegetables are tender.
3. Stir the mixture and serve.

NUTRITIONS

- *Calories: 204 Cal*
- *Carbohydrates: 35 g*
- *Sugar: 4 g*
- *Fiber: 4 g*
- *Fat: 3 g*
- *Saturated Fat: 0 g*
- *Protein: 7 g*
- *Sodium: 229 mg*

109. BALSAMIC BEEF AND MUSHROOMS MIX

PREPARATION	COOKING	SERVES
5 MIN	8 HOURS	4

INGREDIENTS

- 2 pounds' beef, cut into strips
- ¼ cup balsamic vinegar
- 2 cups beef stock
- 1 tablespoon ginger, grated
- Juice of ½ lemon
- 1 cup brown mushrooms, sliced
- A pinch of salt and black pepper
- 1 teaspoon ground cinnamon

DIRECTIONS

1. In your slow cooker, mix all the ingredients, cover and cook on low for 8 hours.
2. Divide everything between plates and serve.

NUTRITIONS

- Calories: 446
- Fat: 14g
- Fiber: 0.6g
- Carbs: 2.9 g
- Protein: 70g

110. SIMPLE BEEF ROAST

PREPARATION	COOKING	SERVES
10 MIN	8 HOURS	8

INGREDIENTS

- 5 pounds' beef roast
- 2 tablespoons Italian seasoning
- 1 cup beef stock
- 1 tablespoon sweet paprika
- 3 tablespoons olive oil

DIRECTIONS

1. In your slow cooker, mix all the ingredients, cover and cook on low for 8 hours.
2. Carve the roast, divide it between plates and serve.

NUTRITIONS

- *Calories: 587*
- *Fat: 24.1g*
- *Fiber: 0.3g*
- *Carbs: 0.9g*
- *Protein: 86.5g*

111. CAULIFLOWER CURRY

PREPARATION	COOKING	SERVES
5 MIN	5 HOURS	4

INGREDIENTS

- 1 cauliflower head, florets separated
- 2 carrots, sliced
- 1 red onion, chopped
- ¾ cup of coconut milk
- 2 garlic cloves, minced
- 2 tablespoons curry powder
- A pinch of salt and black pepper
- 1 tablespoon red pepper flakes
- 1 teaspoon garam masala

DIRECTIONS

1. In your slow cooker, mix all the ingredients.
2. Cover, cook on high for 5 hours, divide into bowls and serve.

NUTRITIONS

- Calories: 160
- Fat: 11.5g
- Fiber: 5.4g
- Carbs: 14.7g
- Protein: 3.6g

112. PORK AND PEPPERS CHILI

PREPARATION	COOKING	SERVES
5 MIN	8 H 5 MIN	4

INGREDIENTS

- 1 red onion, chopped
- 2 pounds' pork, ground
- 4 garlic cloves, minced
- 2 red bell peppers, chopped
- 1 celery stalk, chopped
- 25 ounces' fresh tomatoes, peeled, crushed
- ¼ cup green chilies, chopped
- 2 tablespoons fresh oregano, chopped
- 2 tablespoons chili powder
- A pinch of salt and black pepper
- A drizzle of olive oil

DIRECTIONS

1. Heat a sauté pan with the oil over medium-high heat and add the onion, garlic and meat. Mix and brown for 5 minutes, then transfer to your slow cooker.
2. Add the rest of the ingredients, toss, cover and cook on low for 8 hours.
3. Divide everything into bowls and serve.

NUTRITIONS

- *Calories: 448*
- *Fat: 13g*
- *Fiber: 6.6g*
- *Carbs: 20.2g*
- *Protein: 63g*

113. GREEK STYLE QUESADILLAS

PREPARATION	COOKING	SERVES
10 MIN	10 MIN	4

INGREDIENTS

- 4 whole-wheat tortillas
- 1 cup Mozzarella cheese, shredded
- 1 cup fresh spinach, chopped
- 2 tablespoon Greek yogurt
- 1 egg, beaten
- ¼ cup green olives, sliced
- 1 tablespoon olive oil
- 1/3 cup fresh cilantro, chopped

DIRECTIONS

1. In the bowl, combine Mozzarella cheese, spinach, yogurt, egg, olives, and cilantro.
2. Then pour olive oil into the skillet.
3. In the skillet, Place one tortilla and spread it with Mozzarella mixture.
4. Top it with the second tortilla and spread it with cheese mixture again.
5. Then place the third tortilla and spread it with all remaining cheese mixture.
6. Cover it with the last tortilla and fry it for 5 minutes from each side over medium heat.

NUTRITIONS

- Calories: 193
- Fat: 7.7g
- Fiber: 3.2g
- Carbs: 23.6g
- Protein: 8.3g

114. MEDITERRANEAN BURRITO

PREPARATION	COOKING	SERVES
10 MIN	0 MIN	2

INGREDIENTS

- 2 wheat tortillas
- 2 oz. red kidney beans, canned, drained
- 2 tablespoons hummus
- 2 teaspoons tahini sauce
- 1 cucumber
- 2 lettuce leaves
- 1 tablespoon lime juice
- 1 teaspoon olive oil
- ½ teaspoon dried oregano

DIRECTIONS

1. Mash the red kidney beans until you get a puree.
2. Then spread the wheat tortillas with beans mash from one side.
3. Add hummus and tahini sauce.
4. Cut the cucumber into the wedges and place them over tahini sauce.
5. Then add lettuce leaves.
6. Make the dressing: mix up together olive oil, dried oregano, and lime juice.
7. Drizzle the lettuce leaves with the dressing and wrap the wheat tortillas in burritos' shape.

NUTRITIONS

- Calories: 288
- Fat: 10.2
- Fiber: 14.6
- Carbs: 38.2
- Protein: 12.5

115. SWEET POTATO BACON MASH

PREPARATION	COOKING	SERVES
10 MIN	20 MIN	4

INGREDIENTS

- 3 sweet potatoes, peeled
- 4 ounces bacon, chopped
- 1 cup chicken stock
- 1 tablespoon butter
- 1 teaspoon salt
- 2 ounces Parmesan, grated

DIRECTIONS

1. Dice sweet potato and put it in the pan.
2. Add chicken stock and close the lid.
3. Boil the vegetables until they are soft.
4. After this, drain the chicken stock.
5. Mash the sweet potato with the help of the potato masher. Add grated cheese and butter.
6. Mix up together salt and chopped bacon. Fry the mixture until it is crunchy (10-15 minutes).
7. Add cooked bacon to the mashed sweet potato and mix up with the help of the spoon.
8. It is recommended to serve the meal warm or hot.

NUTRITIONS

- Calories: 304
- Fat: 18.1
- Fiber: 2.9
- Carbs: 18.8
- Protein: 17
- Ù

116. SAVORY SALMON WITH CILANTRO

PREPARATION	COOKING	SERVES
20 MIN	25 MIN	4

INGREDIENTS

- 4 cups fresh cilantro (divided)
- 2 tablespoons fresh lemon or lime juice
- 2 tablespoons red pepper sauce
- 1 teaspoon cumin
- ½ teaspoon salt
- ½ cup of water
- 2 to 7 ounces raw salmon filets
- 4 cups bell pepper (all colors), seeded and julienned
- ½ teaspoon pepper
- Cooking spray

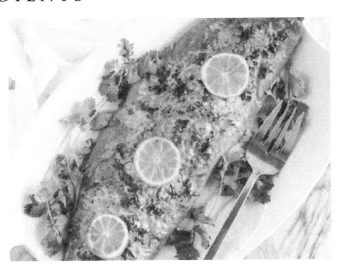

DIRECTIONS

1. Place half the cilantro, lemon juice, red pepper sauce, cumin, salt, and water in a blender. Pulse the blender until smooth. Transfer into a Ziploc bag and place the salmon. Marinate for 1 hour inside the fridge.
2. Preheat the oven to 400F. Arrange the bell peppers in a lightly greased baking dish. Sprinkle with pepper and bake for 10 minutes.
3. Drain the salmon and place on top the pepper slices, and bake for 20 minutes.
4. Garnish with the remaining cilantro.

NUTRITIONS

- Calories per serving: 341;
- Protein: 1 serving of
- lean protein,
- 4 servings of higher carbohydrate,
- Fat: 0,
- Sugar: 0

117. MIDDLE EASTERN SALMON WITH TOMATOES AND CUCUMBER

PREPARATION	COOKING	SERVES
20 MIN	35 MIN	4

INGREDIENTS

- 4 cups sliced cucumber
- 1-pint cherry tomatoes halved
- ¼ cup cider vinegar
- ½ cup fresh dill (chopped)
- Salt and pepper to taste
- 1½ pounds skinless salmon
- tablespoon Za'atar sauce
- lemon wedges for garnish

DIRECTIONS

1. Preheat the oven to 350 0 F
2. Place the cucumber and tomatoes in a bowl. Add in the vinegar, dill, and season with salt and pepper to taste. Toss to coat.
3. Season the salmon with Za'atar on both sides and place on a foil-lined baking sheet. Roast until the internal temperature reaches 145° F.
4. Serve the roasted salmon with cucumber and tomatoes.

NUTRITIONS

- Calories per serving: 282;
- 1   serving of lean protein,
- 2 servings of lower carbohydrate;
- 1 serving of lower carbohydrate,
- No healthy fat servings.

118. CUCUMBER BOWL WITH SPICES AND GREEK YOGURT

PREPARATION	COOKING	SERVES
10 MIN	20 MIN	3

INGREDIENTS

- cucumbers
- ½ teaspoon chili pepper
- ¼ cup fresh parsley (chopped)
- ¾ cup fresh dill (chopped)
- tablespoons lemon juice
- ½ teaspoon salt
- ½ teaspoon ground black pepper
- ¼ teaspoon sage
- ½ teaspoon dried oregano
- 1/3 cup Greek yogurt

DIRECTIONS

1. Make the cucumber dressing: blend the dill and parsley until you get a green mash.
2. Then combine the green mash with lemon juice, salt, ground black pepper, sage, dried oregano, Greek yogurt, and chili pepper.
3. Churn the mixture well.
4. Chop the cucumbers roughly and combine them with cucumber dressing. Mix up well.
5. Refrigerate the cucumber for 20 minutes.

NUTRITIONS

- *Calories: 114*
- *Carbs: 2 servings higher carb*
- *1 serving leaner protein*
- *1 serving lower carb.*

119. STUFFED BELL PEPPERS WITH QUINOA

PREPARATION	COOKING	SERVES
10 MIN	35 MIN	2

INGREDIENTS

- 1 bell peppers
- 1/3 cup quinoa
- 3 oz. chicken stock
- ¼ cup onion (diced)
- ½ teaspoon salt
- ¼ teaspoon tomato paste
- ½ teaspoon dried oregano
- 1/3 cup sour cream
- 1 teaspoon paprika

DIRECTIONS

1. Trim the peppers and remove the seeds
2. Then combine chicken stock and quinoa in the pan.
3. Add salt and boil the ingredients for 10 minutes or until quinoa soaks all liquid.
4. Then combine the cooked quinoa with dried oregano, tomato paste, and onion.
5. Fill the bell peppers with the quinoa mixture and arrange them in the casserole mold.
6. Add sour cream and bake the peppers for 25 minutes at 365° F.
7. Serve the cooked peppers with sour cream sauce from the casserole mold.

NUTRITIONS

- *Calories: 237*
- *1 serving of healthy fat.*
- *1 servings of higher carb*

120. SPAGHETTI SQUASH GRATIN

PREPARATION	COOKING	SERVES
10 MIN	60 MIN	2

INGREDIENTS

- 2 ½ pounds spaghetti squash
- 2 eggs
- 1 cup reduced-fat cheddar cheese (shredded)
- ½ cup plain low-fat Greek yogurt
- 2 cloves garlic (minced)
- Salt and pepper to taste
- ½ cup reduced-fat grated parmesan cheese

DIRECTIONS

1. Preheat the oven to 400° F.
2. Halve the spaghetti squash and scoop out the seeds. Put squash face down on a baking sheet lined with foil. Place in the oven and cook for 30 minutes. Allow cooling before scooping the meat and placing it in a large bowl.
3. In another bowl, combine the remaining ingredients. Mix well until well combined.
4. Spread in a casserole dish and bake for 30 more minutes in the oven.

NUTRITIONS

- *Calories per serving: 503*
- *2 servings higher carb*
- *1 serving leanest protein*
- *1 serving leaner protein.*

121. SALMON FLORENTINE

PREPARATION	COOKING	SERVES
10 MIN	30 MIN	2

INGREDIENTS

- ½ cup chopped green onion
- 1 teaspoon olive oil
- 2 garlic cloves (minced)
- 1 12 oz. packaged frozen chopped spinach
- 1 ½ cups chopped celery
- ¼ teaspoon crushed red pepper flakes
- Salt and pepper to taste
- ½ cup part-skim ricotta cheese
- ½ ounces wild salmon filets

DIRECTIONS

1. Preheat the oven to 350° F.
2. Heat skillet over medium flame and cook the green onions and olive oil. Add the garlic and cook for another 30 seconds. Stir in the spinach, celery, red pepper flakes, and season with salt and pepper to taste. Stir for 3 minutes until the spinach has wilted. Turn off the heat and set it aside to cool slightly.
3. Mix the ricotta cheese into the cooked spinach. Mix until it's well-combined.
4. Place the salmon on a parchment-lined baking sheet. Top the salmon with the ricotta and spinach mixture.
5. Place in the oven for 30 minutes.

NUTRITIONS

- *Calories per serving: 145;*
- *2 servings lean protein*
- *1 serving higher carb*
- *2 servings healthy fat.*

122. CHEESEBURGER SOUP

PREPARATION	COOKING	SERVES
20 MIN	25 MIN	4

INGREDIENTS

- ¼ cup of chopped onion
- 1 quantity of 14.5 oz. can have diced tomato
- 1 lb. of 90% lean ground beef
- ¾ cup of diced celery
- 2 teaspoon of Worcestershire sauce
- 3 cups of low sodium chicken broth
- ¼ teaspoon of salt
- 1 teaspoon of dried parsley
- 7 cups of baby spinach
- ¼ teaspoon of ground pepper
- 1 oz. of reduced-fat shredded cheddar cheese

DIRECTIONS

1. Get a large soup pot and cook the beef until it becomes brown. Add the celery, onion, and sauté until it becomes tender. Remove from the fire and drain excess liquid.
2. Stir in the broth, tomatoes, parsley, Worcestershire sauce, pepper, and salt. Cover and allow it to simmer on low heat for about 20 minutes
3. Add spinach and leave it to cook until it becomes wilted in about 1-3 minutes. Top each of your servings with 1 ounce of cheese.

NUTRITIONS

- *Calories: 400;*
- *2 servings lean protein,*
- *2 servings higher carb*
- *1 serving moderate carb.*

123. BRAISED COLLARD GREENS IN PEANUT SAUCE WITH PORK TENDERLOIN

PREPARATION	COOKING	SERVES
20 MIN	1 H 12 MIN	4

INGREDIENTS

- 2 cups of chicken stock
- 12 cups of chopped collard greens
- 5 tablespoon of powdered peanut butter
- 3 cloves of garlic (crushed)
- 1 teaspoon of salt
- ½ teaspoon of all-spice
- ½ teaspoon of black pepper
- 2 teaspoon of lemon juice
- ¾ teaspoon of hot sauce
- 1 ½ lb. of pork tenderloin

DIRECTIONS

1. Get a pot with a tight-fitting lid and combine the collards with the garlic, chicken stock, hot sauce, and half of the pepper and salt. Cook on low heat for about 1 hour or until the collards become tender.
2. Once the collards are tender, stir in the all-spice, lemon juice and powdered peanut butter. Keep it warm.
3. Season the pork tenderloin with the remaining pepper and salt, and broil in a toaster oven for 10 minutes until you have an internal temperature of 145° F. Make sure to turn the tenderloin every 2 minutes to achieve an even browning all over. After that, you can take away the pork from the oven and allow it to rest for like 5 minutes.
4. Slice the pork as you will

NUTRITIONS

- *Calories: 320;*
- *1 serving healthy fat,*
- *2 servings lean protein,*
- *1 serving higher carb.*

124. TENDER LAMB CHOPS

PREPARATION	COOKING	SERVES
10 MIN	6 HOURS	8

INGREDIENTS

- 8 lamb chops
- ½ teaspoon dried thyme
- 1 onion (sliced)
- 1 teaspoon dried oregano
- 2 garlic cloves (minced)
- Pepper and salt

DIRECTIONS

1. Add sliced onion into the slow cooker.
2. Combine thyme, oregano, pepper, and salt. Rub over lamb chops.
3. Place lamb chops on a low-heat cooker and top it with garlic.
4. Pour ¼ cup water around the lamb chops.
5. Cover and cook on low heat for 6 hours.
6. Serve and enjoy.

NUTRITIONS

- *Calories: 40;*
- *1 serving lean protein,*
- *1 serving higher carb.*

125. SMOKY PORK & CABBAGE

PREPARATION	COOKING	SERVES
10 MIN	8 HOURS	6

INGREDIENTS

- lbs. pork roast
- 1/2 cabbage head, chopped
- 1 cup of water
- 1/3 cup liquid smoke
- tablespoon kosher salt

DIRECTIONS

1. Rub the pork with kosher salt and place it into the crockpot.
2. Pour liquid smoke over the pork and add water.
3. Cover and cook on low heat for 7 hours.
4. Remove pork from the crockpot and add cabbage to the bottom of the crockpot.
5. Place pork on top of the cabbage.
6. Cover again and cook for 1 more hour.
7. Shred pork with a fork and serve.

NUTRITIONS

- *Calories: 484;*
- *1 serving lean protein,*
- *1 serving moderate carb.*

126. SEASONED PORK CHOPS

PREPARATION	COOKING	SERVES
10 MIN	4 HOURS	4

INGREDIENTS

- 4 pork chops
- 2 garlic cloves (minced)
- 1 cup chicken broth
- 1 tablespoon poultry seasoning
- 1/4 cup olive oil
- Pepper and salt

DIRECTIONS

1. In a bowl, whisk together olive oil, poultry seasoning, garlic, broth, pepper, and salt.
2. Pour olive oil mixture into the slow cooker, then place pork chops into the crockpot.
3. Cover and cook on high heat for 4 hours.
4. Serve and enjoy.

NUTRITIONS

- *Calories: 386;*
- *2 servings lean protein,*
- *1 serving healthy fat.*

127. SHRIMP AND CAULIFLOWER GRITS

PREPARATION	COOKING	SERVES
20 MIN	25 MIN	4

INGREDIENTS

- 1-pound raw shrimps, peeled and deveined
- ½ tablespoon Cajun seasoning
- Cooking spray
- 1 tablespoon lemon juice
- ¼ cup chicken broth
- 1 tablespoon butter
- 2 ½ cups cauliflower, grated or minced finely
- ½ cup unsweetened cashew milk
- ¼ teaspoon salt
- 2 tablespoons sour cream
- 1/3 cup reduced-fat shredded cheddar cheese
- ¼ cup sliced scallions

DIRECTIONS

1. Place the shrimps and Cajun seasonings into a Ziploc bag and close the bag. Toss to coat the shrimps evenly with the seasoning.
2. Spray a skillet with cooking spray and cook the seasoned shrimps until pink. It will take about 2 to 3 minutes per side. Add the lemon juice and chicken broth. Make sure to scrape the bottom to remove the browned bits. Set aside.
3. In another skillet, heat butter over medium flame and add the rice cauliflower. Cook for 5 minutes and add the milk and salt. Cook for another 5 minutes. Remove from the heat and add the sour cream and cheese. Stir until well-combined.
4. Serve the shrimps on top of the cauliflower grits.
5. Garnish with scallions.

NUTRITIONS

- Calories per serving: 456;
- 2 servings leanest
- protein,
- 2 servings healthy fat,
- 1 serving higher carb,
- 1 serving moderate carb.

128. TUNA NIÇOISE SALAD

PREPARATION	COOKING	SERVES
20 MIN	25 MIN	4

INGREDIENTS

- 4 teaspoons extra virgin olive oil
- 3 tablespoons balsamic vinegar
- 2 garlic cloves (minced)
- 6 cups mixed greens
- 2 cups string beans (steamed)
- 1 cup cherry tomatoes (halved)
- 6 hard-boiled eggs (sliced)
- 2 7oz. can of tuna, packed in water and drained

DIRECTIONS

1. Mix the oil, vinegar, and garlic in a bowl until well combined.
2. Place the remaining ingredients in a bowl and drizzle with the prepared sauce.

NUTRITIONS

- *Calories per serving: 392;*
- *serving higher carb,*
- *servings lower carb,*
- *1 serving healthy fat,*
- *servings leanest*
- *protein.*

129. VEGGIE DIPS AND BUFFALO DIP

PREPARATION	COOKING	SERVES
20 MIN	25 MIN	4

INGREDIENTS

- 1 tablespoon olive oil
- 2 teaspoons lemon juice
- ½ teaspoon salt
- ½ teaspoon pepper
- ½ teaspoon rosemary
- 4 cups sliced yellow squash
- 3 cups sliced zucchini
- 4 light spreadable cheese wedges
- 1 ½ cup plain low-fat Greek yogurt
- ¼ cup light ranch dressing

DIRECTIONS

1. Preheat the oven to 400°F.
2. Put the oil, lemon juice, salt, pepper, rosemary, and vegetables in a bowl. Toss to coat the vegetables.
3. Arrange the vegetables on a baking sheet in a single layer.
4. Bake for 20 minutes until crisp.
5. Meanwhile, place the remaining ingredients in a bowl. Whisk to combine the dip.
6. Serve the crispy vegetables with the dip.

NUTRITIONS

- *Calories per serving: 140;*
- *1 serving moderate*
- *carb,*
- *1 healthy fat serving,*
- *2 servings higher*
- *carb,*
- *1 serving lean protein.*

130. GRILLED TEMPEH WITH EGGPLANTS AND WATERCRESS

PREPARATION	COOKING	SERVES
20 MIN	35 MIN	4

INGREDIENTS

- 20 ounces tempeh, sliced into large chunks
- 4 ½ cups diced eggplants
- ½ tablespoons rice vinegar
- ½ teaspoon ground black pepper
- ½ teaspoon salt (divided)
- 1 ½ cups watercress
- ¼ cup minced scallions
- ½ cup fresh tomatoes (sliced)
- ½ tablespoon lemon juice
- 1 ½ tablespoon soy sauce
- 1 teaspoon lime juice

DIRECTIONS

1. Pour boiling water over the tempeh and allow it to soak for 30 minutes.
2. In a bowl, toss the eggplant together with the rice vinegar, pepper, and a quarter of the salt.
3. Fire the grill to 425°F and roast the seasoned eggplants for 30 minutes on all sides until golden brown and tender.
4. Remove the roasted eggplants and allow them to cool.
5. Pat-dry the tempeh and grill for 2 minutes on each side until golden brown. Set aside to cool.
6. Prepare the watercress salad by combining the remaining ingredients in a bowl. Toss to coat.
7. Serve the tempeh, grilled eggplants, and watercress together.

NUTRITIONS

- *Calories per serving: 310;*
- *1 serving higher carb,*
- *1 serving moderate carb,*
- *1 serving lower carb.*

131. MINI MAC IN A BOWL

PREPARATION	COOKING	SERVES
20 MIN	40 MIN	4

INGREDIENTS

- 2 tablespoons diced yellow onion
- 5 ounces 99% lean ground beef
- 2 tablespoons light "Thousand Island" dressing
- 1/8 teaspoon white vinegar
- 1/8 teaspoon onion powder
- 3 cups shredded romaine lettuce
- 2 tablespoons reduced-fat cheddar cheese
- 1 teaspoon sesame seeds

DIRECTIONS

1. Heat a skillet over a medium flame. Grease skillet with cooking spray.
2. Add the onion and sauté for 1 minute. Add the beef and cook until lightly browned.
3. Meanwhile, mix the island dressing, white vinegar, and onion powder. Set aside.
4. Assemble by topping the lettuce with ground beef. Sprinkle cheese on top and garnish with pickle slices and sesame seeds. Drizzle with sauce.

NUTRITIONS

- *Calories per serving: 416;*
- *2 servings healthy fat,*
- *1 serving lean protein,*
- *1 serving lower carb.*

132. PHILLY CHEESESTEAK STUFFED PEPPERS

PREPARATION	COOKING	SERVES
20 MIN	50 MIN	4

INGREDIENTS

- 4 medium green bell peppers, sliced on top and seeded
- 1/3 cup diced yellow onion
- 2 cloves garlic (minced)
- ¼ cup of low sodium bean broth
- 6 ounces baby Bella mushrooms (sliced)
- 1-pound shaved deli roast beef
- 4 tablespoons low-fat cream cheese
- 4 ounces reduced-fat provolone cheese

DIRECTIONS

1. Preheat the oven to 4000 F.
2. Set aside the bell pepper and make sure that they are clean inside.
3. In a skillet, sauté the onion and garlic in broth over medium flame for 5 minutes. Add the mushrooms and deli beef. Stir to cook everything.
4. Remove from skillet and stir in the cream cheese.
5. Line each of the bell pepper with a quarter slice of cheese. Fill an eighth with the roast beef mixture and top with cheese.
6. Place in the oven and bake for 20 minutes.

NUTRITIONS

- *Calories per serving: 486;*
- *1 serving higher carb,*
- *2 servings healthy fat,*
- *1 serving moderate carb,*
- *1 serving lean protein.*

133. EASY SPINACH MUFFINS

PREPARATION	COOKING	SERVES
20 MIN	25 MIN	4

INGREDIENTS

- 10 eggs
- 2 cups spinach (chopped)
- 1/4 tsp. garlic powder
- 1/4 tsp. onion powder
- 1/2 tsp. dried basil
- 1 1/2 cups parmesan cheese (grated)
- Salt

DIRECTIONS

1. Preheat the oven to 400 0 F. Grease muffin tin and set aside.
2. In a large bowl, whisk eggs with basil, garlic powder, onion powder, and salt.
3. Add cheese and spinach and stir well.
4. Pour egg mixture into the prepared muffin tin and bake 15 minutes.
5. Serve and enjoy.

NUTRITIONS

- Calories 110;
- 1 serving lean protein,
- 1 healthy fat.

134. HEALTHY CAULIFLOWER GRITS

PREPARATION	COOKING	SERVES
20 MIN	30 MIN	4

INGREDIENTS

- 6 cups cauliflower rice
- 1/4 tsp. garlic powder
- 1 cup cream cheese
- 1/2 cup vegetable stock
- 1/4 tsp. onion powder
- 1/2 tsp. pepper
- 1 tsp. Salt

DIRECTIONS

1. Add all ingredients into the slow cooker and stir well to combine.
2. Cover and cook on low for 2 hours.
3. Stir and serve.

NUTRITIONS

- *Calories 126;*
- *1 serving higher carb,*
- *1 serving healthy fat,*
- *1 serving moderate carb.*

135. ITALIAN STYLE GENOSE ZUCCHINI

PREPARATION	COOKING	SERVES
5 MIN	25 MIN	4

INGREDIENTS

- 2 medium zucchinis, spiralized
- 2 cups basil leaves
- Juice from 1 lemon, freshly squeezed
- 3 cloves of garlic, minced
- 1/2 cup cashew nuts, soaked in water overnight, then drained
- Salt to taste

DIRECTIONS

1. Place zucchini strips on a plate.
2. Place the rest of the ingredients in a food processor and pulse until smooth.
3. Pour sauce over the zucchini, then serve.

NUTRITIONS

- *Calories per serving: 101;*
- *Protein: 3.1g;*
- *Carbs: 6.6g;*
- *Fat: 7.8g*
- *Sugar: 1g*

136. HEALTHY PEPPERS FLOUNDER MEATBALLS

PREPARATION	COOKING	SERVES
5 MIN	6 MIN	3

INGREDIENTS

- 10 ounces flounder fillet, chopped finely
- 1/3 cup celery stalk, chopped finely
- 1/3 cup red pepper, chopped finely
- 1 tablespoon fresh dill, chopped finely
- 2 teaspoons Dijon mustard
- 2 eggs, slightly beaten
- Salt and pepper to taste

DIRECTIONS

1. Place all ingredients in a bowl. Mix until well-incorporated.
2. Form small patties with your hands and place them on a baking sheet. Allow patties to rest in the fridge for at least 30 minutes.
3. Brush pan with extra virgin olive oil and allow to heat over medium flame.
4. Place individual patties into the pan and cook for 3 minutes on each side.
5. Serve immediately.

NUTRITIONS

- Calories per serving: 380;
- Protein: 28.7g;
- Carbs: 13g;
- Fat: 5.4g
- Sugar: 0.02g

137. A TRIUMPH OF MEAT & VEGETABLES

PREPARATION	COOKING	SERVES
5 MIN	10 MIN	3

INGREDIENTS

- 1/2 teaspoon extra virgin olive oil
- 2 ounces Sirloin steak, 98% lean
- Salt and pepper to taste
- 1 zucchini, cut into long thin strips
- 1 onion, chopped
- 6 ounces asparagus, blanched
- 4 ounces peas, blanched

DIRECTIONS

1. Heat olive oil in a skillet. Season the steak with salt and pepper to taste.
2. Place in the skillet and sear the steak for 5 minutes on each side. Allow resting for five minutes before slicing into strips.
3. Place the remaining ingredients in a bowl and season with salt and pepper to taste
4. Top with steak strips, then toss to combine all ingredients.

NUTRITIONS

- Calories per serving: 174;
- Protein: 4.2g;
- Carbs: 10.3g;
- Fat: 4.1g
- Sugar: 2.1g

138. GARLIC AND OIL - BROCCOLI AND BEEF

PREPARATION	COOKING	SERVES
5 MIN	15 MIN	4

INGREDIENTS

- 4 ounces 95-97% lean ground beef
- 1/4 cup Roma tomatoes, chopped
- 1/4 teaspoon garlic powder
- 1/4 teaspoon onion powder
- 1 1/4 cup broccoli, cut into bite-sized pieces
- A pinch of red pepper flakes
- 1-ounce low-sodium cheddar cheese, shredded

DIRECTIONS

1. Place 3 tablespoons of water in a pan and heat over medium flame. Water sauté the beef and tomatoes for 5 minutes until the tomatoes are wilted. Add in the garlic and onion powder and stir for another 3 minutes.
2. Add the broccoli and close the lid. Cook for another 5 minutes.
3. Garnish with red pepper flakes and cheddar cheese on top.

NUTRITIONS

- *Calories per serving: 97;*
- *Protein:9.9 g;*
- *Carbs: 2.6g;*
- *Fat: 1.7g*
- *Sugar:0.9 g*

444

139. MEAT IN THE WOODS

PREPARATION	COOKING	SERVES
5 MIN	7 MIN	6

INGREDIENTS

- 1 pound 98% lean ground beef
- A pinch of salt
- 1/4 teaspoon black pepper
- 8 ounces Romaine lettuce, torn
- 1 cup cherry tomatoes, halved
- 1/2 cup pickles, diced
- 1/4 cup cheddar cheese, shredded

DIRECTIONS

1. Season the beef with salt and pepper.
2. Heat a non-stick pan and sauté the white beef, constantly stirring for 7 minutes. Set aside and allow to slightly cool.
3. Place the lettuce, tomatoes, pickles, and cheese. Sprinkle the cooked beef on top.
4. Toss to mix all ingredients.

NUTRITIONS

- Calories per serving: 186;
- Protein: 21g;
- Carbs: 8.7g;
- Fat: 3.1g
- Sugar: 0.8g

140. TURKEY ON A BOAT

PREPARATION	COOKING	SERVES
5 MIN	20 MIN	8

INGREDIENTS

- 4 medium zucchinis
- 2 tablespoons extra virgin olive oil
- 1-pound lean ground turkey
- 3 cloves of garlic, minced
- 1/2 onion, chopped
- 1/2 green pepper, seeded and chopped
- 1/2 cup skimmed mozzarella cheese, shredded

DIRECTIONS

1. Prepare the zucchini by slicing them in half lengthwise. Scoop the meat out. Chopped the scooped-up zucchini meat and set it aside.
2. Heat oil in a saucepan over medium flame. Stir in the turkey and garlic and sauté for 5 minutes.
3. Stir in the onions halfway while the turkey is cooking. Add in the green pepper and zucchini meat. Cook for another 3 minutes. Set aside to cool completely.
4. Once cooled, stir in the mozzarella cheese.
5. Fill the hollowed-out zucchini with the meat mixture.
6. Place in a 3600F preheated oven and bake for 10 minutes.

NUTRITIONS

- *Calories per serving: 115;*
- *Protein: 13.2g;*
- *Carbs: 6.3g;*
- *Fat: 1.4g*
- *Sugar: 0.5g*

141. WEDDING OF BROCCOLI AND TOMATOES

PREPARATION	COOKING	SERVES
5 MIN	2 MIN	3

INGREDIENTS

- 1 head broccoli, cut into florets then blanched
- 1/4 cup tomatoes, diced
- Salt and pepper to taste
- Chopped parsley for garnish

DIRECTIONS

1. Place all ingredients in a bowl.
2. Toss to coat all ingredients.
3. Serve.

NUTRITIONS

- Calories per serving: 52;
- Protein: 1.1g;
- Carbs: 3.2g;
- Fat: 0.1g
- Sugar: 0.2g

447

142. HAMBURGER SALAD

PREPARATION	COOKING	SERVES
5 MIN	7 MIN	6

INGREDIENTS

- 1 pound 98% lean ground beef
- A pinch of salt
- 1/4 teaspoon black pepper
- 8 ounces Romaine lettuce, torn
- 1 cup cherry tomatoes, halved
- 1/2 cup pickles, diced
- 1/4 cup cheddar cheese, shredded

DIRECTIONS

1. Season the beef with salt and pepper.
2. Heat a non-stick pan and sauté the white beef, constantly stirring for 7 minutes. Set aside and allow to slightly cool.
3. Place the lettuce, tomatoes, pickles, and cheese. Sprinkle the cooked beef on top.
4. Toss to mix all ingredients.

NUTRITIONS

- Calories per serving: 186;
- Protein: 21g;
- Carbs: 8.7g;
- Fat: 3.1g
- Sugar: 0.8g

143. GREEN BUDDHA SMILE

PREPARATION	COOKING	SERVES
5 MIN	10 MIN	6

INGREDIENTS

- 2 pounds boneless and skinless chicken breast
- 2 tablespoons lemon juice, freshly squeezed
- Salt and pepper to taste
- 1-pound Brussels sprouts, trimmed and halved
- 3 cloves of garlic, minced
- 3/4 cup plain Greek yogurt
- 1 teaspoon stone-ground mustard
- 1/4 cup balsamic vinegar

- 2 cups cooked quinoa
- 1 cup chopped red apple, cored, and chopped
- 1/4 cup pepitas
- 1 avocado, sliced
- 1 1/2 cup arugula
- 1 tablespoon fresh basil

DIRECTIONS

1. Place chicken and lemon juice in a bowl. Season with salt and pepper to taste. Allow marinating in the fridge for at least 30 minutes.
2. Fire up the grill to 3750F and cook the chicken for 6 minutes on each side. Add in the Brussels sprouts and cook for 3 minutes on each side. Set the chicken and Brussels sprouts aside.
3. In a bowl, mix the garlic, yogurt, mustard, and vinegar. Season with salt to taste. Set aside.
4. On a bowl, place the quinoa and top with apple, pepitas, avocado, and arugula. Top with grilled chicken and Brussels sprouts.
5. Drizzle with the sauce and garnish with basil.

NUTRITIONS

- Calories total: 411;
- Protein: 44.2g;
- Carbs: 40.4g;
- Fat: 4g
- Sugar: 3g

144. ZUCCHINI FETTUCCINE WITH MEXICAN TACO

PREPARATION	COOKING	SERVES
5 MIN	20 MIN	6

INGREDIENTS

- 1 tablespoon olive oil
- 1-pound lean ground turkey
- 1 clove garlic, minced
- 1/2 small onion, chopped
- 1 tablespoon chili powder
- 1/4 teaspoon garlic powder
- 1/4 teaspoon onion powder
- 1/4 teaspoon dried oregano
- 1 1/2 teaspoon ground cumin
- 1/4 cup water
- 1/4 cup diced tomatoes

- 2 large zucchinis, spiralized
- 1/2 cup shredded cheddar cheese

DIRECTIONS

1. Place oil in a pot and heat over medium flame.
2. Sauté the turkey for 2 minutes before adding the garlic and onions. Stir for another minute.
3. Season with chili powder, garlic powder, onion powder, oregano, and ground cumin.
4. Sauté for another minute before adding the water and tomatoes.
5. Close the lid and allow to simmer for 7 minutes.
6. Add in the zucchini and cheese and allow to cook for 3 more minutes.

NUTRITIONS

- *Calories per serving: 145;*
- *Protein: 15g;*
- *Carbs: 8.5g;*
- *Fat:2.1 g*
- *Sugar: 0.5g*

145. ONION GREEN BEANS

PREPARATION	COOKING	SERVES
5 MIN	12 MIN	2

INGREDIENTS

- 11 oz. green beans
- 1 tablespoon of onion powder 1 tablespoon of olive oil
- 1/2 teaspoon of salt
- 1/4 teaspoon of red pepper flakes

DIRECTIONS

1. Wash the green beans thoroughly and put them in the bowl.
2. Sprinkle the green beans with lion's powder, salt, chilies, and olive oil.
3. Shake the green bean carefully.
4. Preheat the 400F air refrigerator.
5. Place the green beans in the deep fryer and cook for 8 minutes.
6. Next, shake the green beans and cook them for 4 minutes or more at 400 F. 7. When time remains: shake the green beans.
7. Serve them with joy!

NUTRITIONS

- Calories total: 302
- Fat: 7.2g
- Fiber: 5.5g
- Carbohydrates: 13.9g
- Protein: 3.2g

146. CREAM OF MUSHROOMS SATAY

PREPARATION	COOKING	SERVES
5 MIN	6 MIN	2

INGREDIENTS

- 7 oz. cremini mushrooms
- 2 tablespoon coconut milk
- 1 tablespoon butter
- 1 teaspoon chili flakes
- ½ teaspoon balsamic vinegar
- ½ teaspoon curry powder
- ½ teaspoon white pepper

DIRECTIONS

1. Wash the mushrooms carefully.
2. Then sprinkle the mushrooms with chili flakes, curry powder, and white pepper.
3. Preheat the air fryer to 400 F.
4. Toss the butter in the air fryer basket and melt it.
5. Put the mushrooms in the air fryer and cook for 2 minutes.
6. Shake the mushrooms well and sprinkle with the coconut milk and balsamic vinegar.
7. Cook the mushrooms for 4 minutes more at 400 F.
8. Then skewer the mushrooms on the wooden sticks and serve.
9. Enjoy!

NUTRITIONS

- Calories per serving: 116
- Fat: 9.5g
- Fiber: 1.3g
- Carbs: 5.6g
- Protein: 3g

147. TORTORETO MUSHROOMS WITH CHEDDAR

PREPARATION	COOKING	SERVES
5 MIN	6 MIN	2

INGREDIENTS

- 2 Portobello mushroom hats
- 2 slices Cheddar cheese
- ¼ cup panko breadcrumbs
- ½ teaspoon salt
- ½ teaspoon ground black pepper
- 1 egg
- 1 teaspoon oatmeal
- 2 oz. bacon, chopped cooked

DIRECTIONS

1. Crack the egg into the bowl and whisk it.
2. Combine the ground black pepper, oatmeal, salt, and breadcrumbs in a separate bowl.
3. Dip the mushroom hats in the whisked egg.
4. After this, coat the mushroom hats in the breadcrumb mixture.
5. Preheat the air fryer to 400 F.
6. Place the mushrooms in the air fryer basket tray and cook for 3 minutes.
7. After this, put the chopped bacon and sliced cheese over the mushroom hats and cook the meal for 3 minutes.
8. When the meal is cooked – let it chill gently.
9. Enjoy!

NUTRITIONS

- Calories total: 376
- Fat: 24.1g
- Fiber: 1.8g
- Carbs: 14.6g
- Protein: 25.2g

148. LENTIL TRIUMPH HAMBURGER WITH CARROTS

PREPARATION	COOKING	SERVES
5 MIN	12 MIN	2

INGREDIENTS

- 6 oz. lentils, cooked
- 1 egg
- 2 oz. carrot, grated
- 1 teaspoon semolina
- ½ teaspoon salt
- 1 teaspoon turmeric
- 1 tablespoon butter

DIRECTIONS

1. Crack the egg into the bowl and whisk it.
2. Add the cooked lentils and mash the mixture with the help of the fork.
3. Then sprinkle the mixture with the grated carrot, semolina, salt, and turmeric.
4. Mix it up and make the medium burgers.
5. Put the butter into the lentil burgers. It will make them juicy.
6. Preheat the air fryer to 360 F.
7. Put the lentil burgers in the air fryer and cook for 12 minutes.
8. Flip the burgers into another side after 6 minutes of cooking.
9. Then chill the cooked lentil burgers and serve them.
10. Enjoy!

NUTRITIONS

- Calories total: 404
- Fat: 9g
- Fiber: 26.9g
- Carbs: 56g
- Protein: 25.3g

149. STIR-FRIED SWEET POTATOES WITH PARMESAN

PREPARATION	COOKING	SERVES
5 MIN	35 MIN	2

INGREDIENTS

- 2 sweet potatoes, peeled
- ½ yellow onion, sliced
- ½ cup cream
- ¼ cup spinach
- 2 oz. Parmesan cheese, shredded
- ½ teaspoon salt
- 1 tomato
- 1 teaspoon olive oil

DIRECTIONS

1. Chop the sweet potatoes, tomato and spinach.
2. Spray the air fryer tray with the olive oil.
3. Then place on the layer of the chopped sweet potato.
4. Add the layer of the sliced onion.
5. After this, sprinkle the sliced onion with the chopped spinach and tomatoes.
6. Sprinkle the casserole with salt and shredded cheese.
7. Pour cream.
8. Preheat the air fryer to 390 F.
9. Cover the air fryer tray with the foil.
10. Cook the casserole for 35 minutes.
11. When the casserole is cooked – serve it.
12. Enjoy!

NUTRITIONS

- Calories per serving: 93
- Fat: 1.8g
- Fiber: 3.4g
- Carbs: 20.3g
- Protein: 1.8g

150. CHICKEN GOULASH WITH GREEN PEPPERS

PREPARATION	COOKING	SERVES
5 MIN	17 MIN	6

INGREDIENTS

- 4 oz. chive stems
- 2 green peppers, chopped
- 1 teaspoon olive oil
- 14 oz. ground chicken
- 2 tomatoes
- ½ cup chicken stock
- 2 garlic cloves, sliced
- 1 teaspoon salt
- 1 teaspoon ground black pepper
- 1 teaspoon mustard

DIRECTIONS

1. Chop chives roughly.
2. Spray the air fryer basket tray with the olive oil.
3. Preheat the air fryer to 365 F.
4. Put the chopped chives in the air fryer basket tray.
5. Add the chopped green pepper and cook the vegetables for 5 minutes.
6. Add the ground chicken.
7. Chop the tomatoes into small cubes and add them to the air fryer mixture too.
8. Cook the mixture for 6 minutes more.
9. Add the chicken stock, sliced garlic cloves, salt, ground black pepper, and mustard.
10. Mix well to combine.
11. Cook the goulash for 6 minutes more.

NUTRITIONS

- *Calories per serving: 161*
- *Fat: 6.1g*
- *Carbs: 6g*
- *Protein: 20.3g*

151. LETTUCE SALAD WITH BEEF STRIPS

PREPARATION	COOKING	SERVES
5 MIN	12 MIN	5

INGREDIENTS

- 2 cup lettuce
- 10 oz. beef brisket
- 2 tablespoon sesame oil
- 1 tablespoon sunflower seeds
- 1 cucumber
- 1 teaspoon ground black pepper
- 1 teaspoon paprika
- 1 teaspoon Italian spices
- 2 teaspoon butter
- 1 teaspoon dried dill
- 2 tablespoon coconut milk

DIRECTIONS

1. Cut the beef brisket into strips.
2. Sprinkle the beef strips with the ground black pepper, paprika, and dried dill.
3. Preheat the air fryer to 365 F.
4. Put the butter in the air fryer basket tray and melt it.
5. Then add the beef strips and cook them for 6 minutes on each side.
6. Meanwhile, tear the lettuce and toss it in a big salad bowl.
7. Crush the sunflower seeds and sprinkle them over the lettuce.
8. Chop the cucumber into small cubes and add to the salad bowl.
9. Then combine the sesame oil and Italian spices. Stir the oil.
10. Combine the lettuce mixture with the coconut milk and stir it using 2 wooden spatulas.
11. When the meat is cooked – let it chill to room temperature.
12. Add the beef strips to the salad bowl.
13. Stir it gently and sprinkle the salad with the sesame oil dressing.
14. Serve the dish immediately.

NUTRITIONS

- Calories per serving: 199
- Fat: 12.4g
- Carbs: 3.9g
- Protein: 18.1g

152. CAULIFLOWER SPRINKLED WITH CURRY

PREPARATION	COOKING	SERVES
5 MIN	5 HOURS	4

INGREDIENTS

- 1 cauliflower head, florets separated
- 2 carrots, sliced
- 1 red onion, chopped
- ¾ cup of coconut milk
- 2 garlic cloves, minced
- 2 tablespoons curry powder
- A pinch of salt and black pepper
- 1   tablespoon red pepper flakes
- 1 teaspoon garam masala

DIRECTIONS

1. In your slow cooker, mix all the ingredients.
2. Cover, cook on high for 5 hours, divide into bowls and serve.

NUTRITIONS

- *Calories per serving: 160*
- *Fat: 11.5g*
- *Fiber: 5.4g*
- *Carbs: 14.7g*
- *Protein: 3.6g*

153. PORK STEW WITH GREEN CHILLI

PREPARATION	COOKING	SERVES
5 MIN	20 MIN	4

INGREDIENTS

- 2 scallions, chopped
- 2 cloves of garlic
- 1 lb. tomatillos, trimmed and chopped
- 8 large romaine or green lettuce leaves, divided
- 2 serrano chilies, seeds, and membranes
- ½ tsp of dried Mexican oregano (or you can use regular oregano)
- 1 ½ lb. of boneless pork loin, to be

- cut into bite-sized cubes
- ¼ cup of cilantro, chopped
- ¼ tablespoon (each) salt and paper
- 1 jalapeno, seeds and membranes to be removed and thinly sliced
- 1 cup of sliced radishes
- 4 lime wedges

DIRECTIONS

1. Combine scallions, garlic, tomatillos, 4 lettuce leaves, serrano chilies, and oregano in a blender. Then puree until smooth
2. Put pork and tomatillo mixture in a medium pot. 1-inch of puree should cover the pork; if not, add water until it covers it. Season with pepper & salt, and cover it simmers. Simmer on the heat for approximately 20 minutes.
3. Now, finely shred the remaining lettuce leaves.
4. When the stew is done cooking, garnish with cilantro, radishes, finely shredded lettuce, sliced jalapenos, and lime wedges.

NUTRITIONS

- *Calories total: 370*
- *Protein: 36g*
- *Carbohydrate: 14g*
- *Fat: 19 g*

154. ROSEMARY SCENT CAULIFLOWER BUNDLES

PREPARATION	COOKING	SERVES
5 MIN	30 MIN	3

INGREDIENTS

- 1/3 cup of almond flour
- 4 cups of riced cauliflower
- 1/3 cup of reduced-fat, shredded mozzarella or cheddar cheese
- 2 eggs
- 2 tablespoons of fresh rosemary, finely chopped
- ½ teaspoon of salt

DIRECTIONS

1. Preheat your oven to 400°F
2. Combine all the listed ingredients in a medium-sized bowl
3. Scoop cauliflower mixture into 12 evenly-sized rolls/biscuits onto a lightly-greased and foil-lined baking sheet.
4. Bake until it turns golden brown, which should be achieved in about 30 minutes.

NUTRITIONS

- *Calories per serving: 254*
- *Protein: 24g*
- *Carbohydrate: 7g*
- *Fat: 8 g*

155. CHICKEN STIR FRY

PREPARATION	COOKING	SERVES
5 MIN	25 MIN	2

INGREDIENTS

- ½ cup chicken broth, low sodium
- 12 ounces skinless chicken breasts, cut into strips
- 1 cup red bell pepper, seeded and chopped
- 8 ounces (1 cup) broccoli, cut into florets
- One teaspoon crushed red pepper

DIRECTIONS

1. Place a small amount of chicken broth in a saucepan. Heat over medium flame and stir in the chicken. Water sauté the chicken for at least 5 minutes while stirring constantly.
2. Place the rest of the ingredients and stir.
3. Cover the pan with a lid and cook for another 5 minutes.

NUTRITIONS

- Calories per serving: 137
- Protein: 15g
- Carbs: 15.4g
- Fat: 1.2g
- Sugar: 0.6g

156. CAULIFLOWER SALAD

PREPARATION	COOKING	SERVES
5 MIN	3 MIN	2

INGREDIENTS

- 1 cup cauliflower florets
- ¼ cup apple cider vinegar
- One tablespoon Tuscan seasoning

DIRECTIONS

1. Add all fixings into a bowl and toss to combine.
2. Allow resting in the fridge for at least 30 minutes before serving.

NUTRITIONS

- *Calories per serving: 41*
- *Protein: 1.3g*
- *Carbs: 8.7g*
- *Fat: 0.1g*
- *Sugar: 2g*

157. GARLIC CHICKEN WITH ZOODLES

PREPARATION	COOKING	SERVES
5 MIN	1MIN	5

INGREDIENTS

- 1 ½ pound boneless and skinless chicken breasts, it should be cut into bite-sized pieces
- 6 slices sun-dried tomatoes
- One teaspoon chopped garlic
- 1 cup low fat plain Greek yogurt
- ½ cup chicken broth, low sodium
- ½ teaspoon garlic powder
- ½ teaspoon Italian seasoning
- 1 cup spinach, chopped
- 1 ½ cup zucchini, cut into thin noodles

DIRECTIONS

1. Place two tablespoons water in a pan and heat over low-medium flame. Water sauté the chicken for 3 minutes while constantly stirring until the sides are slightly golden.
2. Stir in the tomatoes and garlic and stir for another 3 minutes. Add in the yogurt, chicken broth, garlic powder, and Italian seasoning. Cover the pan with its lid and just wait for it to simmer for at least 7 minutes.
3. Stir in the spinach last. Cook for another 2 minutes.
4. Place the zucchini noodles in a deep dish and pour over the chicken. Toss the noodles to coat with the sauce.
5. Serve immediately.

NUTRITIONS

- Calories per serving: 205
- Protein: 33.3g
- Carbs: 6g
- Fat: 2g
- Sugar: 1.2g

158. "MACARONI"

PREPARATION	COOKING	SERVES
5 MIN	10 MIN	4

INGREDIENTS

- Two tablespoons yellow onion, diced
- 5 ounces 95-97% lean ground beef
- Two tablespoons light thousand island dressing
- 1/8 teaspoon apple cider vinegar
- 1/8 teaspoon onion powder
- 3 cups Romaine lettuce, shredded
- Two tablespoons low-fat cheddar cheese, shredded
- 1-ounce dill pickle slices
- One teaspoon sesame seed

DIRECTIONS

1. Pour three tablespoons of water into a pan and heat over a medium-low flame. Water sauté the onions for 30 seconds before adding the beef. Sauté the meat for 4 minutes while stirring constantly.
2. Add in the thousand island dressing, apple cider vinegar, and onion powder. Close the lid and keep on cooking for 5 minutes. Remove the cover and allow to simmer until the sauce thickens. Turn off the heat and allow the beef to rest and cool.
3. Place the lettuce at the bottom and pour in the beef—layer with cheddar cheese and pickles in a bowl. Sprinkle with sesame on top.

NUTRITIONS

- *Calories per serving:119*
- *Protein: 10.8g*
- *Carbs: 4.4g*
- *Fat: 2.1g*
- *Sugar: 2.5g*

159. BROCCOLI TACO

PREPARATION	COOKING	SERVES
5 MIN	15 MIN	4

INGREDIENTS

- 4 ounces 95-97% lean ground beef
- ¼ cup Roma tomatoes, chopped
- ¼ teaspoon garlic powder
- ¼ teaspoon onion powder
- One ¼ cup broccoli, cut into bite-sized pieces
- A pinch of red pepper flakes
- 1-ounce low-sodium cheddar cheese, shredded

DIRECTIONS

1. Place three tablespoons of water in a pan and heat over medium flame. Water sauté the beef and tomatoes for 5 minutes until the tomatoes are wilted. Add in the garlic and onion powder, then stir for another 3 minutes.
2. Add the broccoli and close the lid. Cook for another 5 minutes.
3. Garnish with red pepper flakes and cheddar cheese on top.

NUTRITIONS

- Calories per serving:97
- Protein:9.9 g
- Carbs: 2.6g
- Fat: 1.7g
- Sugar:0.9 g

160. CRUNCHY CHICKEN TACOS

PREPARATION	COOKING	SERVES
20 MIN	25 MIN	4

INGREDIENTS

- ½ cup low sodium chicken stock
- Two chicken breasts, minced
- One red onion, chopped
- One clove of garlic, minced
- Three plum tomatoes, chopped
- One teaspoon cumin powder
- One teaspoon cinnamon powder
- One teaspoon ground coriander
- One red onion, chopped
- ½ red chili, chopped
- One tablespoon lime juice
- Meat from 1 ripe avocado
- One cucumber, sliced into thick rounds

DIRECTIONS

1. Place a tablespoon of chicken stock in a pan and heat over medium flame. Water sauté the chicken, onion, garlic, and tomatoes for 4 minutes or until the tomatoes have wilted.
2. Season with cumin, cinnamon, and coriander. Lessen the heat to low and cook for another 5 minutes. Set aside and allow to cool.
3. In a bowl, mix together the onion, chili, lime juice, and mashed avocado. It is the salsa.
4. Scoop the salsa and top on sliced cucumber. Top with cooked chicken.

NUTRITIONS

- Calories per serving: 313
- Protein: 31.8g
- Carbs: 14.9 g
- Fat: 3.8g
- Sugar: 5g

161. CAULIFLOWER WITH KALE PESTO

PREPARATION	COOKING	SERVES
5 MIN	2 MIN	6

INGREDIENTS

DIFFICULT: EASY

- 3 cups cauliflower, cut into florets
- 3 cups raw kale, stems removed
- 2 cups fresh basil
- Two tablespoons extra virgin olive oil
- Three tablespoons lemon juice
- Three cloves of garlic
- ¼ teaspoon salt

DIRECTIONS

1. Put an adequate amount of water in the pan and bring to a boil over medium flame. Blanch the cauliflower for 2 minutes. Drain, then place in a bowl of ice-cold water for 5 minutes. Drain again.
2. In a blender, add the rest of the ingredients. Pulse until smooth.
3. Pour over the pesto over the cooked cauliflower.

NUTRITIONS

- *Calories per serving: 41*
- *Protein: 1.8g*
- *Carbs: 5g*
- *Fat: 5.3g*
- *Sugar: 1.4g*

162. CHICKEN CHILI

PREPARATION	COOKING	SERVES
5 MIN	45 MIN	6

INGREDIENTS

- 1-pound boneless skinless chicken breast, chopped
- One teaspoon ground cumin
- 1 cup chopped poblano pepper
- ½ cup chopped onion
- One clove of garlic, minced
- 2 cups low-sodium chicken broth
- 1 cup rehydrated pinto beans
- 1 cup chopped tomatoes
- Two tablespoons minced cilantro

DIRECTIONS

1. Make sure to put all fixings except the cilantro in a pressure cooker.
2. Close the lid and set the vent to the sealing position.
3. Cook on high for 45 minutes until the beans are soft.
4. Garnish with cilantro before serving.

NUTRITIONS

- Calories per serving: 229
- Protein: 26.1g
- Carbs: 23.9g
- Fat: 2g
- Sugar: 2.2g

163. AVOCADO, CITRUS, AND SHRIMP SALAD

PREPARATION	COOKING	SERVES
5 MIN	4 MIN	4

INGREDIENTS

- One head green leaf lettuce
- One avocado
- ½ pound wild-caught shrimp
- Two tablespoons olive oil
- Juice of 1 lemon

DIRECTIONS

1. Put the lettuce in a dish, then top with mashed avocado meat.
2. Clean the shrimps by deveining and removing the head.
3. Heat oil in a skillet using medium-low heat and heat the oil. Cook the shrimps for 2 minutes on each side.
4. Place the shrimps on top of mashed avocado and drizzle with lemon juice.

NUTRITIONS

- Calories per serving: 359
- Protein: 10.6g
- Carbs: 50.1g
- Fat: 7.5g
- Sugar: 2.8g

164. BROCCOLI ALFREDO

PREPARATION	COOKING	SERVES
5 MIN	2 MIN	5

INGREDIENTS

- Two heads of broccoli, cut into florets
- Two tablespoons lemon juice, freshly squeezed
- ½ cup cashew, soaked for 2 hours in water then drained
- Two tablespoons white miso, low sodium
- Two teaspoon Dijon mustard
- Freshly cracked black pepper

DIRECTIONS

1. Boil water in a pot using a medium flame. Blanch the broccoli for 2 minutes, then place it in a bowl of iced water. Drain.
2. In a food processor, place the remaining ingredients and pulse until smooth.
3. Pour the alfredo sauce over the broccoli. Toss to coat with the sauce.

NUTRITIONS

- *Calories per serving: 359*
- *Protein: 10.6g*
- *Carbs: 50.2 g*
- *Fat: 8.4g*
- *Sugar: 2.4g*

165. STEAK MACHINE

PREPARATION	COOKING	SERVES
5 MIN	10 MIN	3

INGREDIENTS

- 1/2 teaspoon extra virgin olive oil
- 2 ounces Sirloin steak, 98% lean
- Salt and pepper to taste
- One zucchini, cut into long thin strips
- One onion, chopped
- 6 ounces asparagus, blanched
- 4 ounces peas, blanched

DIRECTIONS

1. Heat olive oil in a skillet. If desired, you may season the steak with salt and pepper to taste.
2. Place in the skillet and sear the steak for 5 minutes on each side. Let the meal rest for five minutes before cutting it into strips.
3. Place the remaining ingredients in a bowl and season with salt and pepper to taste
4. Top with steak strips, then toss to combine all ingredients.

NUTRITIONS

- Calories per serving:174
- Protein: 4.2g
- Carbs: 10.3g
- Fat: 4.1g
- Sugar: 2.1g

166. GARLIC SHRIMP ZUCCHINI NOODLES

PREPARATION	COOKING	SERVES
5 MIN	4 MIN	5

INGREDIENTS

- 16 ounces uncooked shrimps, shelled and deveined
- One tablespoon olive oil
- 1 cup cherry tomatoes, cut in half
- 8 cups zucchini strips
- Two tablespoons minced garlic
- One teaspoon dried oregano
- ½ teaspoon chili powder
- ½ teaspoon salt

DIRECTIONS

1. Brush the shrimps with olive oil. Place on a skillet and cook for 2 minutes on all sides or until pink. Set aside.
2. Place the rest of the fixings in a bowl and add the shrimps. Season with salt, then toss to coat the ingredients.

NUTRITIONS

- *Calories per serving: 142*
- *Protein: 19.7g*
- *Carbs: 6.3g*
- *Fat: 4.2g*
- *Sugar: 3.8g*

167. CROCKPOT CHILI

PREPARATION	COOKING	SERVES
5 MIN	45 MIN	8

INGREDIENTS

- 1-pound boneless skinless chicken breasts, cut into strips
- ½ cup chopped onion
- Two teaspoons ground cumin
- One teaspoon minced garlic
- ½ teaspoon chili powder
- Salt and pepper to taste
- 1 ½ cups water
- One can green enchilada sauce
- ½ cup dried beans, soaked overnight

DIRECTIONS

1. Place all ingredients in a pot.
2. Mix all ingredients until combined.
3. Close the lid and change the heat to medium.
4. Bring to a boil and allow to simmer for 45 minutes or until the beans are cooked.
5. Serve with chopped cilantro on top.

NUTRITIONS

- *Calories per serving: 84*
- *Protein: 13.4g*
- *Carbs: 3.6 g*
- *Fat: 1.7g*
- *Sugar: 0.8g*

168. TOMATILLO AND GREEN CHILI PORK STEW

PREPARATION	COOKING	SERVES
10 MIN	20 MIN	4

INGREDIENTS

DIFFICULTY: MEDIUM

- Two scallions, chopped
- Two cloves of garlic
- 1 lb. tomatillos, trimmed and chopped
- Eight large romaine or green lettuce leaves, divided
- Two serrano chilies, seeds, and membranes
- ½ tsp of dried Mexican oregano (or you can use regular oregano)
- 1 ½ lb. of boneless pork loin, to be cut into bite-sized cubes
- ¼ cup of cilantro, chopped
- ¼ tablespoon (each) salt and paper
- One jalapeno, seeds and membranes to be removed and thinly sliced
- 1 cup of sliced radishes
- Four lime wedges

DIRECTIONS

1. Combine scallions, garlic, tomatillos, four lettuce leaves, serrano chilies, and oregano in a blender. Then puree until smooth
2. Put pork and tomatillo mixture in a medium pot. 1-inch of puree should cover the pork; if not, add water until it covers it. Season with pepper & salt, and cover it simmers. Simmer on the heat for approximately 20 minutes.
3. Now, finely shred the remaining lettuce leaves.
4. When the stew is done cooking, garnish with cilantro, radishes, finely shredded lettuce, sliced jalapenos, and lime wedges.

NUTRITIONS

- *Calories: 370*
- *Protein: 36g*
- *Carbohydrate: 14g*
- *Fat: 19 g*

169. AVOCADO LIME SHRIMP SALAD

PREPARATION	COOKING	SERVES
15 MIN	0 MIN	2

INGREDIENTS

- 14 ounces of jumbo cooked shrimp, peeled and deveined; chopped
- 4 ½ ounces of avocado, diced
- 1 ½ cup of tomato, diced
- ¼ cup of chopped green onion
- ¼ cup of jalapeno with the seeds removed, diced fine
- One teaspoon of olive oil
- Two tablespoons of lime juice
- 1/8 teaspoon of salt
- One tablespoon of chopped cilantro

DIRECTIONS

1. Get a small bowl and combine green onion, olive oil, lime juice, pepper, and salt pinch. Wait for about 5 minutes for all of them to marinate and mellow the flavor of the onion.
2. Get a large bowl and combined chopped shrimp, tomato, avocado, jalapeno. Combine all of the ingredients, add cilantro, and gently toss.
3. Add pepper and salt as desired.

NUTRITIONS

- *Calories: 314*
- *Protein: 26g*
- *Carbs: 15g*
- *Fiber: 9g*

170. ROSEMARY CAULIFLOWER ROLLS

PREPARATION	COOKING	SERVES
10 MIN	30 MIN	6

INGREDIENTS

- 1/3 cup of almond flour
- 4 cups of riced cauliflower
- 1/3 cup of reduced-fat, shredded mozzarella or cheddar cheese
- Two eggs
- Two tablespoons of fresh rosemary, finely chopped
- ½ teaspoon of salt

DIRECTIONS

1. Preheat your oven to 400°F
2. Combine all the listed ingredients in a medium-sized bowl
3. Scoop cauliflower mixture into 12 evenly-sized rolls/biscuits onto a lightly-greased and foil-lined baking sheet.
4. Bake until it turns golden brown, which should be achieved in about 30 minutes.

NUTRITIONS

- Calories: 254
- Protein: 24g
- Carbohydrate: 7g
- Fat: 8 g

171. MEDITERRANEAN CHICKEN SALAD

PREPARATION	COOKING	SERVES
5 MIN	25 MIN	4

INGREDIENTS

For Chicken:
- One ¾ lb. boneless, skinless chicken breast
- ¼ teaspoon each of pepper and salt (or as desired)
- 1 ½ tablespoon of butter, melted

For Mediterranean salad:
- 1 cup of sliced cucumber
- 6 cups of romaine lettuce that is torn or roughly chopped
- 10 pitted Kalamata olives

- 1 pint of cherry tomatoes
- 1/3 cup of reduced-fat feta cheese
- ¼ teaspoon each of pepper and salt (or lesser)
- One small lemon juice (it should be about two tablespoons)

DIRECTIONS

1. Prewarm your oven or grill to about 350°F.
2. Season the chicken with salt, butter, and black pepper
3. Roast or grill chicken until it reaches an internal temperature of 165°F in about 25 minutes. Once your chicken breasts are cooked, remove and keep aside to rest for about 5 minutes before you slice it.
4. Combine all the salad ingredients you have and toss everything together very well
5. Serve the chicken with Mediterranean salad

NUTRITIONS

- *Calories: 340*
- *Protein: 45g*

- *Carbohydrate: 9g*
- *Fat: 4 g*

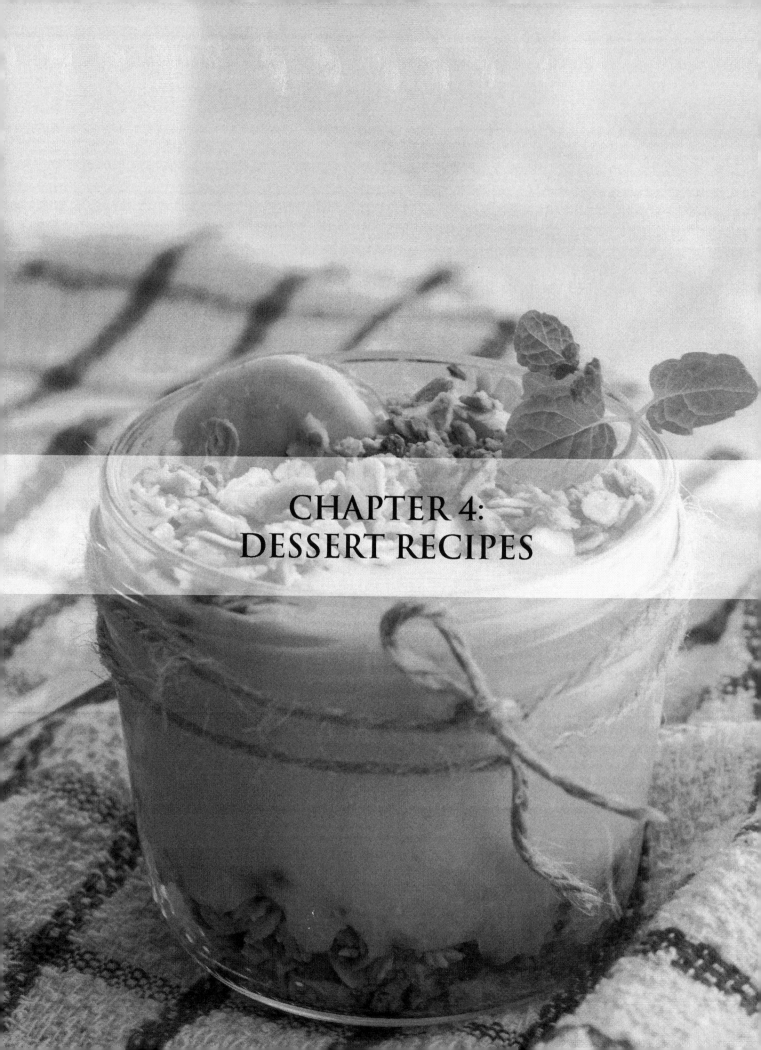

CHAPTER 4:
DESSERT RECIPES

172. ASPARAGUS GREEN SCRAMBLE

PREPARATION	COOKING	SERVES
5 MIN	6 MIN	2

INGREDIENTS

- 3 eggs
- 1 Portobello mushroom, chopped
- 2 garlic cloves, chopped
- 1/2 cup spinach
- 4 asparagus, trimmed, diced
- Sea salt to taste
- Cayenne pepper to taste
- 1 tbsp olive oil

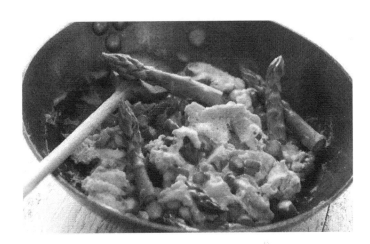

DIRECTIONS

1. In a bowl, whisk the eggs with salt and cayenne pepper.
2. In a skillet, add the oil and pour in the egg mix.
3. Cook for 1 minute.
4. Add the spinach, mushroom, asparagus, and garlic.
5. Stir for 4 minutes. Serve.

NUTRITIONS

- *Carbohydrates: 3 g*
- *Fat: 6 g*
- *Protein: 13 g*

173. CRANBERRY SALAD

PREPARATION	COOKING	SERVES
5 MIN	5 MIN	2

INGREDIENTS

- 1 Sugar-free cranberry jell pack (1/2 cup for snacks allowed)
- 1/2 cup celery chopped (1 green)
- 7 Half Cut Walnut (1 snack)

DIRECTIONS

1. Mix Jell-O according to the instructions of the box.
2. Add walnuts and celery.
3. Allow setting.
4. Shake until serving.
5. Requires servings in 4-1/2 cups.

NUTRITIONS

- Fats: 11 g
- Sodium: 73 mg
- Potassium: 212 mg
- Carbohydrates: 54 g
- Protein: 4.1 g

174. CHICKEN SALAD WITH PINEAPPLE AND PECANS

PREPARATION	COOKING	SERVES
10 MIN	5 MIN	4

INGREDIENTS

- (6-ounce) Boneless, skinless, cooked and cubed chicken breast
- Tablespoons of celery hacked
- Cut 1/4 cup of pineapple
- 1/4 cup orange peeled segments
- Tablespoon of pecans hacked
- 1/4 cup seedless grapes
- Salt and black chili pepper, to taste
- Cups cut from roman lettuce

DIRECTIONS

1. Put chicken, celery, pineapple, grapes, pecans, and raisins in a medium dish.
2. Kindly blend until mixed with a spoon, then season with salt and pepper.
3. Create a bed of lettuce on a plate.
4. Cover with a mixture of chicken and serve.

NUTRITIONS

- *Calories: 386 Cal*
- *Carbohydrates: 20 g*
- *Fat: 19 g*
- *Protein: 25 g*

175. ZUCCHINI FRITTERS

PREPARATION	COOKING	SERVES
10 MIN	15 MIN	4

INGREDIENTS

- 1 1/2 pound of grated zucchini
- 1 Tsp. of salt
- 1/4 cup of grated Parmesan
- 1/4 cup of flour
- 2 cloves of minced garlic
- 2 Tbsp of olive oil
- 1 large egg
- Freshly ground black pepper and kosher salt to taste

DIRECTIONS

1. Put the grated zucchini into a colander over the sink
2. Add your salt and toss it to mix properly, then leave it to settle for about 10 minutes.
3. Next, use a clean cheesecloth to drain the zucchini completely.
4. Combine drained zucchini, Parmesan, garlic, flour, and the beaten egg in a large bowl, mix, and season with pepper and salt.
5. Next, heat the olive oil in a skillet applying medium-high heat.
6. Use a tablespoon to scoop batter for each cake, put in the oil, and flatten using a spatula.
7. Allow to cook until the underside is richly golden brown, then flip over to the other side and cook.
8. Your delicious Zucchini fritters are ready to be served.

NUTRITIONS

- Total Fat: 12.0 g
- Cholesterol: 101.9 mg
- Sodium: 728.9 mg
- Total Carbohydrate: 11.9 g
- Dietary Fiber: 1.9 g
- Sugars: 4.6 g
- Protein: 8.6 g

176. HEALTHY BROCCOLI SALAD

PREPARATION	COOKING	SERVES
5 MIN	25 MIN	6

INGREDIENTS

- 3 cups broccoli, chopped
- 1 tbsp apple cider vinegar
- 1/2 cup Greek yogurt
- 2 tbsp sunflower seeds
- 3 bacon slices, cooked and chopped
- 1/3 cup onion, sliced
- 1/4 tsp. stevia

DIRECTIONS

1. In a mixing bowl, mix broccoli, onion, and bacon.
2. In a small bowl, mix yogurt, vinegar, and stevia and pour over broccoli mixture.
3. Stir to combine.
4. Sprinkle sunflower seeds on top of the salad.
5. Store salad in the refrigerator for 30 minutes.
6. Serve and enjoy.

NUTRITIONS

- *Calories: 90 Cal*
- *Fat: 4.9 g*
- *Carbohydrates: 5.4 g*
- *Sugar: 2.5 g*
- *Protein: 6.2 g*
- *Cholesterol: 12 mg*

177. DELICIOUS ZUCCHINI QUICHE

PREPARATION	COOKING	SERVES
15 MIN	60 MIN	8

INGREDIENTS

- 6 eggs
- 2 medium zucchinis, shredded
- 1/2 tsp. dried basil
- 2 garlic cloves, minced
- 1 tbsp dry onion, minced
- 2 tbsp parmesan cheese, grated
- 2 tbsp fresh parsley, chopped
- 1/2 cup olive oil
- 1 cup cheddar cheese, shredded
- 1/4 cup coconut flour
- 3/4 cup almond flour
- 1/2 tsp. salt

DIRECTIONS

1. Preheat the oven to 350°F.
2. Grease a 9-inch pie dish and set aside.
3. Squeeze out excess liquid from zucchini.
4. Add all ingredients into the large bowl and mix until well combined.
5. Pour into the prepared pie dish.
6. Bake in preheated oven for 45-60 minutes or until set.
7. Remove from the oven and let it cool completely.
8. Slice and serve.

NUTRITIONS

- *Calories: 288 Cal*
- *Fat: 26.3 g*
- *Carbohydrates: 5 g*
- *Sugar: 1.6 g*
- *Protein: 11 g*
- *Cholesterol: 139 mg*

178. COBB SALAD WITH BLUE CHEESE DRESSING

PREPARATION	COOKING	SERVES
15 MIN	30 MIN	6

INGREDIENTS

Dressing:
- 1/2 cup buttermilk
- 1 cup mayonnaise
- 2 tbsp Worcestershire sauce
- 1/2 cup sour cream
- 1 1/2 cup crumbled blue cheese
- Salt and black pepper to taste
- 2 tbsp chopped chives

Salad:
- 6 eggs
- 2 chicken breasts, boneless and skinless
- 5 strips bacon
- 1 iceberg lettuce, cut into chunks
- 1 romaine lettuce, chopped
- 1 bibb lettuce, cored and leaves removed
- 2 avocados, pitted and diced
- 2 large tomatoes, chopped
- 1/2 cup crumbled blue cheese
- 2 scallions, chopped

DIRECTIONS

1. In a bowl, whisk the buttermilk, mayonnaise, Worcestershire sauce, and sour cream.
2. Stir in the blue cheese, salt, black pepper, and chives. Place in the refrigerator to chill until ready to use.
3. Bring the eggs to boil in salted water over medium heat for 10 minutes.
4. Once ready, drain the eggs and transfer them to the ice bath. Peel and chop the eggs. Set aside.
5. Preheat the grill pan over high heat. Season the chicken with salt and pepper.
6. Grill for 3 minutes on each side. Remove to a plate to cool for 3 minutes, and cut into bite-size chunks.
7. Fry the bacon in another pan set over medium heat until crispy, about 6 minutes. Remove, let cool for 2 minutes, and chop.
8. Arrange the lettuce leaves in a salad bowl and add the avocado, tomatoes, eggs, bacon, and chicken in single piles.
9. Sprinkle the blue cheese over the salad as well as the scallions and black pepper.
10. Drizzle the blue cheese dressing on the salad and serve with low carb bread.

NUTRITIONS

- *Calories: 122 Cal*
- *Fats: 14 g*
- *Carbohydrates: 2 g*
- *Protein: 23 g*

179. VANILLA BEAN FRAPPUCCINO

PREPARATION	COOKING	SERVES
3 MIN	6 MIN	4

INGREDIENTS

- 3 cups unsweetened vanilla almond milk, chilled
- 2 tsp. swerve
- 1 1/2 cups heavy cream, cold
- 1 vanilla bean
- 1/4 tsp. xanthan gum
- Unsweetened chocolate shavings to garnish

DIRECTIONS

1. Combine the almond milk, swerve, heavy cream, vanilla bean, and xanthan gum in the blender and process on high speed for 1 minute until smooth.
2. Pour into tall shake glasses, sprinkle with chocolate shavings, and serve immediately.

NUTRITIONS

- Calories: 193 Cal
- Fats: 14 g
- Carbohydrates: 6 g
- Protein: 15 g

180. DARK CHOCOLATE MOCHACCINO ICE BOMBS

PREPARATION	COOKING	SERVES
5 MIN	10 MIN	4

INGREDIENTS

- 1/2-pound cream cheese
- 4 tbsp powdered sweetener
- 2 ounces strong coffee
- 2 tbsp cocoa powder, unsweetened
- 1-ounce cocoa butter, melted
- 2 1/2 ounces dark chocolate, melted

DIRECTIONS

1. Combine cream cheese, sweetener, coffee, and cocoa powder in a food processor.
2. Roll 2 tbsp of the mixture and place on a lined tray.
3. Mix the melted cocoa butter and chocolate, and coat the bombs with it.
4. Freeze for 2 hours.

NUTRITIONS

- *Calories: 127 Cal*
- *Fats: 13g*
- *Carbohydrates: 1.4 g*
- *Protein: 1.9 g*

181. CHOCOLATE BARK WITH ALMONDS

PREPARATION	COOKING	SERVES
5 MIN	10 MIN	12

INGREDIENTS

- 1/2 cup toasted almonds, chopped
- 1/2 cup butter
- 10 drops stevia
- 1/4 tsp. salt
- 1/2 cup unsweetened coconut flakes
- 4 ounces dark chocolate

DIRECTIONS

1. Melt together the butter and chocolate in the microwave for 90 seconds.
2. Remove and stir in stevia.
3. Line a cookie sheet with waxed paper and spread the chocolate evenly.
4. Scatter the almonds on top, coconut flakes, and sprinkle with salt.
5. Refrigerate for one hour.

NUTRITIONS

- *Calories: 161 Cal*
- *Fats: 15.3 g*
- *Carbohydrates: 1.9 g*
- *Protein: 1.9 g*

182. PROTEIN BROWNIES

PREPARATION	COOKING	SERVES
10 MIN	40 MIN	8

INGREDIENTS

- Almond milk (1/2 cup)
- Egg whites (1/2 cup, chocolate flavored)
- Apple sauce (1/2 cup, unsweetened)
- Yogurt (1/2 cup+1 tbsp, nonfat, Greek)
- Flour (1 cup, oat)
- Chocolate protein (2-3 scoops, powdered)
- Cocoa (3 tbsp, powdered unsweetened)
- Baking powder (1 tsp., baker style)
- Salt (1/2 tsp.)

For the frosting:
- Greek yogurt (1/2 cup, nonfat)
- Cherries (1/4 cup)
- Sweetener (optional)

DIRECTIONS

1. The first step is to heat an oven to 350 degrees Fahrenheit, then lightly spray a baking dish using cooking spray.
2. Add the egg whites and whisk well until beaten lightly.
3. Add the protein powder, oat flour, sweetener, powdered cocoa, and baking powder separately.
4. Stir well until mixed evenly, then pour milk mixture (almond) into the flour mixture.
5. Stir well until thoroughly mixed and set batter aside for approximately 5 minutes.
6. Pour batter into the dish and place into the oven to bake for approximately 25 minutes until thoroughly cooked.
7. Remove brownie from heat, then set aside to cool.
8. Add all the frosting ingredients in a food processor, then process on the highest setting until smooth.
9. Spread frosting over the top of brownies. Serve.

NUTRITIONS

- Carbohydrates: 6 g
- Protein: 16 g
- Fat: 12 g
- Potassium: 4 mg

183. CAESAR SALAD WITH CHICKEN AND PARMESAN

PREPARATION	COOKING	SERVES
20 MIN	1 H 30 MIN	4

INGREDIENTS

- 4 boneless, skinless chicken thighs
- 1/4 cup lemon juice
- 2 garlic cloves, minced
- 4 tbsp olive oil
- 1/2 cup Caesar salad dressing, sugar-free
- 12 bok choy leaves
- 3 Parmesan crisps
- Parmesan cheese, grated for garnishing

DIRECTIONS

1. Mix chicken, lemon juice, 2 tbsp olive oil, and garlic in a Ziploc bag.
2. Seal the bag, shake well, and refrigerate for 1 hour.
3. Preheat the grill to medium and grill the chicken for 4 minutes per side.
4. Cut bok choy lengthwise, and brush with the remaining oil.
5. Grill the bok choy for about 3 minutes.
6. Place in a bowl.
7. Top with chicken and Parmesan; drizzle the dressing over.
8. Top with Parmesan crisps to serve.

NUTRITIONS

- Calories: 529 Cal
- Fat: 39 g
- Carbohydrates: 5 g
- Protein: 33 g

184. RASPBERRY FLAX SEED DESSERT

PREPARATION	COOKING	SERVES
3 MIN	5 MIN	4

INGREDIENTS

- 2 cups raspberries; reserve a few for topping
- 3 cups unsweetened vanilla almond milk
- 1 cup heavy cream
- 1/2 cup chia seeds
- 1/2 cup flaxseeds, ground
- 4 tsp. liquid stevia
- Chopped mixed nuts for topping

DIRECTIONS

1. In a medium bowl, crush the raspberries with a fork until pureed.
2. Pour in the almond milk, heavy cream, chia seeds, and liquid stevia.
3. Mix and refrigerate the pudding overnight.
4. Spoon the pudding into serving glasses, top with raspberries, mixed nuts, and serve

NUTRITIONS

- Calories: 390 Cal
- Fats: 33.5 g
- Carbohydrates: 3 g
- Protein: 13 g

185. POMEGRANATE CHERRY SMOOTHIE BOWL

PREPARATION	COOKING	SERVES
5 MIN	0 MIN	4

INGREDIENTS

- 1 (16-ounce) bag frozen dark sweet cherries
- 1 1/2 cups 2% plain Greek yogurt, plus more if needed
- 3/4 cup pomegranate juice
- 1/3 cup 2% milk, plus more if needed
- 1 teaspoon vanilla extract
- 3/4 teaspoon ground cinnamon
- 6 ice cubes
- 1/2 cup chopped pistachios
- 1/2 cup fresh pomegranate seeds

DIRECTIONS

1. Put the cherries, yogurt, pomegranate juice, milk, vanilla, cinnamon, and ice cubes in a blender. Purée until thoroughly mixed and smooth.
2. You'll want the mixture a little thicker than your average smoothie, but not so thick you can't pour it. If the smoothie is too thick, add another few tablespoon of milk; if it's too thin, add another few tablespoon of yogurt.
3. Pour the smoothie into four bowls. Top each with 2 tablespoons of pistachios and 2 tablespoons of pomegranate seeds, and serve immediately.

NUTRITIONS

- *Calories: 212 Cal*
- *Total Fat: 7 g*
- *Saturated Fat: 3 g*
- *Cholesterol: 18 mg*
- *Sodium: 53 mg*
- *Total Carbohydrates:*
- *35 g*
- *Fiber: 3 g*
- *Protein: 4 g*

186. CUSTARD CREAM

PREPARATION	COOKING	SERVES
15 MIN	30 MIN	4

INGREDIENTS

- 200 unsalted butter, chopped
- 200g milk chocolate buttons
- 3 eggs, lightly whisked
- 1 cup white sugar
- 2/3 cup plain flour
- 1/3 cup cocoa powder
- 12 custard cream biscuits

DIRECTIONS

1. Preheat oven to 400F/ 350F
2. Line a 2ocm rectangular cake pan with baking paper, allowing 2 facets to overhang.
3. Place the butter and chocolate in a heatproof bowl over a saucepan of simmering water. Don't let the bowl touch the water.
4. Stir with a metal spoon until melted.
5. Remove from heat. Set aside to cool slightly.
6. Stir the eggs, sugar, flour, and cocoa powder into the butter mixture until just combined.
7. Pour into the prepared pan.
8. Bake for 20 minutes
9. Remove from the oven and arrange the biscuits on top.
10. Bake for a further 25 minutes or until a skewer inserted in the center comes out with moist crumbs clinging.
11. Set aside to cool completely.
12. Cut into squares to serve.

NUTRITIONS

- Cholesterol: 19 mg
- Sodium: 540 mg
- Fats: 20g
- Carbohydrates: 20 g
- Protein: 15 g

187. CHOCOLATE BARS

PREPARATION	COOKING	SERVES
10 MIN	20 MIN	6

INGREDIENTS

- 15 oz cream cheese, softened
- 15 oz unsweetened dark chocolate
- 1 tsp vanilla
- 10 drops liquid stevia

DIRECTIONS

1. Grease an 8-inch square dish and set aside.
2. In a saucepan, dissolve chocolate over low heat.
3. Add stevia and vanilla and stir well.
4. Remove pan from heat and set aside.
5. Add cream cheese into the blender and blend until smooth.
6. Add melted chocolate mixture into the cream cheese and blend until just combined.
7. Transfer mixture into the prepared dish and spread evenly, and place in the refrigerator until firm.
8. Slice and serve.

NUTRITIONS

- Calories: 230
- Fat: 24 g
- Carbs: 7.5 g
- Sugar: 0.1 g
- Protein: 6 g
- Cholesterol: 29 mg

188. BLUEBERRY MUFFINS

PREPARATION	COOKING	SERVES
15 MIN	35 MIN	12

INGREDIENTS

- 2 eggs
- 1/2 cup fresh blueberries
- 1 cup heavy cream
- 2 cups almond flour
- 1/4 tsp lemon zest
- 1/2 tsp lemon extract
- 1 tsp baking powder
- 5 drops stevia
- 1/4 cup butter, melted

DIRECTIONS

1. heat the cooker to 350 F. Line muffin tin with cupcake liners and set aside.
2. Add eggs into the bowl and whisk until mix.
3. Add remaining ingredients and mix to combine.
4. Pour mixture into the prepared muffin tin and bake for 25 minutes.
5. Serve and enjoy.

NUTRITIONS

- Calories: 190
- Fat: 17 g
- Carbs: 5 g
- Sugar: 1 g
- Protein: 5 g
- Cholesterol: 55 mg

189. CHIA PUDDING

PREPARATION	COOKING	SERVES
20 MIN	0 MIN	2

INGREDIENTS

- 4 tbsp chia seeds
- 1 cup unsweetened coconut milk
- 1/2 cup raspberries

DIRECTIONS

1. Add raspberry and coconut milk into a blender and blend until smooth.
2. Pour mixture into the glass jar.
3. Add chia seeds in a jar and stir well.
4. Seal the jar with a lid and shake well and place in the refrigerator for 3 hours.
5. Serve chilled and enjoy.

NUTRITIONS

- Calories: 360
- Fat: 33 g
- Carbs: 13 g
- Sugar: 5 g
- Protein: 6 g
- Cholesterol: 0 mg

190. AVOCADO PUDDING

PREPARATION	COOKING	SERVES
20 MIN	0 MIN	8

INGREDIENTS

- 2 ripe avocados, pitted and cut into pieces
- 1 tbsp fresh lime juice
- 14 oz can of coconut milk
- 2 tsp liquid stevia
- 2 tsp vanilla

DIRECTIONS

1. Inside the blender, add all ingredients and blend until smooth.
2. Serve immediately and enjoy.

NUTRITIONS

- *Calories: 317*
- *Fat: 30 g*
- *Carbs: 9 g*
- *Sugar: 0.5 g*
- *Protein: 3 g*
- *Cholesterol: 0 mg*

191. DELICIOUS BROWNIE BITES

PREPARATION	COOKING	SERVES
20 MIN	0 MIN	13

INGREDIENTS

- 1/4 cup unsweetened chocolate chips
- 1/4 cup unsweetened cocoa powder
- 1 cup pecans, chopped
- 1/2 cup almond butter
- 1/2 tsp vanilla
- 1/4 cup monk fruit sweetener
- 1/8 tsp pink salt

DIRECTIONS

1. Add pecans, sweetener, vanilla, almond butter, cocoa powder, and salt into the food processor and process until well combined.
2. Transfer brownie mixture into the large bowl. Add chocolate chips and fold well.
3. Make small round shape balls from brownie mixture and place onto a baking tray.
4. Place in the freezer for 20 minutes.
5. Serve and enjoy.

NUTRITIONS

- Calories: 108
- Fat: 9 g
- Carbs: 4 g
- Sugar: 1 g
- Protein: 2 g
- Cholesterol: 0 mg

192. PUMPKIN BALLS

PREPARATION	COOKING	SERVES
15 MIN	0 MIN	18

INGREDIENTS

- 1 cup almond butter
- 5 drops liquid stevia
- 2 tbsp coconut flour
- 2 tbsp pumpkin puree
- 1 tsp pumpkin pie spice

DIRECTIONS

1. Mix pumpkin puree in a large bowl and almond butter until well combined.
2. Add liquid stevia, pumpkin pie spice, and coconut flour and mix well.
3. Make small balls from the mixture and place them onto a baking tray.
4. Place in the freezer for 1 hour.
5. Serve and enjoy.

NUTRITIONS

- Calories: 96
- Fat: 8 g
- Carbs: 4 g
- Sugar: 1 g
- Protein: 2 g
- Cholesterol: 0 mg

193. SMOOTH PEANUT BUTTER CREAM

PREPARATION	COOKING	SERVES
10 MIN	0 MIN	8

INGREDIENTS

- 1/4 cup peanut butter
- 4 overripe bananas, chopped
- 1/3 cup cocoa powder
- 1/4 tsp vanilla extract
- 1/8 tsp salt

DIRECTIONS

1. In the blender, add all the listed ingredients and blend until smooth.
2. Serve immediately and enjoy.

NUTRITIONS

- Calories: 101
- Fat: 5 g
- Carbs: 14 g
- Sugar: 7 g
- Protein: 3 g
- Cholesterol: 0 mg

194. VANILLA AVOCADO POPSICLES

PREPARATION	COOKING	SERVES
20 MIN	0 MIN	6

INGREDIENTS

- 2 avocadoes
- 1 tsp vanilla
- 1 cup almond milk
- 1 tsp liquid stevia
- 1/2 cup unsweetened cocoa powder

DIRECTIONS

1. In the blender, add all the listed ingredients and blend smoothly.
2. Pour blended mixture into the Popsicle molds and place in the freezer until set.
3. Serve and enjoy.

NUTRITIONS

- *Calories: 130*
- *Fat: 12 g*
- *Carbs: 7 g*
- *Sugar: 1 g*
- *Protein: 3 g*
- *Cholesterol: 0 mg*

195. CHOCOLATE POPSICLE

PREPARATION	COOKING	SERVES
20 MIN	10 MIN	6

INGREDIENTS

- 4 oz unsweetened chocolate, chopped
- 6 drops liquid stevia
- 1 1/2 cups heavy cream

DIRECTIONS

1. Add heavy cream into the microwave-safe bowl and microwave until it just begins the boiling.
2. Add chocolate into the heavy cream and set aside for 5 minutes.
3. Add liquid stevia into the heavy cream mixture and stir until chocolate is melted.
4. Pour mixture into the Popsicle molds and place in freezer for 4 hours or until set.
5. Serve and enjoy.

NUTRITIONS

- *Calories: 198*
- *Fat: 21 g*
- *Carbs: 6 g*
- *Sugar: 0.2 g*
- *Protein: 3 g*
- *Cholesterol: 41 mg*

196. RASPBERRY ICE CREAM

PREPARATION	COOKING	SERVES
10 MIN	0 MIN	2

INGREDIENTS

- 1 cup frozen raspberries
- 1/2 cup heavy cream
- 1/8 tsp stevia powder

DIRECTIONS

1. Blend all the listed ingredients in a blender until smooth.
2. Serve immediately and enjoy.

NUTRITIONS

- Calories: 144
- Fat: 11 g
- Carbs: 10 g
- Sugar: 4 g
- Protein: 2 g
- Cholesterol: 41 mg

197. CHOCOLATE FROSTY

PREPARATION	COOKING	SERVES
20 MIN	0 MIN	4

INGREDIENTS

- 2 tbsp unsweetened cocoa powder
- 1 cup heavy whipping cream
- 1 tbsp almond butter
- 5 drops liquid stevia
- 1 tsp vanilla

DIRECTIONS

1. Add cream into the medium bowl and beat using the hand mixer for 5 minutes.
2. Add remaining ingredients and blend until thick cream forms.
3. Pour in serving bowls and place them in the freezer for 30 minutes.
4. Serve and enjoy.

NUTRITIONS

- *Calories: 137*
- *Fat: 13 g*
- *Carbs: 3 g*
- *Sugar: 0.5 g*
- *Protein: 2 g*
- *Cholesterol: 41 mg*

198. CHOCOLATE ALMOND BUTTER BROWNIE

PREPARATION	COOKING	SERVES
10 MIN	16 MIN	4

INGREDIENTS

- 1 cup bananas, overripe
- 1/2 cup almond butter, melted
- 1 scoop protein powder
- 2 tbsp unsweetened cocoa powder

DIRECTIONS

1. Preheat the air fryer to 325 F. Grease air fryer baking pan and set aside.
2. Blend all ingredients in a blender until smooth.
3. Pour batter into the equipped pan then place in the air fryer basket, and cook for 16 minutes.
4. Serve and enjoy.

NUTRITIONS

- Calories: 82
- Fat: 2 g
- Carbs: 11 g
- Sugar: 5 g
- Protein: 7 g
- Cholesterol: 16 mg

199. PEANUT BUTTER FUDGE

PREPARATION	COOKING	SERVES
10 MIN	10 MIN	20

INGREDIENTS

- 1/4 cup almonds, toasted and chopped
- 12 oz smooth peanut butter
- 15 drops liquid stevia
- 3 tbsp coconut oil
- 4 tbsp coconut cream
- Pinch of salt

DIRECTIONS

1. Line baking tray with parchment paper.
2. Melt coconut oil in a pan over low heat. Add peanut butter, coconut cream, stevia, and salt in a saucepan. Stir well.
3. Pour fudge mixture into the prepared baking tray and sprinkle chopped almonds on top.
4. Place the tray in the refrigerator for 1 hour or until set.
5. Slice and serve.

NUTRITIONS

- *Calories: 131*
- *Fat: 12 g*
- *Carbs: 4 g*
- *Sugar: 2 g*
- *Protein: 5 g*
- *Cholesterol: 0 mg*

200. ALMOND BUTTER FUDGE

PREPARATION	COOKING	SERVES
10 MIN	10 MIN	18

INGREDIENTS

- 3/4 cup creamy almond butter
- 1 1/2 cups unsweetened chocolate chips

DIRECTIONS

1. Line 8*4-inch pan with parchment paper and set aside.
2. Add chocolate chips and almond butter into the double boiler and cook over medium heat until the chocolate-butter mixture is melted. Stir well.
3. Place mixture into the prepared pan and place in the freezer until set.
4. Slice and serve.

NUTRITIONS

- *Calories: 197*
- *Fat: 16 g*
- *Carbs: 7 g*
- *Sugar: 1 g*
- *Protein: 4 g*
- *Cholesterol: 0 mg*

201. BOUNTY BARS

PREPARATION	COOKING	SERVES
20 MIN	0 MIN	12

INGREDIENTS

- 1 cup coconut cream
- 3 cups shredded unsweetened coconut
- 1/4 cup extra virgin coconut oil
- 1/2 teaspoon vanilla powder
- 1/4 cup powdered erythritol
- 1 1/2 oz. cocoa butter
- 5 oz. dark chocolate

DIRECTIONS

1. Heat the oven at 350 °F and toast the coconut in it for 5-6 minutes. Remove from the oven once toasted and set aside to cool.
2. Take a medium-sized bowl and add coconut oil, coconut cream, vanilla, erythritol, and toasted coconut. Mix the ingredients well to prepare a smooth mixture.
3. Make 12 bars of equal size with your hands from the prepared mixture and adjust in the tray lined with parchment paper.
4. Place the tray in the fridge for around one hour and, in the meantime, put the cocoa butter and dark chocolate in a glass bowl.
5. Heat a cup of water in a saucepan over medium heat and place the bowl over it to melt the cocoa butter and the dark chocolate.
6. Remove from the heat once melted properly, mix well until blended and set aside to cool.
7. Take the coconut bars and coat them with dark chocolate mixture one by one using a wooden stick. Adjust on the tray lined with parchment paper and drizzle the remaining mixture over them.
8. Refrigerate for around one hour before you serve the delicious bounty bars.

NUTRITIONS

- Calories: 230
- Fat: 25 g
- Carbohydrates: 5 g
- Protein: 32 g

202. BANANA BREAD

PREPARATION	COOKING	SERVES
5 MIN	40 MIN	6

INGREDIENTS

- ¾ cup of sugar
- 1/3 cup butter
- 1 tbsp. vanilla extract
- 1 egg
- 2 bananas
- 1 tbsp. baking powder
- 1 and ½ cups flour
- ½ tbsp. baking soda
- 1/3 cup milk
- 1 and ½ tbsp. cream of tartar
- Cooking spray

DIRECTIONS

1. Mix in milk with cream of tartar, vanilla, egg, sugar, bananas and butter in a bowl and turn whole.
2. Mix in flour with baking soda and baking powder.
3. Blend the 2 mixtures, turn properly, move into an oiled pan with cooking spray, put into the air fryer and cook at 320°F for 40 minutes.
4. Remove bread, allow to cool, slice. Serve.

NUTRITIONS

- *Calories: 540*
- *Total Fat: 16g*
- *Total carbs: 28g*

203. MINI LAVA CAKES

PREPARATION	COOKING	SERVES
5 MIN	20 MIN	3

INGREDIENTS

- 1 egg
- 4 tbsp. sugar
- 2 tbsp. olive oil
- 4 tbsp. milk
- 4 tbsp. flour
- 1 tbsp. Cocoa powder
- ½ tbsp. Baking powder
- ½ tbsp. orange zest

DIRECTIONS

1. Mix in egg with sugar, flour, salt, oil, milk, orange zest, baking powder and cocoa powder, turn properly. Move it to oiled ramekins.
2. Put ramekins in the air fryer and cook at 320°F for 20 minutes.
3. Serve warm.

NUTRITIONS

- Calories: 329
- Total Fat: 8.5g
- Total carbs: 12.4g

204. GINGER CHEESECAKE

PREPARATION	COOKING	SERVES
20 MIN	20 MIN	6

INGREDIENTS

- 2 tbsp. butter
- ½ cup ginger cookies
- 16 oz. cream cheese
- 2 eggs
- ½ cup sugar
- 1 tbsp. rum
- ½ tbsp. vanilla extract
- ½ tbsp. nutmeg

DIRECTIONS

1. Spread pan with the butter and sprinkle cookie crumbs on the bottom.
2. Whisk cream cheese with rum, vanilla, nutmeg and eggs, beat properly and sprinkle the cookie crumbs.
3. Put in the air fryer and cook at 340° F for 20 minutes.
4. Allow cheesecake to cool in the fridge for 2 hours before slicing.
5. Serve.

NUTRITIONS

- *Calories: 312*
- *Total Fat: 9.8g*
- *Total carbs: 18g*

205. PUDDING PIES

PREPARATION	COOKING	SERVES
10 MIN	25 MIN	8

INGREDIENTS

For the crust
- 5 1/3 tbsp unsalted butter
- 65 vanilla wafers

For the pie
- Two bananas

For the pudding
- 2 tsp vanilla extract
- ½ cup of sugar
- ¼ tsp salt
- 1/3 cup flour
- 2 cups of milk
- Four egg yolks

For the whipped cream
- 1 tsp vanilla extract
- 2 tbsp confectioner's sugar
- 1 cup cream

DIRECTIONS

Crust making
1. Crush vanilla wafers in a blender and blend with butter. Save some wafer powder for topping.
2. Take a pie plate and spread the dough on it, and bake in a preheated oven at 350 degrees for 12 mins
3. Let it cool

Making pudding
4. Mix flour, salt, and sugar in a saucepan on medium heat.
5. Add milk to the mixture and mix till it becomes thick.
6. Separate egg yolk in a bowl and pour 3 tbsp of milk mixture while hot and mix.
7. Pour this egg mixture into a saucepan and stir till it gets thickened.
8. Turn off the flame and add vanilla while stirring.

Assembly
9. Divide bananas into two portions.
10. Organize the first one-half of banana slices on the crust.
11. Pour pudding mixture (half) over the layer of bananas.
12. Spread leftover powdered wafers over the pudding and topped it with leftover bananas.
13. Then again, pour the pudding over the top of the second layer of bananas.
14. To fully cool it, place the pot in the fridge.

Whipped cream
15. Blend vanilla, sugar, and heavy cream and make it frothy.
16. Spread the frothy cream over the chilled pudding and serve.

NUTRITIONS

- *567 kcal: Calories;*
- *65 g: Carbohydrates*
- *165 mg Cholesterol;*
- *16 g Fat;*
- *6 g Protein;*
- *1g: fiber.*

206. PANCAKE CINNAMON ROLL

PREPARATION	COOKING	SERVES
30 MIN	20 MIN	8

INGREDIENTS

Pancakes
- Two tablespoons white vinegar
- One teaspoon baking powder
- 1 cup flour
- ½ teaspoon baking soda
- 1 1/2 teaspoons vanilla extract
- Two tablespoons sugar
- ½ teaspoon salt
- ¾ cup milk
- Two tablespoons butter
- One egg

Cinnamon Swirl Filling
- 1 1/2 teaspoons cinnamon
- ¼ cup butter
- 5 ½ tablespoons sugar

Cream Cheese Icing
- ¾ cup confectioners' sugar
- 2 oz. cream cheese
- ¼ cup butter
- ½ tsp vanilla extract

DIRECTIONS

1. Sour the milk by adding vinegar to it. Keep it aside for a few minutes.
2. Combine butter, vanilla extract, and eggs in sour milk.
3. Take a large bowl, add sugar, baking powder, salt, baking soda, and flour and mix them well.
4. Gradually pour sour milk solution into the dry mixture and mix until a smooth batter is formed.
5. Take another bowl, mix cinnamon, butter, and sugar in it.
6. Put this mixture in a cone-shaped container and refrigerate.
7. In a small bowl, blend cream cheese and butter until they get smooth.
8. Then add confectioners' sugar and half tsp of vanilla into the mixture and mix. Icing is ready.
9. On medium heat, place skillet sprayed with cooking oil and place two-third of batter on it.
10. Cook the batter. After 3 minutes' bubbles begin to rise.
11. Take out the cone-shaped container from the fridge and swirl the mixture over the pancake. Be careful that the mixture should not touch the skillet.
12. Turn the pancake upside down and cook the other side for the next three minutes.
13. Spread the icing on the pancake and serve.

NUTRITIONS

- Calories 327 kcal;
- 3.9 g Protein;
- 37.9 g Carbohydrates;
- 18.1 g Fat;
- 71 mg Cholesterol

207. CHOCOLATE CHIP COFFEE CAKE MUFFINS

PREPARATION	COOKING	SERVES
20 MIN	25 MIN	15

INGREDIENTS

- 1 cup of chocolate chips
- 1/2 cup sugar
- 2 cups flour (all-purpose)
- 2 tsp baking powder
- 2 tsp coffee granules (instant)
- 1 tsp cinnamon (powdered)
- 1/4 tsp salt
- One egg
- 1/2 cup brown sugar
- 1 cup milk
- 1 tsp vanilla extract

- 1/2 cup butter

Topping
- 1/4 cup brown sugar
- 1/4 cup butter
- 1/2 tsp cinnamon (powdered)
- tsp flour (all-purpose)

DIRECTIONS

1. In a medium-sized bowl, whisk vanilla, butter, egg, and milk.
2. In another large bowl, mix sugar, baking powder, coffee, salt, cinnamon, and flour and add with mixing the egg mixture. Spread chocolate chips and toss,
3. In greased muffins molds, fill the batter
4. Combine sugar (brown), cinnamon, and flour in a bowl and add butter and whisk until a smooth thick, smooth solution is formed. Topping is ready
5. Spread it on the batter.
6. Put the baking pan with batter in it in a preheated oven at 375 degrees for 25 minutes.
7. After baking, let it cool and serve.

NUTRITIONS

- *Calories 291 kcal,*
- *Fat 14 grams,*
- *Cholesterol 41 milligram,*
- *Carbohydrate 41 grams*

208. ZUCCHINI BREAD

PREPARATION	COOKING	SERVES
20 MIN	50 MIN	24

INGREDIENTS

- 1 cup walnuts (sliced)
- 3 cups flour
- 3 tsp vanilla extract
- 1 tsp baking soda
- 1 tsp cinnamon
- Two 1/4 cups sugar
- 1 tsp salt
- 2 cups zucchini
- Three eggs
- 1 tsp baking powder
- 1 cup oil

DIRECTIONS

1. Whisk baking powder and soda, cinnamon, salt, and flour in a container.
2. Whisk oil, sugar, egg, and vanilla in a large container. Add dry ingredients and whisk well. Put nuts with zucchini and mix well.
3. Pour smooth without lumps batter in baking pan.
4. Place the pan in a preheated oven at 325 degrees for 50 minutes.
5. After baking, cool it and serve.

NUTRITIONS

- *Calories 255 kcal;*
- *3.3 grams' protein;*
- *13.1 grams' fat;*
- *23.3 grams Cholesterol;*
- *32.1 grams*

Carbohydrates.

209. HAYSTACKS

PREPARATION	COOKING	SERVES
10 MIN	0 MIN	15

INGREDIENTS

- 4 cups chow mien noodle
- 12 oz. chocolate chips
- 11 oz. butterscotch chips

DIRECTIONS

1. In a bowl, whisk butterscotch chips and chocolate chips and use a microwave to melt them to make a smooth flowy liquid.
2. Put noodles in the liquid and toss them so that they are coated with chocolate chip syrup.
3. Pour full spoon batter over butter paper and place the tray in the fridge to cool them for 20 minutes and serve.

NUTRITIONS

- 267 kcal Calories;
- 2 grams' protein;
- 38 grams
- Carbohydrates;
- 11 grams Fat;
- 3-milligram
- Cholesterol

210. VANILLA CUSTARD

PREPARATION	COOKING	SERVES
10 MIN	20 MIN	4

INGREDIENTS

- 1/3 cup sugar
- 1 cup milk
- 1 Vanilla Bean
- 1 tbsp corn flour
- Four yolks of egg
- 1 cup cream

DIRECTIONS

1. Take a saucepan, add cream, vanilla beans, and its seeds and milk in it and cook on medium flame with continuous stirring until it boils and remove beans for it.
2. In a bowl, mix corn flour, egg yolk, and sugar.
3. Pour hot milk solution over an egg mixture with constant stirring.
4. Place the bowl on low flame and cook with continuous stirring until the solution gets thickens.
5. Cool it down and serve with pancakes or fruits.

NUTRITIONS

- 1570 kcal Calories;
- Protein 5 grams,
- Carbohydrates 23 grams;
- Fat 29 grams,
- 0-milligram Cholesterol.

211. CHOCOLATE CHEESECAKE SHAKE

PREPARATION	COOKING	SERVES
10 MIN	0 MIN	4

INGREDIENTS

- Six scoops of ice cream (chocolate flavor)
- 8 oz. cream cheese
- 2 cups of milk

DIRECTIONS

1. Make a smooth solution of milk (one cup) and cream cheese in a blender.
2. Then make a smooth mixture of ice cream and milk (one cup).
3. Fill the serving glass with milk and cream solution and then pour ice cream smoothie and serve.

NUTRITIONS

- Calories 227 kcal;
- 15.6 grams' fat;
- 7.3 grams' protein;
- 51.3 grams Cholesterol;
- 15.3 grams Carbohydrates.

212. PISTACHIO MILK-SHAKE

PREPARATION	COOKING	SERVES
5 MIN	0 MIN	4

INGREDIENTS

- 1 tsp vanilla extract
- 5 cups ice cream (pistachio)
- 4 tbsp pistachios
- Pinch of salt
- 1 cup milk

DIRECTIONS

1. Blend salt, ice cream, vanilla extract, and milk in a blender to make a smooth, fluffy thick solution.
2. Garnish with pistachios and serve.

NUTRITIONS

- 400 kcal Calories;
- 26 grams' fat;
- 140 milligrams cholesterol;
- 31 grams Carbohydrates;
- 9 grams protein.

213. PEANUT BUTTER AND CREAM CHEESE STUFFED BROWNIES

PREPARATION	COOKING	SERVES
30 MIN	25 MIN	12

INGREDIENTS

Base for Brownie
- 1/4 tsp baking soda
- 1/2 cup maple syrup
- 1 tsp vanilla extract
- One egg
- 2 tsp coconut oil
- 6 tbsp cocoa powder
- 1 cup peanut butter

Filling for Peanut Butter Cheesecake
- 2 tsp. vanilla extract
- 2/3 cup maple syrup

- 6 oz. cream cheese
- 1 cup peanut butter

For the Topping
- 7 oz. peanut butter

For the Fudge Sauce
- 2 tbsp. cocoa powder
- 3 tbsp. maple syrup

DIRECTIONS

Brownie Base
1. Take a large bowl, combine all the ingredients for the brownie base and whisk well.
2. Bake for 25 minutes in a preheated oven at 325 degrees. And let it cool.

Fudge Sauce
3. Mix the cocoa powder and maple syrup on medium flame.

Peanut Butter Cheesecake Filling
4. In a blender, blend all the ingredients until a smooth mixture is obtained.
5. Refrigerate the mixture for 10 minutes.
6. At the top of the brownie, spread the filling and place the brownie in the refrigerator overnight with plastic wrap covering.
7. After refrigeration, with peanut butter cubes, garnish the top and pour randomly chocolate sauce and serve.

NUTRITIONS

- *552 kcal calories;*
- *45-gram carbohydrates;*
- *40 milligrams cholesterol;*
- *14 grams' protein;*
- *37 grams' fat.*

214. GRILLED CHEESE TOMATO SANDWICH

PREPARATION	COOKING	SERVES
20 MIN	25 MIN	15

INGREDIENTS

- 2 tsp. mayonnaise
- Two slices tomatoes
- One pinch pepper
- Two slices of Swiss cheese
- 2 tbsp. butter
- One pinch salt
- Two slices of bread
- One pinch of powdered garlic
- One pinch of Italian seasoning

DIRECTIONS

1. Spread mayonnaise over the bread slices.
2. Top one bread with slices of tomato.
3. Drizzle Italian seasoning, salt, and pepper.
4. Place cheese on the tomatoes and place the second bread slice over it.
5. Take a skillet and heat butter and garlic powder on it.
6. Slightly spread butter over both sides of bread and grill both sides until cheese melts and turns brown.

NUTRITIONS

- 559.4 kcal calories;
- 30.5 grams' carbohydrates;
- 19.6 grams' protein;
- 40.3 grams' fat;
- 112.6 grams' cholesterol.

215. PEANUT BUTTER CRUNCH BARS

PREPARATION	COOKING	SERVES
3 MIN	1 MIN	20

INGREDIENTS

- 3 cups of rice cereal
- 1/2 cup maple syrup
- 1 cup peanut butter
- 1 1/2 cups chocolate chips
- 1/4 cup coconut oil

DIRECTIONS

1. Melt all the ingredients except rice cereal in a microwave oven and mix well.
2. Pour the melted mixture over rice cereal in a bowl and toss gently.
3. Spread the mixture in a baking pan lined with butter paper and refrigerate for an hour.
4. Cut into pieces and serve.

NUTRITIONS

- 200 kcal Calories;
- 16 grams Carbohydrates;
- 4 grams' protein;
- 15 grams Cholesterol,
- 0.2 grams Fat

216. MOUSSE TREAT

PREPARATION	COOKING	SERVES
5 MIN	20 MIN	8

INGREDIENTS

- 8 oz. chopped baking semisweet chocolate
- Four egg yolks
- 2 ½ cups whipping cream
- ¼ cup of sugar

DIRECTIONS

1. Blend egg yolks in a blender with slow addition of sugar.
2. At medium flame, heat whipping cream and pour half of the hot whipping cream in the egg mixture and mix well.
3. Pour the egg mixture back to hot whipping cream in a saucepan at low flame and cook for the next five minutes.
4. Add and mix chocolate and cook until chocolate melts.
5. Refrigerate for two hours till it gets chilled.
6. Using a beater, beat cream, and mix in a chocolate mixture.
7. Put one spoon of mixture in each serving dish.

NUTRITIONS

- *430kcal Calories;*
- *175 milligrams cholesterol;*
- *5 grams' protein;*
- *33 grams' fat;*
- *27 grams Carbohydrates.*

217. TIRAMISU MILKSHAKE

PREPARATION	COOKING	SERVES
7 MIN	0 MIN	2

INGREDIENTS

- 2 tsp. espresso powder
- 4 scoops Vanilla Ice Cream
- 1 cup whipped cream
- Four ladyfingers cookies
- 4 tsp. cocoa powder
- 1/2 cup milk

DIRECTIONS

1. In a blender, put espresso powder, ice cream, and milk and blend to get a smooth, fluffy mixture.
2. Pour the shake into glasses and add whipping cream at the top and drizzle cocoa powder.
3. Use ladyfinger cookies for garnishing and serve.

NUTRITIONS

- *257 kcal calories;*
- *6 grams' protein;*
- *83 milligrams cholesterol;*
- *11 grams' fat;*
- *32 grams' carbohydrates.*

218. MAPLE PANCAKES

PREPARATION	COOKING	SERVES
15 MIN	12 MIN	6

INGREDIENTS

- One egg
- 1-1/2 tsp. baking powder
- 1 cup milk
- 1 tbsp maple syrup
- 2 tbsp. oil
- 1 cup flour
- 1/2 tsp. salt

DIRECTIONS

1. Beat oil, milk, egg, and syrup in a bowl.
2. Add and mix salt, baking powder, and flour in another bowl and add egg mixture slowly while stirring.
3. Drop spoonful batter on a heated pan. Cook until bubbles form, and then flip the side and cook another side till turned golden brown.
4. Serve with syrup.

NUTRITIONS

- *Calories 486 kcal;*
- *Carbohydrate 60 g;*
- *Protein 14g;*
- *Fat 21 g;*
- *Cholesterol 123 mg*

219. PIZZA BREAD

PREPARATION	COOKING	SERVES
5 MIN	40 MIN	4

INGREDIENTS

- Four chopped garlic cloves
- One large loaf of Italian bread
- 2 oz. Parmigiano-Reggiano
- 4 tbsp. olive oil
- 3 tbsp. butter
- 1/2 tsp oregano
- 1/4 cup parsley
- pinch of red pepper flakes
- 14.5 oz. tomatoes mashed
- Kosher salt
- 8 oz. mozzarella cheese grated

DIRECTIONS

1. In a saucepan, melt butter, add olive oil, stir fry garlic and oregano, and red pepper flakes.
2. Later add salt and parsley and turn off the flame.
3. Take cut bread pieces and press to reduce its height to two-third, and spread garlic paste (cooked in step one) over the cut side of bread with the help of a brush.
4. Afterward, cook tomatoes and leftover garlic paste in a saucepan at medium flame.
5. Reduce the flame to low at put a pan on simmer for 15 minutes and add salt later.
6. Place mozzarella cheese over bread (prepared in step three) and bake until cheese melts. It will take almost 6-8 minutes.
7. When the sauce is cooked, spread over baked bread, place leftover mozzarella cheese, and bake for the next 8-10 minutes until cheese melts. Drizzle parmigiana-Reggiano after taking it out of the oven. Sprinkle leftover parsley and olive oil and serve when cool down.

NUTRITIONS

- 152 kcal calories;
- 7 grams 'protein;
- 14 milligrams cholesterol;
- 5 grams' fat;
- 18 grams' carbohydrates

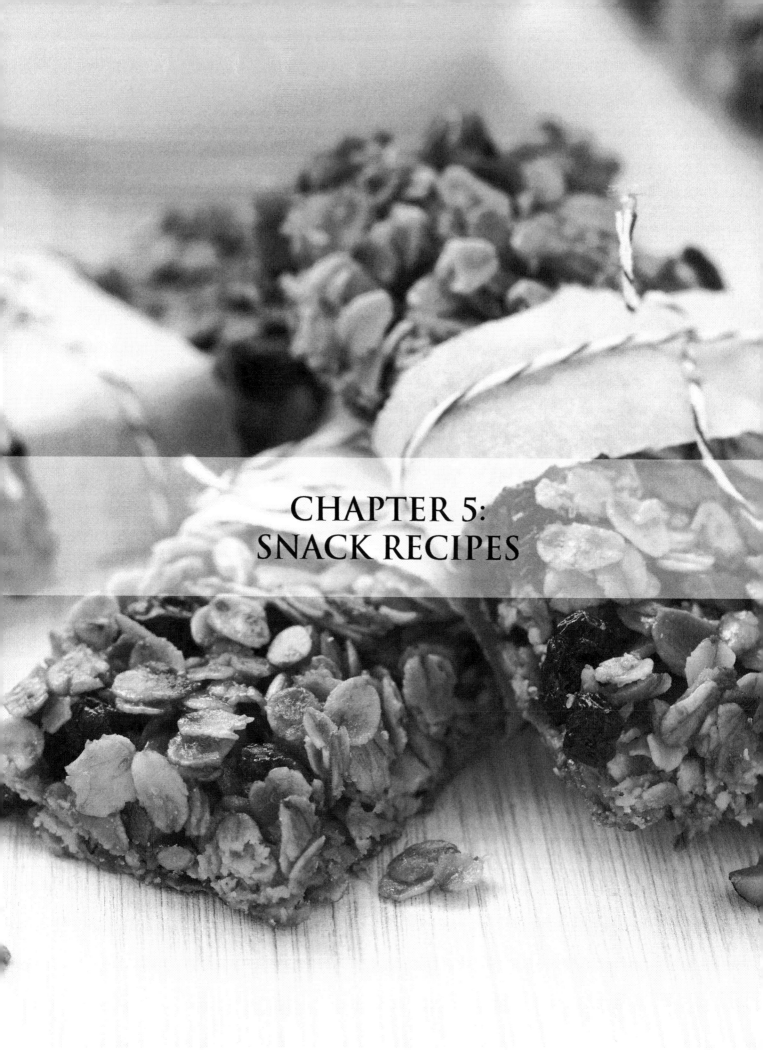

CHAPTER 5:
SNACK RECIPES

220. BROCCOLI SALAD

PREPARATION	COOKING	SERVES
5 MIN	25 MIN	1

INGREDIENTS

- 1/3 tablespoons sherry vinegar
- 1/24 cup olive oil
- 1/3 teaspoons fresh thyme, chopped
- 1/6 teaspoon Dijon mustard
- 1/6 teaspoon honey
- Salt to taste
- 1 1/3 cups broccoli florets
- 1/3 red onions
- 1/12 cup Parmesan cheese shaved
- 1/24 cup pecans

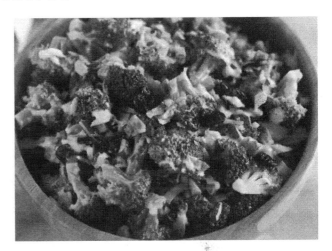

DIRECTIONS

1. Mix the sherry vinegar, olive oil, thyme, mustard, honey, and salt in a bowl.
2. In a serving bowl, blend the broccoli florets and onions.
3. Drizzle the dressing on top.
4. Sprinkle with the pecans and Parmesan cheese before serving.

NUTRITIONS

- Calories 199
- Fat 17.4 g
- Saturated fat 2.9 g
- Carbohydrates 7.5 g
- Fiber 2.8 g
- Protein 5.2 g

221. POTATO CARROT SALAD

PREPARATION	COOKING	SERVES
15 MIN	10 MIN	1

INGREDIENTS

- Water
- One potato, sliced into cubes
- 1/2 carrots, cut into cubes
- 1/6 tablespoon milk
- 1/6 tablespoon Dijon mustard
- 1/24 cup mayonnaise
- Pepper to taste
- 1/3 teaspoons fresh thyme, chopped
- 1/6 stalk celery, chopped
- 1/6 scallions, chopped
- 1/6 slice turkey bacon, cooked crispy and crumbled

DIRECTIONS

1. Fill your pot with water.
2. Place it over medium-high heat.
3. Boil the potatoes and carrots for 10 to 12 minutes or until tender.
4. Drain and let cool.
5. In a bowl, mix the milk mustard, mayo, pepper, and thyme.
6. Stir in the potatoes, carrots, and celery.
7. Coat evenly with the sauce.
8. Cover and refrigerate for 4 hours.
9. Top with the scallions and turkey bacon bits before serving.

NUTRITIONS

- *Calories 106*
- *Fat 5.3 g*
- *Saturated fat 1 g*
- *Carbohydrates 12.6 g*
- *Fiber 1.8g*
- *Protein 2 g*

222. MARINATED VEGGIE SALAD

PREPARATION	COOKING	SERVES
4 H 30 MIN	3 MIN	1

INGREDIENTS

- One zucchini, sliced
- Four tomatoes, sliced into wedges
- ¼ cup red onion, sliced thinly
- One green bell pepper, sliced
- Two tablespoons fresh parsley, chopped
- Two tablespoons red-wine vinegar
- Two tablespoons olive oil
- One clove garlic, minced
- One teaspoon dried basil
- Two tablespoons water
- Pine nuts, toasted and chopped

DIRECTIONS

1. In a bowl, combine the zucchini, tomatoes, red onion, green bell pepper, and parsley.
2. Pour the vinegar and oil into a glass jar with a lid.
3. Add the garlic, basil, and water.
4. Seal the jar and stir well to combine.
5. Pour the dressing into the vegetable mixture.
6. Cover the bowl.
7. Marinate in the refrigerator for 4 hours.
8. Garnish with the pine nuts before serving.

NUTRITIONS

- Calories 65
- Fat 4.7 g
- Saturated fat 0.7 g
- Carbohydrates 5.3 g
- Fiber 1.2 g
- Protein 0.9 g

223. MEDITERRANEAN SALAD

PREPARATION	COOKING	SERVES
20 MIN	5 MIN	1

INGREDIENTS

- One teaspoon balsamic vinegar
- 1/2 tablespoon basil pesto
- 1/2 cup lettuce
- 1/8 cup broccoli florets, chopped
- 1/8 cup zucchini, chopped
- 1/8 cup tomato, chopped
- 1/8 cup yellow bell pepper, chopped
- 1/2 tablespoons feta cheese, crumbled

DIRECTIONS

1. Arrange the lettuce on a serving platter.
2. Top with the broccoli, zucchini, tomato, and bell pepper.
3. In a bowl, mix the vinegar and pesto.
4. Drizzle the dressing on top.
5. Sprinkle the feta cheese and serve.

NUTRITIONS

- *Calories 100*
- *Fat 6 g*
- *Saturated fat 1 g*
- *Carbohydrates 7 g*
- *Protein 4 g*

224. POTATO TUNA SALAD

PREPARATION	COOKING	SERVES
4H 20 MIN	10 MIN	1

INGREDIENTS

- One potato, peeled and sliced into cubes
- 1/12 cup plain yogurt
- 1/12 cup mayonnaise
- 1/6 clove garlic, crushed and minced
- 1/6 tablespoon almond milk
- 1/6 tablespoon fresh dill, chopped
- ½ teaspoon lemon zest
- Salt to taste
- 1 cup cucumber, chopped
- ¼ cup scallions, chopped
- ¼ cup radishes, chopped
- 9 oz. canned tuna flakes
- 1/2 hard-boiled eggs, chopped
- One cups lettuce, chopped

DIRECTIONS

1. Fill your pot with water.
2. Add the potatoes and boil.
3. Cook for 15 minutes or till slightly tender.
4. Drain and let cool.
5. In a bowl, mix the yogurt, mayo, garlic, almond milk, fresh dill, lemon zest, and salt.
6. Stir in the potatoes, tuna flakes, and eggs.
7. Mix well.
8. Chill in the refrigerator for 4 hours.
9. Stir in the shredded lettuce before serving.

NUTRITIONS

- Calories 243
- Fat 9.9 g
- Saturated fat 2 g
- Carbohydrates 22.2 g
- Fiber 4.6 g
- Protein 17.5 g

225. JICAMA AND SPINACH SALAD

PREPARATION	COOKING	SERVES
10 MIN	20 MIN	1

INGREDIENTS

- 2 oz baby spinach, washed and dried
- Grape or cherry tomatoes, cut in half
- 1/2 jicama, washed, peeled, and cut in strips
- Green or Kalamata olives, chopped
- 2 tbsp walnuts, chopped
- 1/2 tsp raw or roasted sunflower seeds
- Maple Mustard Dressing
- 1/2 heaping tbsp Dijon mustard
- Dash cayenne pepper
- 1 tbsp maple syrup
- One garlic clove, minced
- 1 to 2 tbsp water
- ¼ tsp sea salt

DIRECTIONS

1. Divide the baby spinach onto four salad plates. Top each serving with ¼ of the jicama, ¼ of the chopped olives, and four tomatoes. Sprinkle 1 tsp of the sunflower seeds and 2 tsp of the walnuts.
2. In a small mixing bowl, whisk all the ingredients together until emulsified. Check the taste and add more maple syrup for sweetness.
3. Drizzle 1½ tbsp of the dressing over each salad and serve.

NUTRITIONS

- *Calories: 196*
- *Fat: 2 g*
- *Protein: 7 g*
- *Carbs: 28 g*
- *Fiber: 12g*

226. HIGH PROTEIN SALAD

PREPARATION	COOKING	SERVES
5 MIN	5 MIN	1

INGREDIENTS

Salad:
- One 15-oz can green kidney beans
- 1 4 tbsp capers
- 1 4 handfuls arugula
- 1 15-oz can lentils

Dressing:
- 1 1 tbsp caper brine
- 1 1 tbsp tamari
- 1 1 tbsp balsamic vinegar
- 2 2 tbsp peanut butter
- 2 2 tbsp hot sauce

- 2 1 tbsp tahini

DIRECTIONS

For the dressing:
1. In a bowl, stir all the ingredients until they come together to form a smooth dressing.

For the salad:
2. Mix the beans, arugula, capers, and lentils. Top with the dressing and serve.

NUTRITIONS

- Calories: 205
- Fat: 2 g
- Protein: 13 g
- Carbs: 31 g
- Fiber: 17g

227. RICE AND VEGGIE BOWL

PREPARATION	COOKING	SERVES
5 MIN	15 MIN	1

INGREDIENTS

- 1/3 tbsp coconut oil
- 1/2 tsp ground cumin
- 1/2 tsp ground turmeric
- 1/3 tsp chili powder
- One red bell pepper, chopped
- 1/2 tbsp tomato paste
- One bunch of broccolis, cut into bite-sized florets with short stems
- 1/2 tsp salt, to taste
- One large red onion, sliced
- 1/2 garlic cloves, minced
- 1/2 head of cauliflower, sliced into bite-sized florets
- 1/2 cups cooked rice
- Newly ground black pepper to taste

DIRECTIONS

1. Start with warming up the coconut oil over medium-high heat.
2. Stir in the turmeric, cumin, chili powder, salt, and tomato paste.
3. Cook the content for 1 minute. Stir repeatedly until the spices are fragrant.
4. Add the garlic and onion. Fry for 2 to 3 minutes until the onions are softened.
5. Add the broccoli, cauliflower, and bell pepper. Cover then cook for 3 to 4 minutes and stir occasionally.
6. Add the cooked rice. Stir so it will combine well with the vegetables—Cook for 2 to 3 minutes. Stir until the rice is warm.
7. Check the seasoning and change to taste if desired.
8. Lessen the heat and cook on low for 2 to 3 more minutes so the flavors will meld.
9. Serve with freshly ground black pepper.

NUTRITIONS

- Calories: 260
- Fat: 9 g
- Protein: 9 g
- Carbs: 36 g
- Fiber: 5g

228. SQUASH BLACK BEAN BOWL

PREPARATION	COOKING	SERVES
5 MIN	30 MIN	1

INGREDIENTS

- One large spaghetti squash, halved,
- 1/3 cup water (or 2 tbsp olive oil, rubbed on the inside of squash)
- Black bean filling
- 1/2 15-oz can of black beans, emptied and rinsed
- 1/2 cup fire-roasted corn (or frozen sweet corn)
- 1/2 cup thinly sliced red cabbage
- 1/2 tbsp chopped green onion, green and white parts
- ¼ cup chopped fresh cilantro
- ½ lime, juiced or to taste
- Pepper and salt, to taste
- Avocado mash:
- One ripe avocado, mashed
- ½ lime, juiced or to Vtaste
- ¼ tsp cumin
- Pepper and pinch of sea salt

DIRECTIONS

1. Preheat the oven to 400°F.
2. Chop the squash in part and scoop out the seeds with a spoon, like a pumpkin.
3. Fill the roasting pan with 1/3 cup of water. Lay the squash, cut side down, in the pan. Bake for 30 minutes until soft and tender.
4. While this is baking, mix all the ingredients for the black bean filling in a medium-sized bowl.
5. In a small dish, crush the avocado and blend in the ingredients for the avocado mash.
6. Eliminate the squash from the oven and let it cool for 5 minutes. Scrape the squash with a fork so that it looks like spaghetti noodles. Then, fill it with black bean filling and top with avocado mash.
7. Serve and enjoy.

NUTRITIONS

- Calories: 85
- Fat: 0.5 g
- Protein: 4 g
- Carbs: 6 g
- Fiber: 4g

229. PEA SALAD

PREPARATION	COOKING	SERVES
40 MIN	0 MIN	1

INGREDIENTS

- 1/2 cup chickpeas, rinsed and drained
- 1/2 cups peas, divided
- Salt to taste
- One tablespoon olive oil
- ½ cup buttermilk
- Pepper to taste
- 2 cups pea greens
- 1/2 carrots shaved
- 1/4 cup snow peas, trimmed

DIRECTIONS

1. Add the chickpeas and half of the peas to your food processor.
2. Season with the salt.
3. Pulse until smooth. Set aside.
4. In a bowl, toss the remaining peas in oil, milk, salt, and pepper.
5. Transfer the mixture to your food processor.
6. Process until pureed.
7. Transfer this mixture to a bowl.
8. Arrange the pea greens on a serving plate.
9. Top with the shaved carrots and snow peas.
10. Stir in the pea and milk dressing.
11. Serve with the reserved chickpea hummus.

NUTRITIONS

- Calories 214
- Fat 8.6 g
- Saturated fat 1.5 g
- Carbohydrates 27.3 g
- Fiber 8.4 g
- Protein 8 g

230. SNAP PEA SALAD

PREPARATION	COOKING	SERVES
1 HOUR	0 MIN	1

INGREDIENTS

- 1/2 tablespoons mayonnaise
- ¾ teaspoon celery seed
- ¼ cup cider vinegar
- 1/2 teaspoon yellow mustard
- 1/2 tablespoon sugar
- Salt and pepper to taste
- 1 oz. radishes, sliced thinly
- 2 oz. sugar snap peas, sliced thinly

DIRECTIONS

1. In a bowl, combine the mayonnaise, celery seeds, vinegar, mustard, sugar, salt, and pepper.
2. Stir in the radishes and snap peas.
3. Refrigerate for 30 minutes.

NUTRITIONS

- *Calories 69*
- *Fat 3.7 g*
- *Saturated fat 0.6 g*
- *Carbohydrates 7.1 g*
- *Fiber 1.8 g*
- *Protein 2 g*

231. CUCUMBER TOMATO CHOPPED SALAD

PREPARATION	COOKING	SERVES
15 MIN	0 MIN	1

INGREDIENTS

- 1/4 cup light mayonnaise
- 1/2 tablespoon lemon juice
- 1/2 tablespoon fresh dill, chopped
- 1/2 tablespoon chive, chopped
- 1/4 cup feta cheese, crumbled
- Salt and pepper to taste
- 1/2 red onion, chopped
- 1/2 cucumber, diced
- 1/2 radish, diced
- One tomato, diced
- Chives, chopped

DIRECTIONS

1. Combine the mayo, lemon juice, fresh dill, chives, feta cheese, salt, and pepper in a bowl.
2. Mix well.
3. Stir in the onion, cucumber, radish, and tomatoes.
4. Coat evenly.
5. Garnish with the chopped chives.

NUTRITIONS

- Calories 187
- Fat 16.7 g
- Saturated fat 4.1 g
- Carbohydrates 6.7 g
- Fiber 2 g
- Protein 3.3 g

232. ZUCCHINI PASTA SALAD

PREPARATION	COOKING	SERVES
4 MIN	0 MIN	1

INGREDIENTS

- One tablespoon olive oil
- 1/2 teaspoons Dijon mustard
- 1/3 tablespoons red-wine vinegar
- 1/2 clove garlic, grated
- Two tablespoons fresh oregano, chopped
- 1/2 shallot, chopped
- ¼ teaspoon red pepper flakes
- 4 oz. zucchini noodles
- ¼ cup Kalamata olives pitted
- 1 cups cherry tomato, sliced in half
- ¾ cup Parmesan cheese shaved

DIRECTIONS

1. Mix the olive oil, Dijon mustard, red wine vinegar, garlic, oregano, shallot, and red pepper flakes in a bowl.
2. Stir in the zucchini noodles.
3. Sprinkle on top the olives, tomatoes, and Parmesan cheese.

NUTRITIONS

- Calories 299
- Fat 24.7 g
- Saturated fat 5.1 g
- Carbohydrates 11.6 g
- Fiber 2.8 g
- Protein 7 g

233. EGG AVOCADO SALAD

PREPARATION	COOKING	SERVES
10 MIN	0 MIN	1

INGREDIENTS

- 1/2 avocado
- One hard-boiled egg, peeled and chopped
- 1/4 tablespoon mayonnaise
- 1/4 tablespoons freshly squeezed lemon juice
- ¼ cup celery, chopped
- 1/2 tablespoons chives, chopped
- Salt and pepper to taste

DIRECTIONS

1. Add the avocado to a large bowl.
2. Mash the avocado using a fork.
3. Stir in the egg and mash the eggs.
4. Add the mayo, lemon juice, celery, chives, salt, and pepper.
5. Chill in the refrigerator for at least 2o to 30 minutes before serving

NUTRITIONS

- Calories 224
- Fat 18 g
- Saturated fat 3.9 g
- Carbohydrates 6.1 g
- Fiber 3.6 g
- Protein 10.6 g

234. TRIPLE CHOCOLATE CHIP DEEP DISH COOKIES

PREPARATION	COOKING	SERVES
10 MIN	30 MIN	1

INGREDIENTS

- pumpkin (3/4 cup, canned)
- peanut butter (3/4 cup, chocolate)
- chocolate protein (1/2 cup, powdered)
- honey (1/4 cup)
- egg (1, beaten)
- vanilla (1 tsp, pure)
- baking soda (1/2 tsp)
- chocolate chips (1/2 cup, sugar-free)
- Vanilla ice cream (or serving)

DIRECTIONS

1. Add all the ingredients except ice cream and chocolate chips in a bowl
2. Use a mixer (electric) beat until mixed evenly.
3. Heat your oven to 350 degrees Fahrenheit.
4. Gradually add the chocolate chips and gently fold to incorporate.
5. Pour batter into a skillet (medium).
6. Place skillet into a preheated oven to bake for approximately 20 minutes until golden brown.
7. Remove from heat and set aside for roughly 7-10 minutes.
8. Serve using the vanilla ice cream.

NUTRITIONS

- Calories: 502
- Protein: 6 g
- Carbohydrates: 65 g
- Fats: 24 g

235. PROTEIN PUMPKIN SPICED DONUTS

PREPARATION	COOKING	SERVES
10 MIN	15 MIN	1

INGREDIENTS

- oat flour (1 cup)
- xylitol (3/4 cup)
- vanilla protein (1 scoop, powdered)
- flaxseed (1 tbsp, ground)
- cinnamon (1 tbsp, ground)
- baking powder (2 tsp)
- sea salt (1 tsp)
- eggs (3, beaten)
- pumpkin (1/2 cup, canned)
- coconut oil (1 tbsp, melted)
- vanilla (2 tsp, pure)
- apple cider vinegar (1 tsp)
- Ingredients for the frosting:
- cream cheese (1/2 cup, whipped)
- liquid stevia (1/2 tsp)

DIRECTIONS

1. Place the xylitol, oat flour, ground flaxseed, powdered protein, baking powder, ground cinnamon, and a dash of sea salt in a large bowl. Preheat your oven to 350 degrees Fahrenheit.
2. Add the egg (beaten) into another bowl (large) along with the pumpkin (canned), pure vanilla and vinegar and coconut oil (melted),
3. Whisk until mixed (evenly), then pour the mixture into the flour. Stir until thoroughly mixed.
4. Use cooking spray grease a large donut pan.
5. Pour batter into the donut pan (greased).
6. Place batter into the oven and bake for approximately 10 minutes until thoroughly baked.
7. Remove from heat and set donuts onto a wire rack to cool.
8. Add in the cream cheese (whipped) and liquid stevia in a small bowl, whisk until it becomes smooth.
9. Frost donuts using the frosting and serve with a sprinkle of cinnamon (ground) over the top.

NUTRITIONS

- *Calories: 452*
- *Protein: 4.9 g*
- *Carbohydrates: 51 g*
- *Fats: 25 g*

236. HIGH PROTEIN CHIPOTLE CHEDDAR QUESADILLA

PREPARATION	COOKING	SERVES
15 MIN	45 MIN	1

INGREDIENTS

- tortillas (1, low carb)
- cottage cheese (1/2 cups, low sodium)
- cheddar cheese (1/2 cups, low fat, shredded)
- bell pepper (1/4, red, thinly sliced)
- onion (1/4, thinly sliced)
- Portobello mushrooms (1/4 cup, thinly sliced)
- chipotle seasoning (1 tbsp)
- Mild salsa (for dipping)

DIRECTIONS

1. Add the bell pepper (sliced, red), onion (sliced), and mushrooms (sliced) into a large grill pan over medium heat.
2. Cook for approximately 10 minutes until soft. Remove then transfer into a bowl (medium). Set aside.
3. Add the chipotle seasoning and cottage cheese in a small bowl. Stir well to incorporate.
4. Place tortillas onto the grill pan and pour vegetable mixture over tortillas.
5. Sprinkle cottage cheese mixture over the top then top off using the cheddar cheese (shredded).
6. Place an additional tortilla over the top of the filling.
7. Cook for roughly 2 minutes, then flip and continue cooking for the next minute.
8. Repeat process with remaining tortillas and filling. 9. Serve immediately with the salsa (mild).

NUTRITIONS

- Calories: 293
- Protein: 15 g
- Carbohydrates: 24 g
- Fats: 15 g

237. SWEET POTATO CASSEROLE

PREPARATION	COOKING	SERVES
5 MIN	15 MIN	1

INGREDIENTS

- potatoes (1/2 lbs., sweet, peeled, chopped)
- Greek yogurt (1/3 cup, nonfat)
- cinnamon (1/2 tbsp, ground)
- nutmeg (1/8 tsp, ground)
- sea salt (1/4 tsp)
- egg whites (1 tbsp)
- butter (1/4 tbsp, melted)
- pecans (1/2 cup, chopped)
- marshmallows (1/2 cup, miniature)
- sugar (dash, light brown, for sprinkling)

DIRECTIONS

1. Heat your oven to 375 degrees Fahrenheit.
2. Place the potatoes (sweet) into a saucepan (large) over medium-high heat.
3. Cover potatoes using water, then bring to a boil, boil for approximately 30 minutes until soft.
4. Drain potatoes, then place potatoes back into the saucepan.
5. Add the Greek yogurt, cinnamon (ground), nutmeg (ground), and sea salt (dash) into the potatoes.
6. Stir well until coated (evenly).
7. Add in the butter (melted) and egg whites then bring to a stir once more.
8. Transfer potato mixture into a casserole dish (large).
9. Place into the oven then bakes for approximately 30 minutes. Remove from heat then top with the pecans (chopped) and miniature marshmallows.
10. Place back into the oven to bake for an additional 10 minutes until marshmallows are browned.

NUTRITIONS

- *Calories: 86*
- *Protein: 1.6 g*
- *Carbohydrates: 20 g*
- *Fats: 0.1 g*

238. BAKED CHEESY EGGPLANT

PREPARATION	COOKING	SERVES
15 MIN	60 MIN	1

INGREDIENTS

- eggplant (1, fresh)
- tomato (1, 2 can be chopped)
- tomato sauce (1, 2 oz can)
- cheddar cheese (2 oz, shredded)
- onion (1, chopped)
- oregano (dash, dried)
- salt (2 tsp)
- Italian seasoning (dash)
- basil (dried, for taste)
- thyme (dried, for flavor)
- garlic (2-3 tsp, powdered)
- black pepper (1/2 tsp)

DIRECTIONS

1. Slice eggplant (fresh) into thin slices then season using a dash of salt.
2. Next, set aside in a colander for roughly 30 minutes then pat dry using a few paper towels.
3. Rinse under warm running water and thoroughly slice eggplant into quarters.
4. Place a layer of the eggplant (quartered) into a baking dish (large).
5. Cover layer using the tomatoes (chopped) and tomato sauce (1 can).
6. Add ½ of the cheese over the top and repeat layers with the remaining cheese (shredded).
7. Place eggplant into the oven to bake for approximately 45 minutes at 350 degrees Fahrenheit until eggplant is soft.

NUTRITIONS

- *Calories: 336*
- *Protein: 34 g*
- *Carbohydrates: 8.29 g*
- *Fats: 13 g*

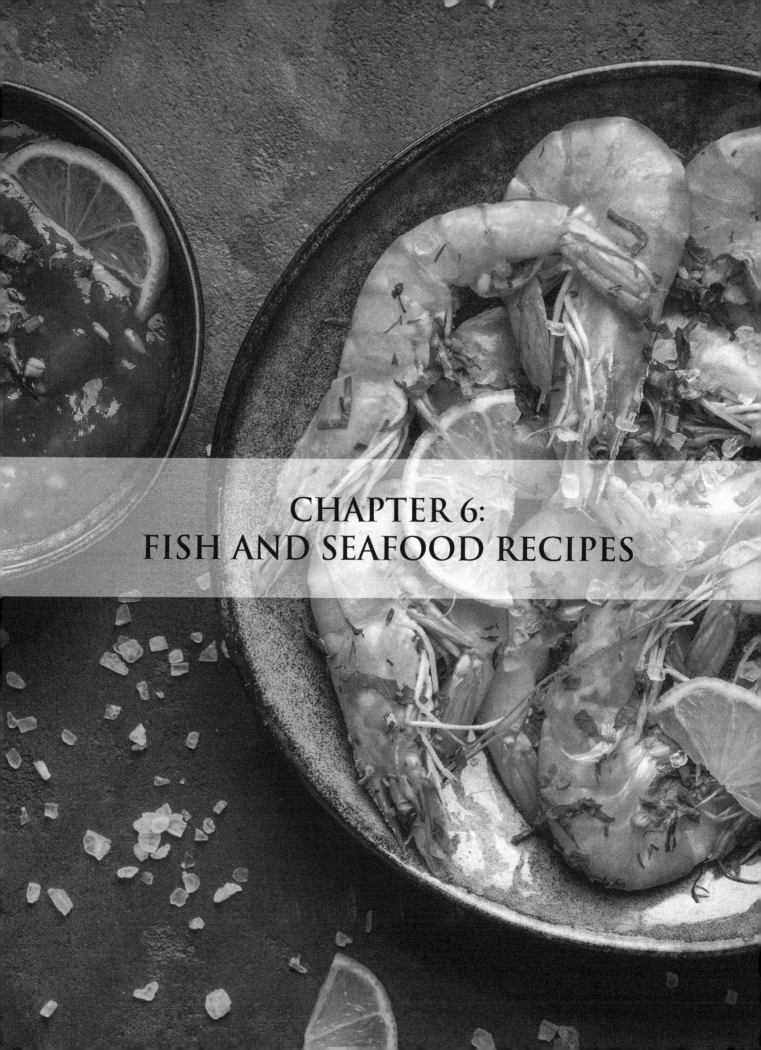

CHAPTER 6:
FISH AND SEAFOOD RECIPES

239. ROASTED TROUT STUFFED WITH VEGGIES

PREPARATION	COOKING	SERVES
10 MIN	25 MIN	2

INGREDIENTS

- 2 (8-ounce) whole trout fillets
- 1 tablespoon extra-virgin olive oil
- ¼ teaspoon salt
- 1/8 teaspoon black pepper
- 1 small onion, thinly sliced
- ½ red bell pepper
- 1 poblano pepper
- 2 or 3 shiitake mushrooms, sliced
- 1 lemon, sliced

DIRECTIONS

1. Set oven to 425°F (220°C). Coat baking sheet with nonstick cooking spray.
2. Rub both trout fillets, inside and out, with the olive oil. Season with salt and pepper.
3. Mix together the onion, bell pepper, poblano pepper, and mushrooms in a large bowl. Stuff half of this mix into the cavity of each fillet. Top the mixture with 2 or 3 lemon slices inside each fillet.
4. Place the fish on the prepared baking sheet side by side. Roast in the preheated oven for 25 minutes
5. Pullout from the oven and serve on a plate.

NUTRITIONS

- *Calories 453,*
- *22g fat,*
- *49g protein*

240. LEMONY TROUT WITH CARAMELIZED SHALLOTS

PREPARATION	COOKING	SERVES
10 MIN	20 MIN	2

INGREDIENTS

Shallots:
- 1 teaspoon almond butter
- 2 shallots, thinly sliced
- Dash salt

Trout:
- 1 tablespoon almond butter
- 2 (4-ounce / 113-g) trout fillets
- 3 tablespoons capers
- ¼ cup freshly squeezed lemon juice
- ¼ teaspoon salt
- Dash freshly ground black pepper
- 1 lemon, thinly sliced

DIRECTIONS

For Shallots
1. Situate skillet over medium heat, cook the butter, shallots, and salt for 20 minutes, stirring every 5 minutes.

For Trout
2. Meanwhile, in another large skillet over medium heat, heat 1 teaspoon of almond butter.
3. Add the trout fillets and cook each side for 3 minutes, or until flaky. Transfer to a plate and set aside.
4. In the skillet used for the trout, stir in the capers, lemon juice, salt, and pepper, then bring to a simmer. Whisk in the remaining 1 tablespoon of almond butter. Spoon the sauce over the fish.
5. Garnish the fish with the lemon slices and caramelized shallots before serving.

NUTRITIONS

- Calories 344,
- 18g fat,
- 21g protein

241. EASY TOMATO TUNA MELTS

PREPARATION	COOKING	SERVES
5 MIN	4 MIN	2

INGREDIENTS

- 1 (5-oz) can chunk light tuna packed in water
- 2 tablespoons plain Greek yogurt
- 2 tablespoons finely chopped celery
- 1 tablespoon finely chopped red onion
- 2 teaspoons freshly squeezed lemon juice
- 1 large tomato, cut into ¾-inch-thick rounds
- ½ cup shredded Cheddar cheese

DIRECTIONS

1. Preheat the broiler to High.
2. Stir together the tuna, yogurt, celery, red onion, lemon juice, and cayenne pepper in a medium bowl.
3. Place the tomato rounds on a baking sheet. Top each with some tuna salad and Cheddar cheese.
4. Broil for 3 to 4 minutes until the cheese is melted and bubbly. Cool for 5 minutes before serving.

NUTRITIONS

- *Calories 244,*
- *10g fat,*
- *30g protein*

242. MACKEREL AND GREEN BEAN SALAD

PREPARATION	COOKING	SERVES
10 MIN	10 MIN	2

INGREDIENTS

- 2 cups green beans
- 1 tablespoon avocado oil
- 2 mackerel fillets
- 4 cups mixed salad greens
- 2 hard-boiled eggs, sliced
- 1 avocado, sliced
- 2 tablespoons lemon juice
- 2 tablespoons olive oil
- 1 teaspoon Dijon mustard
- Salt and black pepper, to taste

DIRECTIONS

1. Cook the green beans in pot of boiling water for about 3 minutes. Drain and set aside.
2. Melt the avocado oil in a pan over medium heat. Add the mackerel fillets and cook each side for 4 minutes.
3. Divide the greens between two salad bowls. Top with the mackerel, sliced egg, and avocado slices.
4. Scourge lemon juice, olive oil, mustard, salt, and pepper, and drizzle over the salad. Add the cooked green beans and toss to combine, then serve.

NUTRITIONS

- *Calories 737,*
- *57g fat,*
- *34g protein*

243. HAZELNUT CRUSTED SEA BASS

PREPARATION	COOKING	SERVES
10 MIN	15 MIN	2

INGREDIENTS

- 2 tablespoons almond butter
- 2 sea bass fillets
- 1/3 cup roasted hazelnuts
- A pinch of cayenne pepper

DIRECTIONS

1. Ready oven to 425°F (220°C). Line a baking dish with waxed paper.
2. Brush the almond butter over the fillets.
3. Pulse the hazelnuts and cayenne in a food processor. Coat the sea bass with the hazelnut mixture, then transfer to the baking dish.
4. Bake in the preheated oven for about 15 minutes. Cool for 5 minutes before serving.

NUTRITIONS

- Calories 468,
- 31g fat,
- 40g protein

244. SHRIMP AND PEA PAELLA

PREPARATION	COOKING	SERVES
20 MIN	60 MIN	2

INGREDIENTS

- 2 tablespoons olive oil
- 1 garlic clove, minced
- ½ large onion, minced
- 1 cup diced tomato
- ½ cup short-grain rice
- ½ teaspoon sweet paprika
- ½ cup dry white wine
- 1¼ cups low-sodium chicken stock
- 8 ounces (227 g) large raw shrimp
- 1 cup frozen peas
- ¼ cup jarred roasted red peppers

DIRECTIONS

1. Heat the olive oil in a large skillet over medium-high heat.
2. Add the garlic and onion and sauté for 3 minutes, or until the onion is softened.
3. Add the tomato, rice, and paprika and stir for 3 minutes to toast the rice.
4. Add the wine and chicken stock and stir to combine. Bring the mixture to a boil.
5. Cover and set heat to medium-low, and simmer for 45 minutes
6. Add the shrimp, peas, and roasted red peppers. Cover and cook for an additional 5 minutes. Season with salt to taste and serve.

NUTRITIONS

Calories 646,
7g fat,

- 42g protein

245. GARLIC SHRIMP WITH ARUGULA PESTO

PREPARATION	COOKING	SERVES
20 MIN	5 MIN	2

INGREDIENTS

- 3 cups lightly packed arugula
- ½ cup lightly packed basil leaves
- ¼ cup walnuts
- 3 tablespoons olive oil
- 3 medium garlic cloves
- 2 tablespoons grated Parmesan cheese
- 1 tablespoon freshly squeezed lemon juice
- 1 (10-ounce) package zucchini noodles
- 8 ounces (227 g) cooked, shelled shrimp
- 2 Roma tomatoes, diced

DIRECTIONS

1. Process the arugula, basil, walnuts, olive oil, garlic, Parmesan cheese, and lemon juice in a food processor until smooth, scraping down the sides as needed. Season
2. Heat a skillet over medium heat. Add the pesto, zucchini noodles, and cooked shrimp. Toss to combine the sauce over the noodles and shrimp, and cook until heated through.
3. Season well. Serve topped with the diced tomatoes.

NUTRITIONS

- Calories 435,
- 30.2g fat,
- 33g protein

246. BAKED OYSTERS WITH VEGETABLES

PREPARATION	COOKING	SERVES
30 MIN	17 MIN	2

INGREDIENTS

- 2 cups coarse salt, for holding the oysters
- 1 dozen fresh oysters, scrubbed
- 1 tablespoon almond butter
- ¼ cup finely chopped scallions
- ½ cup finely chopped artichoke hearts
- ¼ cup finely chopped red bell pepper
- 1 garlic clove, minced
- 1 tablespoon finely chopped fresh parsley
- Zest and juice of ½ lemon

DIRECTIONS

1. Pour the salt into a baking dish and spread to fill the bottom of the dish evenly.
2. Using a shucking knife, insert the blade at the joint of the shell, where it hinges open and shut. Firmly apply pressure to pop the blade in, and work the knife around the shell to open. Discard the empty half of the shell. Using the knife, gently loosen the oyster, and remove any shell particles. Sprinkle salt in the oysters
3. Set oven to 425°F (220°C).
4. Heat the almond butter in a large skillet over medium heat. Add the scallions, artichoke hearts, and bell pepper, and cook for 5 to 7 minutes. Cook garlic
5. Takeout from the heat and stir in the parsley, lemon zest and juice, and season to taste with salt and pepper.
6. Divide the vegetable mixture evenly among the oysters. Bake in the preheated oven for 10 to 12 minutes.

NUTRITIONS

- *Calories 135,*
- *7g fat,*

- *6g protein*

247. CREAMY FISH GRATIN

PREPARATION	COOKING	SERVES
10 MIN	55 MIN	6

INGREDIENTS

- 1 c. heavy cream
- 2 cubed salmon fillets
- 2 cod fillets, cubed
- 2 sea bass fillets, cubed
- 1 celery stalk, sliced
- Salt and pepper
- ½ c. grated Parmesan
- ½ c. crumbled feta cheese

DIRECTIONS

1. Combine the cream with the fish fillets and celery in a deep-dish baking pan.
2. Add salt and pepper to taste then top with the Parmesan and feta cheese.
3. Cook in the preheated oven at 350 F/176 C for 20 minutes.
4. Serve the gratin and enjoy it.

NUTRITIONS

- Calories 301,
- Fat 16.1 g,
- Sat. fat 5 g,
- Fiber 0.2 g,
- Carbs 1.3 g,
- Sugar 0 g,
- Protein 36.9 g,
- Sodium 211 mg

248. MIXED SEAFOOD DISH

PREPARATION	COOKING	SERVES
10 MIN	35 MIN	4

INGREDIENTS

- 12 scrubbed clams, cleaned
- 3 chopped dried chilies, soaked and drained
- 1 lobster, tail separated and halved
- 1 c. water
- ¼ c. flour
- 3 tbsps. olive oil
- 1 ½ lbs. or 700 g. skinless monkfish, boneless and thinly sliced into fillets
- Salt and black pepper
- 35 unpeeled shrimp

- 1 chopped onion
- 4 minced garlic cloves
- 4 grated tomatoes
- 1 baguette slice, toasted
- 30 skinned hazelnuts
- 2 tbsps. chopped parsley
- 1 c. fish stock
- ¼ tsp. smoked paprika
- Lemon wedges
- Crusty bread slices

DIRECTIONS

1. Put the water in a large saucepan, bring to a boil over high heat
2. Add clams, cover and cook for 4 minutes. Take away from heat and discard unopened ones.
3. Heat a skillet with olive oil over medium-high heat.
4. Meantime, put flour on a medium bowl and dredge in fish.
5. Season with salt and pepper.
6. Place fish into the skillet and cook for 3 minutes on each side, after transfer to a plate
7. Add shrimps to the same skillet and cook for about 2 minutes on each side, transfer to a plate.
8. Reduce heat to medium-low, add garlic to the same pan, stir, cook for 1 minute and transfer to a blender.
9. Add onion to the skillet and stir for 3 minutes.
10. Add tomatoes, stir and cook on a low heat for 7 minutes.

NUTRITIONS

- Calories 344,
- 18g fat,

- 21g protein

249. GARLIC SHRIMP WITH OLIVE OIL

PREPARATION	COOKING	SERVES
4 MIN	10 MIN	5

INGREDIENTS

- 1 cup extra-virgin oil
- 4 garlic cloves, minced
- 6 whole dried red chilies
- ¼ cup minced flat-leaf parsley
- 2 pounds shelled and deveined medium shrimp
- Pinch of salt
- Crusty bread, for serving (optional)

DIRECTIONS

1. Warmth olive oil in a large deep skillet until shimmering.
2. Then, add the garlic, chilies, and parsley and cook over moderately high heat for 10 seconds, stirring.
3. Add on the shrimp and cook over high heat, stirring once, until they are pink and curled 3 to 4 minutes.
4. Season with salt and pepper to taste. Transfer to small bowls.
5. Serve with crusty bread. Enjoy!

NUTRITIONS

- Calories:175,
- Fat:2.2g,
- Protein:32g,
- Carbohydrate:8.3g,
- Cholesterol:80mg

250. STEAMED MUSSELS IN TOMATO GARLIC

PREPARATION	COOKING	SERVES
5 MIN	23 MIN	4

INGREDIENTS

- ¼ cup olive oil
- 1 medium-size onion, finely chopped
- 6 cloves garlic, minced
- 3 tablespoons fresh scallions, chopped
- 2 cups canned tomatoes, chopped
- ¼ teaspoon dried thyme
- ¼ teaspoon dried red-pepper flakes
- 4 pounds' mussels, cleaned
- 1/8 teaspoon freshly ground black pepper
- Pinch of salt to taste
- Crusty bread (optional)

DIRECTIONS

1. Prepare a large pot, then heat the oil over moderately low heat.
2. Then put the onion and garlic then cook, stirring occasionally, until the onion is translucent, about 5 minutes.
3. Stir in the scallions, tomatoes, thyme, and red pepper flakes.
4. Reduce the heat and simmer, partially covered, for 15 minutes, stirring occasionally.
5. Add the mussels to the pot. Cover; bring to a boil.
6. Cook, and stir the pot occasionally, just until the mussels open, about 3 minutes. Remove the open mussels.
7. Continue to boil, uncovering the pot as necessary to remove the mussels as soon as their shells open. Discard any that do not open longer.
8. Stir the black pepper into the broth. Add salt to taste.
9. Ladle the broth over the mussels. Serve with crusty bread. Enjoy!

NUTRITIONS

- *Calories:272,*
- *Fat:5.2g,*
- *Protein:35g,*
- *Carbohydrate:12.7g,*
- *Cholesterol:25mg*

251. MEDITERRANEAN-STYLE MUSSELS

PREPARATION	COOKING	SERVES
5 MIN	21 MIN	2

INGREDIENTS

- 1 medium-size onion, chopped
- 5 cloves garlic, minced
- 1 tablespoon extra-virgin olive oil
- 4 ripe tomatoes, plum
- 1 small size bell pepper
- 1 tablespoon capers, drained
- 1 teaspoon dried oregano
- 500g mussels, cleaned

DIRECTIONS

1. Warm oil in a large, wide saucepan with medium heat.
2. Add onion plus garlic. Stirring frequently, cook for 3 min.
3. Temporarily, coarsely chop tomatoes and pepper. Add to the onion along with capers. Sprinkling with seasonings.
4. Stir frequently up until tomatoes start to break down, 5 to 7 min.
5. In the meantime, scrub mussels and pull off beards. Discard any that are open. Stir into a thickened tomato mixture.
6. Cover then cook up until majority of the mussels open, about 6 min. Stir midway through cooking.
7. Remove any mussels that are not open after 6 min. Palate and add salt if desirable.
8. Serve in bowls plus crusty bread. Enjoy!

NUTRITIONS

- Calories:212,
- Fat:8.3g,
- Protein:18.2g,
- Carbohydrate:11.7g,
- Cholesterol:35mg

252. LEEKS AND CALAMARI MIX

PREPARATION	COOKING	SERVES
5 MIN	15 MIN	4

INGREDIENTS

- 2 tablespoons avocado oil
- 2 leeks, chopped
- 1 red onion, chopped
- Salt and black to the taste
- 1-pound calamari rings
- 1 tablespoon parsley, chopped
- 1 tablespoon chives, chopped
- 2 tablespoons tomato paste

DIRECTIONS

1. Heat a pan with the avocado oil over medium heat, add the leeks and the onion, stir and sauté for 5 minutes.
2. Add the rest of the ingredients, toss, simmer over medium heat for 10 minutes, divide into bowls and serve.

NUTRITIONS

- Calories:238,
- Fat:9g,
- Protein:8.4g,
- Carbohydrate:14.4g,
- Cholesterol:95mg

253. SEAFOOD PAELLA

PREPARATION	COOKING	SERVES
5 MIN	35 MIN	4

INGREDIENTS

- 1 tablespoon extra-virgin olive oil
- 4 cloves garlic, minced
- 1 medium-size onion, finely chopped
- 1 red bell pepper, finely chopped
- 300g short or medium grain rice
- ½ teaspoon turmeric
- 1 teaspoon paprika
- 1 14-ounces canned tomatoes, chopped
- 3 cups chicken stock
- 2 pinches of saffron threads
- 12 large shrimp, peeled and deveined
- 12 little neck mussels, thawed
- Handful fresh parsley, roughly chopped
- Lemon wedges

DIRECTIONS

1. In a deep pan with medium-high heat, add olive oil, garlic, onion, and red bell pepper and cook for 3 minutes or until vegetables softened.
2. Then, add rice, turmeric, and paprika and stir well. Then add tomatoes, chicken stock and saffron, stir and bring to a boil.
3. Lower heat to simmer and cover and cook for another 20 minutes. Spread shrimp, mussels, and green peas on top.
4. Cover then cook for additional 10-15 minutes, until mussels have opened and shrimps are pink.
5. Turn off the heat and sprinkle with parsley on top. Serve with lemon wedges on top. Enjoy!

NUTRITIONS

- Calories:233,
- Fat:5.2g,
- Protein:13g,
- Carbohydrate:33g,
- Cholesterol:18mg

254. BAKED SALMON IN GARLIC PEPPER

PREPARATION	COOKING	SERVES
10 MIN	25 MIN	3

INGREDIENTS

- 4 (6-ounce) salmon fillets
- 4 tablespoons unsalted butter
- 1 tablespoon garlic, minced
- 3 tablespoons capers, drained
- Fresh herbs like parsley, chives or dill
- Salt and Pepper
- Lemon quartered

DIRECTIONS

1. Heat the oven to 325 degrees Fahrenheit. Season each sides of the salmon thru salt and pepper.
2. Thaw the butter in a wide oven-safe skillet over medium heat.
3. When the butter is sparkling, stirring in the garlic plus the capers. Cook, stirring, till warm, about 1 minute.
4. Take away the skillet off of the heat. Put the salmon fillets, skin-side down, to the skillet.
5. Slant the pan so that butter pools on one side then spoon garlic caper butter over each fillet.
6. Cover the frying pan with a sheet of aluminum foil or conceal with parchment paper by lightly tucking it around the salmon.
7. Bake the salmon, enclosed, for 15 minutes. Bare then spoon extra of the butter over the salmon.
8. Remain to roast, open, until your chosen doneness, 5 to 10 minutes more, depending on how thick the salmon is. Tip: We cook salmon until an instant-read thermometer reads 125 degrees Fahrenheit when inserted into the thickest part.
9. On the other hand, finish cooking the salmon with the broiler for some additional color on top. Watch thoroughly so the fish does not burn.
10. Squash fresh lemon juice over the baked salmon, sprinkle with lots of fresh herbs.
11. Serve with additional spoonful of the garlic caper butter on top. Enjoy!

NUTRITIONS

- Calories:294,
- Fat:11.3g,
- Protein:28.2g,
- Carbohydrate:1.7g,
- Cholesterol:85mg

255. SAUTEED OCTOPUS

PREPARATION	COOKING	SERVES
5 MIN	1 H 10 MIN	4

INGREDIENTS

- 2 pounds' whole octopus, cleaned and cooked ahead (see the Directions below)
- 2 tablespoons extra-virgin olive oil
- 2 medium-size green chili
- 2 plum tomatoes, sliced
- ¼ pitted olives
- 2 tablespoons fresh oregano leaves, chopped
- 2 teaspoons cider vinegar

DIRECTIONS

1. How to cook the whole octopus:
2. All frozen octopus is pre-cleaned, and if buying fresh, you can ask the fishmonger to clean it for you.
3. In a large pot, let water to boil and then diminish to a simmer. Put the whole octopus, and simmer for 1 hour.
4. Take away the octopus from boiling water, and let cool at room temperature for 15 minutes.
5. To Sauté: Cut the tentacles from the head, and discard the head. Chop the tentacles into small pieces.
6. Heat a large sauté pan with olive oil over medium heat, add the octopus, green chili, tomatoes, olives, oregano, and vinegar.
7. Sauté for 10 minutes. Serve immediately.

NUTRITIONS

- Calories:274,
- Fat:8.3g,
- Protein:35.2g,
- Carbohydrate:9.8g,
- Cholesterol:75mg

566

256. GRILLED OCTOPUS

PREPARATION	COOKING	SERVES
40 MIN	1 H 15 MIN	4

INGREDIENTS

- 1 pound of fresh octopus (medium or large), cleaned and cook ahead
- 1/3 cup freshly squeezed lemon juice
- ¼ cup lemon zest
- 2 garlic heads, minced
- 2 tablespoon parsley, minced
- ½ teaspoon dried oregano
- 2/3 cup Olive oil
- Salt and Pepper, to taste

DIRECTIONS

1. Arrange octopus in a pot then cover with enough water. Bring to boil for 40 minutes.
2. Remove the octopus from hot water, rinse it then transfer it in a bowl.
3. Drizzle with olive oil plus the chopped garlic. Let it cool for 30 minutes to 1 hour.
4. Preheat a gas grill to medium-high heat. Slice octopus's tentacles.
5. Grill for 3 or 4 minutes each side until charred. Take away from heat then put it in a bowl.
6. Drizzle with olive oil then add lemon juice. Put salt and pepper.
7. Sprinkle some oregano and parsley on top. Add some garlic (optional).
8. Serve and Enjoy!

NUTRITIONS

- Calories:243,
- Fat:6.3g,
- Protein:38.2g,
- Carbohydrate:4g,
- Cholesterol:0mg

257. SCALLOP SALAD

PREPARATION	COOKING	SERVES
15 MIN	35 MIN	6

INGREDIENTS

- 12 ounces dry sea scallops
- 4 tablespoons olive oil + 2 teaspoons
- 4 teaspoons soy sauce
- 1 ½ cup quinoa, rinsed
- 2 teaspoons garlic, minced
- A pinch of salt
- 3 cups water
- 1 cup snow peas, sliced
- 1 teaspoon sesame oil
- 1/3 cup rice vinegar
- 1 cup scallions, sliced
- 1/3 cup red bell pepper, chopped
- ¼ cup cilantro, chopped

DIRECTIONS

1. In a bowl, mix scallops with 2 teaspoons soy sauce, toss and leave aside for now.
2. Warmth a pan with 1 tablespoon olive oil over medium heat, add quinoa, stir and cook for 8 minutes. Add garlic, stir and cook for 1 more minute.
3. Add water and a pinch of salt, bring to a boil, stir, cover and cook for 15 minutes. Add snow peas, cover and leave for 5 more minutes.
4. Meanwhile, in a bowl, mix 3 tablespoons olive oil with 2 teaspoons soy sauce, vinegar and sesame oil and whisk well.
5. Add quinoa and snow peas to mixture and stir again. Add scallions, bell pepper and stir again.
6. Pat dry the scallions and discard marinade. Heat another pan with 2 teaspoons olive oil over medium high heat, add scallions and cook for 1 minute on each side.
7. Add scallops to quinoa salad, stir gently and serve with chopped cilantro on top.

NUTRITIONS

- Calories:201,
- Fat:5g,
- Fiber:2g,
- Carbs:5g,
- Protein:8g

258. COD & GREEN BEAN RISOTTO

PREPARATION	COOKING	SERVES
4 MIN	40 MIN	2

INGREDIENTS

- ½ cup arugula
- One finely diced white onion
- 4 oz. cod fillet
- 1 cup white rice
- Two lemon wedges
- 1 cup boiling water
- ¼ tsp. black pepper
- 1 cup low sodium chicken broth
- 1 tbsp. extra virgin olive oil
- ½ cup green beans

DIRECTIONS

1. Heat the oil in a large pan on standard heat.
2. Sauté the chopped onion for 5 minutes until soft before adding in the rice and stirring for 1-2 minutes.
3. Combine the broth with boiling water.
4. Add half of the liquid to the pan and stir slowly.
5. Slowly add the rest of the liquid while continuously stirring for up to 20-30 minutes.
6. Stir in the green beans to the risotto.
7. Place the fish on top of the rice, cover, and steam for 10 minutes.
8. Ensure the water does not dry out and keep topping up until the rice is cooked thoroughly.
9. Use your fork to break up the fish fillets and stir into the rice.
10. Sprinkle with freshly ground pepper to serve and a squeeze of fresh lemon.
11. Garnish with the lemon wedges and serve with the arugula.

NUTRITIONS

- Calories 221
- Protein 12 g
- Carbs 29 g
- Fat 8 g
- Sodium (Na) 398 mg
- Potassium (K) 347 mg
- Phosphorus 241 mg

259. MIXED PEPPER STUFFED RIVER TROUT

PREPARATION	COOKING	SERVES
5 MIN	20 MIN	4

INGREDIENTS

- One whole river trout
- 1 tsp. thyme
- ¼ diced yellow pepper
- 1 cup baby spinach leaves
- ¼ diced green pepper
- One juiced lime
- ¼ diced red pepper
- 1 tsp. oregano
- 1 tsp. extra virgin olive oil
- 1 tsp. black pepper

DIRECTIONS

1. Preheat the broiler /grill on high heat.
2. Lightly oil a baking tray.
3. Mix all of the fixings apart from the trout and lime.
4. Slice the trout lengthways (there should be an opening here from where it was gutted) and stuff the mixed ingredients inside.
5. Squeeze the lime juice over the fish and then place the lime wedges on the tray.
6. Place under the broiler on the baking tray and broil for 15-20 minutes or until fish is thoroughly cooked through and flakes easily.
7. Enjoy alone or with a side helping of rice or salad.

NUTRITIONS

- Calories 290
- Protein 15 g
- Carbs 0 g
- Fat 7 g
- Sodium (Na) 43 mg
- Potassium (K) 315 mg
- Phosphorus 189 mg

260. HADDOCK & BUTTERED LEEKS

PREPARATION	COOKING	SERVES
5 MIN	15 MIN	2

INGREDIENTS

- 1 tbsp. unsalted butter
- One sliced leek
- ¼ tsp. black pepper
- 2 tsp. Chopped parsley
- 6 oz. haddock fillets
- ½ juiced lemon

DIRECTIONS

1. Preheat the oven to 375°F/Gas Mark 5.
2. Add the haddock fillets to baking or parchment paper and sprinkle with the black pepper.
3. Squeeze over the lemon juice and wrap into a parcel.
4. Bake the parcel on a baking tray for 10-15 minutes or until the fish is thoroughly cooked through.
5. Meanwhile, heat the butter over medium-low heat in a small pan.
6. Add the leeks and parsley and sauté for 5-7 minutes until soft.
7. Serve the haddock fillets on a bed of buttered leeks and enjoy!

NUTRITIONS

- Calories 124
- Protein 15 g
- Carbs 0 g
- Fat 7 g
- Sodium (Na) 161 mg
- Potassium (K) 251 mg
- Phosphorus 220 mg

261. THAI SPICED HALIBUT

PREPARATION	COOKING	SERVES
5 MIN	20 MIN	2

INGREDIENTS

- 2 tbsps. coconut oil
- 1 cup white rice
- ¼ tsp. black pepper
- ½ diced red chili
- 1 tbsp. fresh basil
- 2 pressed garlic cloves
- 4 oz. halibut fillet
- One halved lime
- Two sliced green onions
- One lime leaf

DIRECTIONS

1. Preheat oven to 400°F/Gas Mark 5.
2. Add half of the ingredients into baking paper and fold into a parcel.
3. Repeat for your second parcel.
4. Add to the oven for 15-20 minutes or until fish is thoroughly cooked through.
5. Serve with cooked rice.

NUTRITIONS

- Calories 311
- Protein 16 g
- Carbs 17 g
- Fat 15 g
- Sodium (Na) 31 mg
- Potassium (K) 418 mg
- Phosphorus 257 mg

262. HOMEMADE TUNA NIÇOISE

PREPARATION	COOKING	SERVES
5 MIN	10 MIN	2

INGREDIENTS

- One egg
- ½ cup green beans
- ¼ sliced cucumber
- One juiced lemon
- 1 tsp. black pepper
- ¼ sliced red onion
- 1 tbsp. olive oil
- 1 tbsp. capers
- 4 oz. drained canned tuna
- Four iceberg lettuce leaves
- 1 tsp. chopped fresh cilantro

DIRECTIONS

1. Prepare the salad by washing and slicing the lettuce, cucumber, and onion.
2. Add to a salad bowl.
3. Mix 1 tbsp oil with the lemon juice, cilantro, and capers for a salad dressing. Set aside.
4. Boil a pan of water on high heat, then lower to simmer and add the egg for 6 minutes. (Steam the green beans over the same pan in a steamer/colander for 6 minutes).
5. Remove the egg and rinse under cold water.
6. Peel before slicing in half.
7. Mix the tuna, salad, and dressing together in a salad bowl.
8. Toss to coat.
9. Top with the egg and serve with a sprinkle of black pepper.

NUTRITIONS

- Calories 199
- Protein 19 g
- Carbs 7 g
- Fat 8 g
- Sodium (Na) 466 mg
- Potassium (K) 251 mg
- Phosphorus 211 mg

263. MONK-FISH CURRY

PREPARATION	COOKING	SERVES
5 MIN	20 MIN	2

INGREDIENTS

- One garlic clove
- Three finely chopped green onions
- 1 tsp. grated ginger
- 1 cup of water.
- 2 tsp. Chopped fresh basil
- 1 cup cooked rice noodles
- 1 tbsp. coconut oil
- ½ sliced red chili
- 4 oz. Monk-fish fillet
- ½ finely sliced stick lemon-grass
- 2 tbsps. chopped shallots

DIRECTIONS

1. Slice the monkfish into bite-size pieces.
2. By means of a pestle, also mortar or food processor, crush the basil, garlic, ginger, chili, and lemon-grass to form a paste.
3. Heat the oil in a pan over medium-high heat and add the shallots.
4. Now add the water to the pan and bring to a boil.
5. Add the Monk-fish, lower the heat and cover to simmer for 10 minutes or until cooked through.
6. Enjoy with rice noodles and scatter with green onions to serve.

NUTRITIONS

- Calories 249
- Protein 12 g
- Carbs 30 g
- Fat 10 g
- Sodium (Na) 32 mg
- Potassium (K) 398 mg
- Phosphorus 190 mg

CONCLUSION

Thank you for reaching the end of this book; I hope this had helped you through your journey.

Let us just remember some important information about Mediterranean Diet:

- Consume lots of garlic! It is a great add-on to your diet and is very healthy. Garlic is known to have antibiotic properties as it helps reduce coughs, infections, acne and even toothaches. The best part about garlic is that it has no side effects and can be included in every meal of the day.

Overdose can include things like diarrhea, vomiting, abdominal pain or even an increased heart rate.

- Olive oil is very commonly referred to as "Liquid gold" for a reason; it has many health benefits especially in preventing heart problems like stroke or heart attack. A study was conducted on more than 20,000 people which showed that olive oil prevents cardiovascular diseases on a regular basis. It contains high levels of oleic acid which lowers bad cholesterol and increases good cholesterol by reducing LDL cholesterol and increasing HDL Cholesterol. Olive oil also helps prevent colon cancer; it contains polyphenols which are phytochemicals that prevent cell mutations by the cancer causing agents called free radicals that include pollutants like pesticides or herbicides used in farming and radiation from the sun among others.

It is best to use extra virgin olive oil in order to get the benefits of its nutrients; it also contains lots of antioxidants that are anti-inflammatory in nature. It can be used to cook or simply add a dash of it while eating salads, vegetables, bread and even omelets; it can also be used as a substitute for butter.

A couple of things you should keep in mind about olive oil is that it has a low smoking point so when cooking it is recommended not to heat it above 300 degrees Fahrenheit and keep the heat at medium or low temperature. Another thing is that store bought olive oil should be stored in a cool dark place as light and heat deteriorate its quality.

Make sure to avoid packaged oils; instead always buy a reputable brand made from fresh olives as they tend to last longer before going bad than the packaged ones. Always read the label on the bottle you plan on buying; look for extra virgin olive oil which has no additives with no more than 1% acidity level and contains lots of polyphenols mostly oleuropein.

- Be sure to include fruit in your diet as much as possible. It is a great source of vitamins and minerals; including a lot of antioxidants. Orange, apple, grapefruit, apricot and cantaloupe are some of the best choices for you. Fresh fruit is also a great source of natural sugars which can be converted into energy by the body or consumed as simple sugars to fuel blood sugar levels.

- Beans are especially good for those who want to lower blood pressure levels and even help those who struggle with constipation; one cup cooked beans contain about 50 calories with very little fat content. Black beans have the highest amount of fiber (about 6 grams) among all bean types while chickpeas have about 4 grams per cup serving which is why it is the most recommended type among others.

- Leafy greens are very healthy dietary choice because they are rich source for vitamins and minerals like vitamin A , C, E, K as well as iron and folate; they also contain beta-carotene which helps maintain the immune system.

INDEX RECIPES

1. BEEF WITH BROCCOLI PLUS CAULIFLOWER RICE 304

2. GRILLED CHICKEN POWER BOWL WITH GREEN GODDESS DRESSING 305

3. BACON CHEESEBURGER 306

4. CHEESEBURGER PIE 307

5. CRISPY APPLES 308

6. TURKEY CAPRESE MEATLOAF CUPS 309

7. ZUCCHINI NOODLES WITH CREAMY AVOCADO PESTO 310

8. AVOCADO CHICKEN SALAD 311

9. RICOTTA RAMEKINS 312

10. CHICKEN LO MEIN 313

11. PANCAKES WITH BERRIES 314

12. OMELETTE À LA MARGHERITA 315

13. OMELET WITH TOMATOES AND SPRING ONIONS 316

14. COCONUT CHIA PUDDING WITH BERRIES 317

15. EEL ON SCRAMBLED EGGS AND BREAD 318

16. CHIA SEED GEL WITH POMEGRANATE AND NUTS 319

17. LAVENDER BLUEBERRY CHIA SEED PUDDING 320

18. YOGURT WITH GRANOLA AND PERSIMMON 321

19. SMOOTHIE BOWL WITH SPINACH, MANGO AND MUESLI 322

20. ALKALINE BLUEBERRY SPELT PANCAKES 323

21. ALKALINE BLUEBERRY MUFFINS 324

22. CRUNCHY QUINOA MEAL 325

23. COCONUT PANCAKES 326

24. QUINOA PORRIDGE 327

25. AMARANTH PORRIDGE 328

26. BANANA BARLEY PORRIDGE 329

27. ZUCCHINI MUFFINS 330

28. MILLET PORRIDGE 331

29. JACKFRUIT VEGETABLE FRY 332

30. ZUCCHINI PANCAKES 333

31. SQUASH HASH 334

32. HEMP SEED PORRIDGE 335

33. PUMPKIN SPICE QUINOA 336

34. SCRAMBLED EGGS WITH SOY SAUCE AND BROCCOLI SLAW 337

35. MANGO COCONUT OATMEAL 338

36. WHOLE-WHEAT BLUEBERRY MUFFINS 339

37. WALNUT CRUNCH BANANA BREAD 340

38. PLANT-POWERED PANCAKES 341

39. BOK CHOY WITH TOFU STIR FRY 344

40. SALMON WITH VEGETABLES 345

41. EASIEST TUNA COBBLER EVER 346

42. DELICIOUSLY HOMEMADE PORK BUNS 347

43. PEPPER PESTO LAMB	348	69. ASPARAGUS SALMON FILLETS	374
44. CHICKEN GOULASH	349	70. CRISPY BAKED CHICKEN	375
45. GRILLED MAHI MAHI WITH JICAMA SLAW	350	71. SOUR AND SWEET FISH	376
46. PORK CACCIATORE	351	72. CREAMY CHICKEN	377
47. PORK WITH TOMATO & OLIVES	352	73. PAPRIKA BUTTER SHRIMP	378
48. PORK ROAST	353	74. ALMOND FLOUR BURGER WITH GOAT CHEESE	379
49. SALMON BURGERS	354	75. SAUSAGE SKILLET WITH CABBAGE	380
50. SEARED SCALLOPS	355	76. AIR FRYER ASPARAGUS	382
51. BLACK COD	356	77. AVOCADO FRIES	383
52. MISO-GLAZED SALMON	357	78. BELL-PEPPER CORN WRAPPED IN TORTILLA	384
53. CUCUMBER-BASIL SALSA ON HALIBUT POUCHES	358	79. CAULIFLOWER RICE	385
54. CURRY SALMON WITH MUSTARD	359	80. STUFFED MUSHROOMS	386
55. DIJON MUSTARD AND LIME MARINATED SHRIMP	360	81. ZUCCHINI OMELET	387
56. WW SALAD IN A JAR	361	82. CHEESY CAULIFLOWER FRITTERS	388
57. YUMMY SMOKED SALMON	362	83. ZUCCHINI PARMESAN CHIPS	389
58. ASPARAGUS FRITTATA RECIPE	363	84. JALAPENO CHEESE BALLS	390
59. AVOCADOS STUFFED WITH SALMON	364	85. COCONUT BATTERED CAULIFLOWER BITES	391
60. ONION AND ZUCCHINI PLATTER	365	86. CRISPY JALAPENO COINS	392
61. LEMON FLAVORED SPROUTS	366	87. CRISPY ROASTED BROCCOLI	393
62. AVOCADO AND CAPRESE SALAD	367	88. TURKEY STUFFED BELL PEPPERS	394
63. CILANTRO AND KIDNEY BEANS	368	89. LEAN CROCKPOT PULLED PORK	395
64. GINGER SOUP	369	90. EASY CREAMY CAJUN SHRIMP PASTA	396
65. SCALLOPS IN BACON SAUCE	370	91. FALL CHICKEN NOODLE STIR FRY	397
66. FISH TACO BOWLS	371	92. HEALTHY SALMON CHOWDER	398
67. BUTTERY GARLIC SHRIMP	372	93. FLAT IRON STEAK FAJITA BOWLS	399
68. SALMON STEW	373		

94. REAL SIMPLE AND CLEAN MEATBALLS 400

95. HIGH PROTEIN LOW CARB SHRIMP CEVICHE 401

96. BAKED RICOTTA WITH PEARS 402

97. PESTO ZUCCHINI NOODLES 403

98. STEWED HERBED FRUIT 404

99. HERBED WILD RICE 405

100. BUFFALO CHICKEN SLIDERS 406

101. HIGH PROTEIN CHICKEN MEATBALLS 407

102. BARLEY RISOTTO 408

103. RISOTTO WITH GREEN BEANS, SWEET POTATOES, AND PEAS 409

104. MAPLE LEMON TEMPEH CUBES 410

105. BOK CHOY WITH TOFU STIR-FRY 411

106. THREE-BEAN MEDLEY 412

107. HERBED GARLIC BLACK BEANS 413

108. QUINOA WITH VEGETABLES 414

109. BALSAMIC BEEF AND MUSHROOMS MIX 415

110. SIMPLE BEEF ROAST 416

111. CAULIFLOWER CURRY 417

112. PORK AND PEPPERS CHILI 418

113. GREEK STYLE QUESADILLAS 419

114. MEDITERRANEAN BURRITO 420

115. SWEET POTATO BACON MASH 421

116. SAVORY SALMON WITH CILANTRO 422

117. MIDDLE EASTERN SALMON WITH TOMATOES AND CUCUMBER 423

118. CUCUMBER BOWL WITH SPICES AND GREEK YOGURT 424

119. STUFFED BELL PEPPERS WITH QUINOA 425

120. SPAGHETTI SQUASH GRATIN 426

121. SALMON FLORENTINE 427

122. CHEESEBURGER SOUP 428

123. BRAISED COLLARD GREENS IN PEANUT SAUCE WITH PORK TENDERLOIN 429

124. TENDER LAMB CHOPS 430

125. SMOKY PORK & CABBAGE 431

126. SEASONED PORK CHOPS 432

127. SHRIMP AND CAULIFLOWER GRITS 433

128. TUNA NIÇOISE SALAD 434

129. VEGGIE DIPS AND BUFFALO DIP 435

130. GRILLED TEMPEH WITH EGGPLANTS AND WATERCRESS 436

131. MINI MAC IN A BOWL 437

132. PHILLY CHEESESTEAK STUFFED PEPPERS 438

133. EASY SPINACH MUFFINS 439

134. HEALTHY CAULIFLOWER GRITS 440

135. ITALIAN STYLE GENOSE ZUCCHINI 441

136. HEALTHY PEPPERS FLOUNDER MEATBALLS 442

137. A TRIUMPH OF MEAT & VEGETABLES 443

138. GARLIC AND OIL - BROCCOLI AND BEEF 444

139. MEAT IN THE WOODS 445

140. TURKEY ON A BOAT 446

141. WEDDING OF BROCCOLI AND TOMATOES 447

142. HAMBURGER SALAD — 448

143. GREEN BUDDHA SMILE — 449

144. ZUCCHINI FETTUCCINE WITH MEXICAN TACO — 450

145. ONION GREEN BEANS — 451

146. CREAM OF MUSHROOMS SATAY — 452

147. TORTORETO MUSHROOMS WITH CHEDDAR — 453

148. LENTIL TRIUMPH HAMBURGER WITH CARROTS — 454

149. STIR-FRIED SWEET POTATOES WITH PARMESAN — 455

150. CHICKEN GOULASH WITH GREEN PEPPERS — 456

151. LETTUCE SALAD WITH BEEF STRIPS — 457

152. CAULIFLOWER SPRINKLED WITH CURRY — 458

153. PORK STEW WITH GREEN CHILLI — 459

154. ROSEMARY SCENT CAULIFLOWER BUNDLES — 460

155. CHICKEN STIR FRY — 461

156. CAULIFLOWER SALAD — 462

157. GARLIC CHICKEN WITH ZOODLES — 463

158. "MACARONI" — 464

159. BROCCOLI TACO — 465

160. CRUNCHY CHICKEN TACOS — 466

161. CAULIFLOWER WITH KALE PESTO — 467

162. CHICKEN CHILI — 468

163. AVOCADO, CITRUS, AND SHRIMP SALAD — 469

164. BROCCOLI ALFREDO — 470

165. LEAN AND GREEN STEAK MACHINE — 471

166. GARLIC SHRIMP ZUCCHINI NOODLES — 472

167. CROCKPOT CHILI — 473

168. TOMATILLO AND GREEN CHILI PORK STEW — 474

169. AVOCADO LIME SHRIMP SALAD — 475

170. ROSEMARY CAULIFLOWER ROLLS — 476

171. MEDITERRANEAN CHICKEN SALAD — 477

172. ASPARAGUS GREEN SCRAMBLE — 480

173. CRANBERRY SALAD — 481

174. CHICKEN SALAD WITH PINEAPPLE AND PECANS — 482

175. ZUCCHINI FRITTERS — 483

176. HEALTHY BROCCOLI SALAD — 484

177. DELICIOUS ZUCCHINI QUICHE — 485

178. COBB SALAD WITH BLUE CHEESE DRESSING — 486

179. VANILLA BEAN FRAPPUCCINO — 487

180. DARK CHOCOLATE MOCHACCINO ICE BOMBS — 488

181. CHOCOLATE BARK WITH ALMONDS — 489

182. PROTEIN BROWNIES — 490

183. CAESAR SALAD WITH CHICKEN AND PARMESAN — 491

184. RASPBERRY FLAX SEED DESSERT — 492

185. POMEGRANATE CHERRY SMOOTHIE BOWL — 493

186. CUSTARD CREAM — 494

187. CHOCOLATE BARS — 495

188. BLUEBERRY MUFFINS — 496

189. CHIA PUDDING — 497

190. AVOCADO PUDDING — 498

191. DELICIOUS BROWNIE BITES — 499

192. PUMPKIN BALLS — 500

193. SMOOTH PEANUT BUTTER CREAM — 501

194. VANILLA AVOCADO POPSICLES — 502

195. CHOCOLATE POPSICLE — 503

196. RASPBERRY ICE CREAM — 504

197. CHOCOLATE FROSTY — 505

198. CHOCOLATE ALMOND BUTTER BROWNIE — 506

199. PEANUT BUTTER FUDGE — 507

200. ALMOND BUTTER FUDGE — 508

201. BOUNTY BARS — 509

202. BANANA BREAD — 510

203. MINI LAVA CAKES — 511

204. GINGER CHEESECAKE — 512

205. PUDDING PIES — 513

206. PANCAKE CINNAMON ROLL — 514

207. CHOCOLATE CHIP COFFEE CAKE MUFFINS — 515

208. ZUCCHINI BREAD — 516

209. HAYSTACKS — 517

210. VANILLA CUSTARD — 518

211. CHOCOLATE CHEESECAKE SHAKE — 519

212. PISTACHIO MILK-SHAKE — 520

213. PEANUT BUTTER AND CREAM CHEESE STUFFED BROWNIES — 521

214. GRILLED CHEESE TOMATO SANDWICH — 522

215. PEANUT BUTTER CRUNCH BARS — 523

216. MOUSSE TREAT — 524

217 TIRAMISU MILKSHAKE — 525

218. MAPLE PANCAKES — 526

219. PIZZA BREAD — 527

220. BROCCOLI SALAD — 530

221. POTATO CARROT SALAD — 531

222. MARINATED VEGGIE SALAD — 532

223. MEDITERRANEAN SALAD — 533

224. POTATO TUNA SALAD — 534

225. JICAMA AND SPINACH SALAD — 535

226. HIGH PROTEIN SALAD — 536

227. RICE AND VEGGIE BOWL — 537

228. SQUASH BLACK BEAN BOWL — 538

229. PEA SALAD — 539

230. SNAP PEA SALAD — 540

231. CUCUMBER TOMATO CHOPPED SALAD — 541

232. ZUCCHINI PASTA SALAD — 542

233. EGG AVOCADO SALAD — 543

234. TRIPLE CHOCOLATE CHIP DEEP DISH COOKIES — 544

235. ROASTED TROUT STUFFED WITH VEGGIES — 545

236. LEMONY TROUT WITH CARAMELIZED SHALLOTS — 546

237. EASY TOMATO TUNA MELTS — 547

238. MACKEREL AND GREEN BEAN SALAD — 548

239. HAZELNUT CRUSTED SEA BASS — 550

240. SHRIMP AND PEA PAELLA — 551

241. GARLIC SHRIMP WITH ARUGULA PESTO — 552

242. BAKED OYSTERS WITH VEGETABLES — 553

243. CREAMY FISH GRATIN — 554

244. PROTEIN PUMPKIN SPICED DONUTS — 555

245. HIGH PROTEIN CHIPOTLE CHEDDAR QUESADILLA — 556

246. SWEET POTATO CASSEROLE — 557

247. BAKED CHEESY EGGPLANT — 558

248. MIXED SEAFOOD DISH — 559

249. GARLIC SHRIMP WITH OLIVE OIL — 560

250. STEAMED MUSSELS IN TOMATO GARLIC — 561

251. MEDITERRANEAN-STYLE MUSSELS — 562

252. LEEKS AND CALAMARI MIX — 563

253. SEAFOOD PAELLA — 564

254. BAKED SALMON IN GARLIC PEPPER — 565

255. SAUTEED OCTOPUS — 566

256. GRILLED OCTOPUS — 567

257. SCALLOP SALAD — 568

258. COD & GREEN BEAN RISOTTO — 569

259. MIXED PEPPER STUFFED RIVER TROUT — 570

260. HADDOCK & BUTTERED LEEKS — 571

261. THAI SPICED HALIBUT — 572

262. HOMEMADE TUNA NIÇOISE — 573

263. MONK-FISH CURRY — 574

Printed in Great Britain
by Amazon